Community Dental Health

Community Dental Health

Edited by

ANTHONY W. JONG, D.D.S., M.P.H., D.Sc.

Professor and Chairperson, Department of Dental Care Management,
Associate Dean for Academic Affairs, Goldman School of Graduate Dentistry,
Boston University; Associate Professor, Department of Socio-Medical Sciences and
Community Medicine, School of Medicine, Boston University Medical Center;
Lecturer, Department of Dental Care Administration, School of Dental Medicine,
Harvard University, Boston, Massachusetts

SECOND EDITION

with 37 illustrations

The C. V. Mosby Company

ST. LOUIS • WASHINGTON, D.C. • TORONTO   1988

MOSBY

A TRADITION OF PUBLISHING EXCELLENCE

Editor: Donna Saya Sokolowski
Assistant editor: Maureen Slaten
Project manager: Carlotta Seely
Editing/production: Jeanne A. Gulledge
Book design: Gail Morey Hudson
Cover design: John Rokusek

SECOND EDITION

The C.V. Mosby Company
11830 Westline Industrial Drive, St. Louis, Missouri 63146

Library of Congress Cataloging-in-Publication Data

Community dental health.

   Rev. ed. of: Dental public health and community
dentistry. 1981.
   Includes bibliographies and index.
   1.   Dental public health.   2.   Community dental
services.   3.   Dental public health—United States.
I.   Jong, Anthony W.   II.   Dental public health and
community dentistry.   [DNLM: 1.   Public Health Dentistry—
United States.   WU 113 C734]
RK52.C665 1987   362.1'976'00973   87-7973
ISBN 0-8016-2576-9

AC/D/D   9 8 7 6 5 4   02/D/236

Contributors

LESTER E. BLOCK, D.D.S., M.P.H.

Associate Professor, Public Health Administration, School of Public Health, University of Minnesota, Minneapolis, Minnesota

JOSEPH BOFFA, D.D.S., M.P.H.

Associate Professor, Department of Dental Care Management, Boston University Medical Center, Goldman School of Graduate Dentistry, Boston, Massachusetts

MITCHELL BUREK, M.Ed., Ph.D.

Associate Professor, Department of Dental Care Management, Boston University Medical Center, Goldman School of Graduate Dentistry, Boston, Massachusetts

VIRGINIA A. CALLANEN, M.S., M.P.H.

Project Director, Division of Dental Health, Massachusetts Department of Public Health, Boston, Massachusetts

MARIANNE B. DeSOUZA, R.D.H., B.A., M.S.

Department of Dental Care Management, Boston University Medical Center, Goldman School of Graduate Dentistry, Boston, Massachusetts

JEAN MARIE DOHERTY, D.M.D., M.P.H., D.Sc.

Chief, Geriatric Dentistry Section, Veterans Administration West Side Medical Center, Chicago, Illinois; Clinical Assistant Professor, Geriatric Dentistry, Department of Oral Diagnosis, University of Illinois, Chicago, Illinois

JANE L. FORREST, R.D.H., M.S.

Mapleshade, New Jersey

PAULA K. FRIEDMAN, D.D.S.

Associate Professor, Department of Dental Care Management, Assistant Dean for Administration, Boston University Medical Center, Goldman School of Graduate Dentistry; Assistant Attending Dental Surgeon, Beth Israel Hospital, Boston, Massachusetts

GEORGE M. GLUCK, D.D.S., M.P.H.

Professor and Chairperson, Department of Community Dentistry, Fairleigh S. Dickinson, Jr., College of Dental Medicine, Fairleigh Dickinson University, Hackensack, New Jersey

JANET L. GOLDEN, M.A.

Cambridge, Massachusetts

LIREKA P. JOSEPH, Dr.P.H.

Rockville, Maryland

DUSHANKA V. KLEINMAN, D.D.S., M.Sc.D.

Washington, D.C.

LINDA B. LAKIN, R.D.H., M.S.

Coordinator of Geriatric Dentistry, Department of Community Dentistry, Fairleigh S. Dickinson, Jr., College of Dental Medicine, Fairleigh Dickinson University, Hackensack, New Jersey

DENNIS H. LEVERETT. D.D.S., M.P.H.

Chairperson, Department of Community
Dentistry, Eastman Dental Center;
Professor, Department of Dental Research,
University of Rochester, Rochester, New York

MADALYN L. MANN, R.D.H., M.S.

Associate Professor, Department of Dental Care
Management, Boston University Medical Center,
Goldman School of Graduate Dentistry,
Boston, Massachusetts

JANE B. MOOSBRUKER, Ph.D.

Organization Development Consultant,
Bolton, Massachusetts

MAXINE PECK, C.D.A., M.S.

Director, Dental Assisting Program,
Department of Dental Care Management,
Boston University Medical Center,
Goldman School of Graduate Dentistry,
Boston, Massachusetts

MARY BURNS SHERIDAN, R.D.H., M.S.

LaGrange, Illinois

CHERYL A. TUPPER, C.D.A., M.S.

Berkeley, California

S. GAY WATSON, R.D.H., M.Ed.

Boston, Massachusetts

To my mother
Lily Jong Chin
for the love that has provided me with inspiration
throughout my life

To my wife
Patricia Westwater-Jong
for the understanding and love that has
given me peace of mind

To my daughter
Jessica Westwater Jong
for bringing out the child within me

Preface

The dental health professional will face in the 1990s a world far different from that of the last decade. Growing up in the United States in the 1970s, the emerging professional prepared for a practice in a country that was short of dentists and dental auxiliaries. Labor statistics emphasized the need for more health professionals in a nation with a population explosion and a growing economy. Today the picture is not so clear: Are there too many dentists? Too many dental hygienists? How does the budding professional cope with the present environment? Can we now eliminate dental disease? These are questions we face whether we are involved in private practice or in public health. This book focuses on the role of the dental professional in the evolving socially conscious health field.

In this text we introduce essential concepts in the study of dental care and disease prevention, being ever mindful of the social matrix in which we exist. We cannot talk about sophisticated and expensive restorative dentistry without considering the economic impact on the patient and the community. To the public, health care has become a "right." The Senate Committee on Labor and Public Welfare in 1975 reaffirmed that the availability of high-quality health care to all Americans was a national goal. Although the federal government has been moving inexorably toward the achievement of this goal, progress has been slow and painful. Congressional polemic concerning national health insurance legislation has been raging for many years, and to the weary health professional it seems we are no closer to an equitable solution. Thus the public's expectations of access to quality health care do not necessarily coincide with the practical realities of the nation's economy.

In other countries such as the United Kingdom, New Zealand, and Sweden, the access to health care has been guaranteed by government. However, regardless of the actual implementation of a national program in this country, the new social ethic of responsibility for all has been firmly established. The norms that many health care providers have accepted during their education—that every individual is directly responsible for his or her own personal health care and that professionals determine the needs of society and provide the necessary services—are now being questioned by both professionals and consumers.

As the role of the dentist changes in society from an isolated purveyor of essentially rehabilitative clinical services to an integrated member of a health team concerned with preventive and early diagnostic services, dental education must be modified to provide the student with additional relevant information and skills. The role of consumer groups, the proliferation of third party payment programs, and the emergence of independently practicing dental auxiliaries are affecting the practice of dentistry, and dentistry must respond to these forces. As the prevalence of dental caries decreases in this country, dental public health professionals can direct their efforts toward special population groups who are still in need of their services. The elderly and disabled continue to receive inadequate dental care.

This book, through the contributions of professionals involved in health care delivery, responds to specific need areas such as community dental health education, prevention of dental disease, ethical concerns in dental health care, and so on. The book would not have been possible without the efforts of all the contributors—professionals who are active in teaching and practicing, yet who took the time to write a practical chapter on their field. I would like to thank these contributors and the staff of my department for their interest and help. A special note of appreciation goes to Ellen Wolfe, who edited every chapter and organized my efforts to produce this second edition.

The editor of a book has the rare opportunity to reach a large audience and to put on paper thoughts that for most people must remain as thoughts, never to be seen or heard. I would like to take advantage of this opportunity to thank James M. Dunning, D.D.S., M.P.H., for having guided me on this path of dental public health, a path that over the past 15 years has been rewarding and ever-stimulating. For those readers who find meaning in the words in this book and seek careers in dental public health, my best wishes for a successful career. Not many have trod this path, but those who did have moved the profession a little closer to improving the dental health of the whole community and the society in which we live.

Anthony W. Jong

Contents

Community Dental Health

THE PROVIDERS OF DENTAL SERVICES

Section one introduces the concept of the dental care delivery system in the United States. It focuses on the providers of dental care—the dentist, the dental hygienist, the dental assistant—and their roles in a rapidly changing environment. The way in which we as providers of services integrate ourselves into a system of dental care to promote the health of our patients is the challenge facing members of our profession today. As Dr. Lester Block so aptly states in Chapter 1, "dental public health is a concern for and activity directed toward the improvement and promotion of the dental health of the population as a whole, as well as of individuals within that population."

The methods that governmental agencies use to address the problems of dental disease are treated in this first chapter. Dr. Paula Friedman, in Chapter 2, discusses the forces that are currently affecting the practice of dentistry and introduces alternatives to the traditional one-dentist private practice. In Chapter 3, Ms. Maxine Peck, Ms. Gay Watson, and Ms. Cheryl Tupper attempt to forecast the future for dental auxiliaries in health care delivery by examining the history and current trends in auxiliary education and practice.

Section one will give the student insight into the ecological milieu in which he/she will be practicing in the near future and hopefully will reduce the future shock that recent graduates have incurred. The practice of dentistry is rapidly changing, and the goals and models we had as students may not be achievable in today's world. The greatly accelerated rate of change in society has brought on a dizzying disorientation for many people, health professionals included. The attempt to maintain the status quo will prove futile under the ever-increasing forces of change. As Alvin Toffler cautioned in his timely book, *Future Shock*, "Future shock will not be found in Index Medicus or in any listing of psychological abnormalities. Yet, unless intelligent steps are taken to combat it, millions of human beings will find themselves increasingly disoriented, progressively incompetent to deal rationally with their environments."

DENTAL DISEASE

In order to better understand the public health impact of dental disease, one should keep in mind that dental diseases are not reversible and are not self-curing. Although preventive procedures are highly successful in reducing the major dental diseases (caries and periodontal disease), they have not been able to eliminate them. Therefore in addition to a preventive component, a treatment component is an essential element of any dental public health program.[48]

At least three unique characteristics of the two most common dental diseases of the mouth, dental caries and periodontal disease, are important to consider: (1) they are of universal prevalence; (2) they do not undergo remission or termination if left untreated but accumulate a backlog of unmet needs; and (3) they usually require technically demanding, expensive, and time-consuming professional treatment. The importance of these characteristics is often underestimated by clinicians and nondental public health practitioners.[48]

Almost all individuals are subject to continuously recurring attacks of dental disease. For this reason most people will experience a periodic need for services from the time their teeth erupt. Failure to detect and treat infectious diseases will have little impact on total physician labor requirements since most of those affected will either die or recover spontaneously. Dental disease on the other hand, if left untreated, continues to develop and accumulates a backlog of needs almost always requiring surgical excising of hard or soft tissues and the replacement of diseased, defective, or missing tissues.[48]

Prevalence of dental disease

Studies of the prevalence of dental disease in recent decades have placed problems of dental health in a position of major importance with regard to health needs of the nation. The magnitude of the problem that confronts dental public health is demonstrated by data indicating the incidence and prevalence of dental disease.[21] The National Center for Health Statistics surveyed the U.S. population from 1971 to 1974 and found that 20% of children ages 6 to 11 had at least one untreated decayed primary tooth. This number increased to 31% of children ages 6 to 11 with at least one untreated decayed permanent tooth, 54% of youths ages 12 to 17, and 47% of adults ages 18 to 74. Children between the ages of 12 and 17 averaged 6.2 decayed, missing, filled teeth (DMFT) per person (1.8 were untreated decayed teeth) and adults ages 18 to 74 averaged 16.9 DMFT.[34]

A more recent survey, taken from 1979 to 1980, that included children ages 5 to 17 showed a significant reduction (about one third) from 7.06 decayed, missing, filled surfaces (DMFS) to 4.77. Nearly 37% of children ages 5 to 17 had no caries at all, but 7.7% of the children had 9 or more DMFT.[33]

Periodontal disease affects at least 15% of adults ages 18 to 44, 36% of adults ages 45 to 64, and 50% of adults ages 65 to 74.[32] However, dental disease still remains one of the most common health problems even though the incidence of the disease has been decreasing.

FORMS OF DENTAL HEALTH SERVICES

Historically, dental health services in the United States may be classified into three groups:

1. Services provided by dentists and dental auxiliaries and financed by the patient or source other than the government
2. Services provided by nongovernment dentists and dental auxiliaries partly or entirely remunerated by the government
3. Services provided by dentists and dental auxiliaries employed by the government, such as military personnel[47]

The prevailing philosophy in the United

States places the prime responsibility for health and the acquisition of health services on the individual and not on society, even though there is increased involvement for payment by the federal, state, and local government. In the 1940s the American Dental Association established the Council on Dental Health. One of the fundamental principles formulated by a council subcommittee was that the responsibility for the health of the American people is first of the individual, the community, the state, and the nation and in that order.[45] This attitude that the individual is the first line of responsibility contrasts with an attitude in European countries that suggests that society as a whole is responsible. By the 1970s national state-operated social programs were the norm in Europe. It has been suggested that the catastrophic events that befell Europe, primarily the effects of two wars in the first half of the twentieth century, hastened the development of social welfare programs in European countries. The United States, it must be remembered, largely escaped the physical and social devastation of those wars.[12,43]

Role of federal and state government in public health

Although there is no constitutionally defined role for the federal government in the maintenance of public health and such activities have been the provenance traditionally of the states, nonetheless, over the years there has been a gradual development of a federal presence in the health field. This has come about primarily because of: (1) responsibility for special population groups, such as merchant seamen, members of the armed forces, veterans, and American Indians; (2) the constitutional power to regulate interstate commerce from which most of the regulatory power of the federal government in health is derived; (3) grants-in-aid to states and institutions for a wide variety of activities; and (4) sponsorship and financial partici-

pation in the payment for health services (for example, Medicaid and Medicare).[44]

The Department of Health and Human Services (DHHS) is the major health agency of the federal government and has a budget second only to that of the Department of Defense. It consists of four primary operating agencies:
1. The Public Health Service (PHS), which is under the direction of the Assistant Secretary of Health with the Surgeon General as his/her principal deputy
2. Health Care Financing Administration (HCFA)
3. Social Security Administration (SSA)
4. Office of Human Development Services (HDS)

The Public Health Service consists of five operating agencies:
1. Alcohol, Drug Abuse and Mental Health Administration (ADAMHA)
2. The Centers for Disease Control (CDC)
3. The Food and Drug Administration (FDA)
4. Health Resources and Services Administration (HRSA)
5. National Institutes of Health (NIH)[44]

Dental activities undertaken by the federal government can be placed in two categories and are distributed among the several agencies of the department, which allocates approximately 1.25% of its budget for these activities.[19]

The first group of dental activities consists of programs that seek to improve the nation's capability to provide better oral health protection. These include biological research, disease prevention and control, planning and development programs in dental labor, education and services research, and regulation and compliance functions such as quality assessment. These programs account for about 40% of the department's dental budget. The other 60% is assigned to the second group, which includes those programs concerned with the provision of dental services.[19]

Activities related to dental care in the PHS can be found primarily in the (1) Centers for Disease Control, Center for Prevention Services, and Center for Health Promotion and Education; (2) Health Resources and Services Administration, Bureau of Health Professions, Division of Associated and Dental Health Professions; (3) National Institutes of Health, National Institute of Dental Research (NIDR), which carries out support programs of basic and clinical dental research.[2,17,44] The 1985 appropriation for NIDR was $102.3 million.[5]

The HCFA is responsible for the Medicare and Medicaid programs, including quality and utilization control. The Social Security Administration administers the "social security" program of Old Age, Survivors and Disability Insurance (OASDI), the program of Supplemental Security Income for the Aged, Blind and Disabled (SSI), and the federal-state public assistance program of Aid to Families with Dependent Children (AFDC). The Office of Human Development Services (HDS) contains the Administration on Aging, the Administration on Developmental Disabilities, the Administration for Native Americans, and the Administration for Children, Youth and Families, which oversees the Head Start program with its important dental component.[44]

The PHS provides dental services to specific groups of beneficiaries, with the care usually, but not always, provided by members of the PHS Commissioned Dental Corps. One of the direct care programs is the care provided to the Alaskan Natives and American Indians through the Indian Health Service.[19] Other beneficiaries of dental care by PHS commissioned officers are prisoners in federal penitentiaries, personnel of the Coast Guard, and personnel of the U.S. Merchant Marines. These direct service programs are based on federal responsibility resulting either from treaties, as with the American Indians, or from historical commitments.[19]

State health agencies

The 50 states, Washington, D.C., Guam, Puerto Rico, the Virgin Islands, and the Trust Territories participated in a 1974 study of the programs and expenditures of state health agencies (SHA—an agency or department headed by a state or territorial official). Of the SHAs, 51 reported having some type of dental program. Of the 49 SHAs that reported program activities, 47 noted preventive dental services, with a smaller number reporting restorative and emergency services and screening. Programs in six states provided orthodontic, prosthetic, or cleft palate services in support of crippled children's programs. Health and nutrition education were often provided. Only in one state was hypertension screening a reported service of the dental program.[38]

In 1983, 47 SHAs reported separate dental health programs serving a total of one million persons. These programs screened 870,300 persons for dental diseases, 8100 for oral cancer, and provided outpatient clinical services to 646,000. In addition to the 47 separate dental health programs, all 50 SHAs provided some type of dental service through other personal health programs, including maternal and child, handicapped children's services, SHA operated institutions, and migrant health programs. These programs screened an additional 2.3 million persons for dental disease and 63,400 for oral cancer and provided outpatient care to 837,800.[10]

During the fiscal year 1983, 50 SHAs spent a total of $5.4 billion for their public health programs excluding Medicaid. The $5.4 billion was distributed among program areas as follows: (1) personal health, $4.0 billion; (2) environmental health, $350 million; (3) health resources, $530 million; (4) laboratory programs, $184 million; (5) funds granted to local health departments not allocated to program areas, $78 million. Of the $5.4 billion, 40.1 million, less than 1%, was expended for dental health.[11]

All state and territorial health agencies continue to report the existence of dental health activities of some kind. In 1980 they reported a total expenditure of 32.3 million of which 14.8 million was for prevention. Approximately nine million people received dental health services from official state and territorial health agencies.[9,21]

Maternal and child health services

Since 1935, state health services for women of childbearing age and children to age 21 have been provided federal support through Title V of the Social Security Act. The Maternal and Child Health program (MCH) was responsible for extending and improving health care services for mothers and children through formula grants to state maternal and child health agencies. The grants supported the following activities with dental components: (1) Maternity and Infant Care Projects; (2) Children and Youth Projects; (3) Dental Health Projects for Children; and (4) Crippled Children Services.[25]

The Maternity and Infant Care Projects provided grants to projects serving particular target populations or to areas identifying high-risk mothers and provided necessary health care for prospective mothers and for infants in their first year of life. Emergency dental services were provided at all centers, but only a few offered comprehensive dental care.[24] By 1972 the Children and Youth Projects, started in 1966, provided comprehensive care to about 500,000 children in low-income areas. A program of preventive dental health services and dental care was an essential component of comprehensive child health services and its inclusion was a statutory requirement.[22]

The Child Health Act of 1967 authorized Special Project Grants for Dental Health of Children in essentially low-income areas for school and preschool children. The projects were first funded in 1971 when seven grants were made. By the end of 1974, 19 projects were in opera-

tion. By July 1, 1975, each state's maternal and child health plan had to include at least one of the following projects: maternal and infant care, children and youth, family planning, or dental care.[23]

A major shift in U.S. health policy occurred with the passage of the Omnibus Budget Reconciliation Act of 1981, which included the Maternal and Child Health Block Grant Act. The ammendments consolidated seven grant programs from Title V of the Social Security Act and from the Public Health Service Act into a block grant under a new Title V: Maternal and Child Health Services Block Grant. The consolidated programs are the maternal and child health and crippled childrens programs, genetic disease research, adolescent pregnancy services, sudden infant death syndrome research, hemophilia research, supplemental security income payments to crippled children, and lead-based poisoning research. Dental health is no longer a separate mandatory program under Title V.[42,44]

It is not yet clear what the impact of this major change in Maternal and Child Health policy will be, but to date total funding is not yet back to the levels before block grants and in many states cuts have resulted in the closing of maternal child health clinics. At the same time increased applications for services, because of loss of insurance coverage due to unemployment, has increased the need.[20,44]

The Reagan administration's philosophy of turning social programs back to the states is likely to cause the loss of needed services with the substitution of "block grants" for "categorical grants." When funds are lumped together to be used at a state's discretion, dentistry is likely to suffer and in fact appears to be doing so now. The immediate future for traditional public health programs does not look optimistic, though philosophies may well change when large numbers of people are shown to be unable to get needed care.[12]

Crippled Children Services provides funds that enable states to offer medical, surgical, corrective, and additional services and care to children who are crippled or who are suffering from conditions that lead to crippling. Children may be defined as crippled because of a dental disability or disfiguring condition, for example, cleft lip, cleft palate, or other oral disfigurement.[39] Unfortunately, public financing for the dental care of those with other handicapping conditions such as cerebral palsy and mental retardation has not been readily available. Although some states do have reasonable programs for the treatment of children with handicapping conditions, few have any kind of financing available for the treatment of these persons when they become adults.[12] In some states the term *crippled children* has not been an acceptable one, and in Minnesota, for example, the name of that program has been changed to *Services for Children with Handicaps.*[32]

Head Start

In 1965 Head Start programs were launched by the Office of Economic Opportunity, under the provisions of the Economic Opportunity Act of 1964, in order to provide educational health and social services to preschool children of the needy so that the children would enter school on an equitable basis with their more affluent peers. Each Head Start program is required to provide dental services to enrolled children.[41] Total basic dental services for every enrolled child is the objective of the program, but available funds and lack of dental personnel have been constraints.[14,36] There is evidence that Head Start early education programs are effective. It was demonstrated that in Michigan, children who were assigned to an experimental early education group for 1 year maintained remarkable gains over the control group for 15 years, with half the number of arrests, school dropouts, and teenage pregnancies.[20]

In another follow-up, a 20-year longitudinal study of former Head Start children, it was found that they had a higher employment rate, performed better in school, and rated higher in terms of self-esteem and sense of control of their lives than did other control children of similar disadvantaged backgrounds who did not attend Head Start programs.[28]

Nationally, Head Start faces a cut in coverage from 2 years to 1 year, which means that instead of attending Head Start all through their fourth and fifth years, children will be dropped after a year; this is to happen at a time when the infant mortality rate in certain sections of large metropolitan areas is 25 per 1000 births, a rate that surpasses that of impoverished Trinidad. Head Start financing has barely kept up with inflation and only 18% to 20% of all eligible children from poverty families are enrolled in Head Start programs.[28]

Medicaid and Early Periodic Screening, Diagnosis, and Treatment (EPSDT)

Medicaid (Title XIX of the Social Security Act) was authorized by the Social Security Amendments of 1965 to provide medical assistance to specified groups of needy people. Dental care is an optional benefit under Medicaid.[41] It is mandated under the EPSDT portion of Medicaid that covers children, but this program has never been enforced.[12] Payments made from Medicaid funds reached $14.7 billion in 1976, a 15.5% increase over 1975. An estimated 24.4 million recipients received one or more services during the year. Physicians' services accounted for 9.7% of the 1976 medical dollar and dentists' services accounted for 2.7%. Approximately 55% of the total medical funds were federal general revenue funds, and about 45% were from state and local dollars. Between 1971 and 1976, payment for physicians' services increased from $717 million to $1.4 billion, and payment for dentists' services increased from $181 million to $387 million.[40] In 1977 dental services accounted for approximately 3% of total

Medicaid expenditures, yet they accounted for nearly 80% of all public expenditures for those services. The approximate number of Medicaid recipients increased from over 18 million in 1972 to over 24.6 million in 1976, of whom 4.4 million had received dental services. By 1974, 41 states had exercised the option to provide dental care under Medicaid; of the 25 million recipients of Medicaid financial health services only 3.5 million obtained dental care, and dental fees accounted for only 3% of Medicaid's total vendor payments.[19]

In 1982 government programs accounted for about 4.1% of all expenditures for dental care, while public expenditures were 42.4% of total health care disbursement. Dental care funds under Medicaid had declined from 2.7% of all Medicaid payments in 1972 to 1.7% in 1983 though the overall current dollar amount had increased.[30]

One group that is particularly vulnerable because of lack of third party financing is the elderly. In 1977 persons 65 and older had 3% of their dental expenses covered by health insurance and only 2% by Medicaid. In contrast younger adults had from 12% to 20% covered by insurance and up to 5% covered by Medicaid.[30]

As of 1979, 24 states did not have coverage for denture care under Medicaid, 37 states provided dental benefits to the entire Medicaid eligible population, including adults and children, but in six of these states adult dental benefits were limited to emergency treatment.[4]

Medicaid is the largest federal funding source of health services for children. It was designed primarily to provide services for the needy mothers and children. In fact, needy mothers and children, while constituting 45% of the total recipients, use only 18% of the total dollars since the program has become, primarily, a source of funding for nursing home care for the elderly once they become medically indigent as a result of chronic illness.[20]

Since 1973, the EPSDT program has been more or less operational in all states with Medicaid programs. If offers all Medicaid beneficiaries under 21 the services in its title—a periodic screening for health defects, followed by any necessary diagnosis and treatment.[19,40] The EPSDT program was slow to get off the ground and in 1975 only 4% of the 13 million needy children that it was intended to benefit had actually been screened, let alone been treated. Children in the EPSDT age group and eligible for the program appeared to have a more urgent need for dental care than for medical care. Treated children in the middle 1970s required an average of $90 per child for dental care compared with $35 per child for medical care.[12] Unfortunately, funds have not been available to provide the treatment needed for eligible children. All Medicaid programs are required to provide an EPSDT program in order to receive federal funds, and dental services are mandated for persons under age 21. Under the EPSDT program, state or local agencies must screen all eligible children under age 21, assess the need for health services, and refer those in need to follow-up treatment.[19,40] Thus as part of the Medicaid program, one of the largest sources of funding for health care of poor children, EPSDT has been of limited success in many states. Many children are not covered and there has often been a separation of the diagnostic from the therapeutic, resulting in low rates of follow-through from screening to treatment of conditions found during screening. An amendment to EPSDT regulations, added in 1983, now encourages continuity of care by allowing EPSDT money to be used for payment for treatment as well as screening when an eligible child is under the care of private health care providers or a health center.[20]

Medicare

Medicare (Title XVIII of the Social Security Act) was authorized by the Social Security Amendments of 1965 and covers persons aged

65 and over and certain other disabled persons. Its purpose is to provide insurance protection against the costs of health care.

Part 1 of Medicare is a basic plan for hospital and related care. Payment to dentists for routine dental services is specifically excluded. Services by dental interns or residents in training, where services are ordinarily furnished by a hospital to its in-patients, may be covered, as are payments for the reduction of oral fractures by dentists and physicians. Part 2 is a voluntary supplementary plan for physicians' services and other medical and health services. Routine dental care is not covered and dental procedures are specifically excluded. The need for dental care is great for the population over 65 years of age, and the ability to pay for those services is greatly diminished at that age level. Medicare does virtually nothing to help the elderly with their dental health problems.[13] The dental coverage of Medicare is limited to those services requiring hospitalization, usually for surgical treatment for fractures and cancer and thus constitutes a negligible proportion of the program.[12]

In regard to having dental care covered under Medicare, the American Dental Association has argued before Congress the necessity of a supplemental dental benefits program under Medicare since there are fundamental barriers to dental services for this population. In its testimony the ADA said, "By the end of this decade our population will have increased by one third over what it was when Medicare started. That population will live longer and increasingly be in need of health services. It is time the public at large faced this fact and supported an effective initiative to meet the needs of our citizens."[4,29]

National Health Service Corps

The National Health Service Corps is a federal health labor deployment program established by Public Law 91-623, the Emergency Health Personnel Act of 1970. It authorizes the assignment of commissioned officers and Civil Service personnel of the Public Health Service to areas where health services are inadequate because of critical shortages of health personnel. Physicians, dentists, and nurses, as well as supporting health personnel, may be assigned for 2 years to critical shortage areas designated by the Secretary of Health and Human Services.[35] In 1975 the Corps had 551 health professionals in 268 communities: 325 physicians, 80 dentists, and the balance, physicians assistants, nurse practitioners, or other types of physician extenders. In 1977 there were 97 dentists.[31]

In 1986 a total of 1,109 health practitioners whose training was supported by National Health Services Corps Scholarships were assigned to shortage areas in all 50 states and several other U.S. jurisdictions. Of this number 1,068 were physicians and 24 were dentists. This 1986 total marks a decline in the placement figure that peaked at 1,440 in 1985. The decrease reflects a reduction in the number of scholarships awarded in recent years.[7]

The Bureau of Health Professions defines and designates health manpower shortage areas that are eligible for assignment of National Health Service Corps personnel.[44] Except in unusual cases, state and district dental societies must certify the area's need for a dentist. Patients pay prevailing prices and the dentist is encouraged to stay in the community once the tour of duty is over. Some states have been looking at the problem of labor distribution and are trying to find their own solutions. Some local dental societies have chosen to argue against federal involvement at the expense of the dental needs of the community and the public image of the dental profession.[19]

Veterans Administration

The difference between the Department of Defense (DOD) and the Veterans Administration (VA) is that the DOD primarily serves current and retired members of the armed forces, while the VA serves those with some service connected disability, who have honorably left the service.[44]

In 1980 the VA spent $6.2 billion on medical care. The VA provides some dental care to eligible patients through its system of hospitals and absorbed 12% of all public expenditures for dental care in 1977.[12]

USE OF DENTAL SERVICES

In 1983, Americans visited the dentist more than 400 million times, an average of almost two visits per person. However, nearly one half of all Americans did not visit a dentist in 1983. Persons of higher family incomes were more than twice as likely to visit a dentist as those of low incomes. In every age group, white people were more likely than black people to have had a recent dental visit, with 57% of the whites and 42% of blacks having visited the dentist within the previous year. Among those who did visit the dentist a small percent had a large proportion of the visits. For example, 20% of adolescents had five or more visits. Taking the population as a whole, the average rate of visits for Americans was highest for adolescents ages 12 to 17 years, then in descending order for those ages 35 to 54 years, 18 to 34 years, 55 to 64 years, over 65 years and lowest rate for those ages 2 to 4 years.[27]

GOVERNMENTAL SPENDING FOR DENTAL CARE

Americans spent $425 billion on health care in 1985, including $27.1 billion for dentists' services. Private sector payments accounted for all but $600 million of dental expenditures. Patients paid $17.2 billion directly to dentists, with private insurance paying for $9.3 billion worth of dental care. Of the $600 million spent by the federal, state, and local governments for dental care, approximately $500 million was spent on Medicaid and the rest was spent on dental care in community and migrant health centers and other programs. The estimated $500 million spent on Medicaid dental services in 1984 represented less than 2% of the $39.8 billion spent by Medicaid on health care for needy persons.[6,8] In 1976, of the total amount of $8.6 billion dollars spent for dental care in the United States, the government spent $469 million, or 5%.[18] In 1985 the $600 million governmental agencies spent on dental care was 2.2% of the total dental expenditures, a percentage that has been decreasing from 5.6% in 1975 to 2.9% in 1982, and is projected to further decrease to 1.8% in 1988 and 1.7% in 1990.[6,8]

It is clear that public support for dental health care has been limited to: (1) direct services for selected beneficiaries (for example, military personnel, residents of dental shortage areas, and American Indians); (2) dental research; (3) grants for services to special populations (for example, programs for low-income pregnant women, Crippled Children Services, and Head Start programs); and (4) payment for services for certain low-income populations, such as Medicaid.

Dr. Harold Hillenbrand, former executive director emeritus of the American Dental Association in 1977, stated:

The United States is the only industrially developed country in the world without a coherent, identifiable national health program and has only now reached the stage of making a statement of intent . . . the delivery of dental health care is not now, if it ever was, solely a problem for the dental profession. Real solutions must be found in the unselfish collaboration of dentists, the other health professions, the dental auxiliaries, social and behavioral scientists, epidemiologists, educators, statisticians, government and public health officials, consumers, and a whole host of others. There are enough problems to challenge and plague us all.[26]

Since then little has changed and Dr. Hillenbrand's words are as appropriate in 1987 as they were in 1977. There is still much for dental professionals and dental public health to accomplish in order to meet the dental needs of the people in the United States, and "there are enough problems to challenge and plague us all."

REFERENCES

1. American Board of Dental Public Health: Guidelines for graduate education in dental public health, Ann Arbor, MI, 1970, The Board, p. 10.
2. American Dental Association: No denture care coverage in 24 states, ADA News **10**(13):7, 1979.
3. American Dental Association: Strategic plan report of the American Dental Association's special committee on the future of dentistry: Issue papers on dental research, manpower education, practice and public and professional concerns, Chicago, 1983, The Association.
4. American Dental Association: ADA argues for medicare dental plan, adult care under Medicaid termed 'inadequate,' ADA News **17**(16):2, 1986.
5. American Dental Association: Committee ok's $116.3 million for NIDR, ADA News **17**(5):1, 1986.
6. American Dental Association: U.S. dental spending reaches $27.1 billion, ADA News **17**(17):11, 1986.
7. American Medical Association: 1,109 NHSC aided practitioners placed in U.S. shortage areas; Am. Med. News **29**(36):14, 1986.
8. Arnett, R.H., and others: Projections of health care spending to 1990, Health Care Financing Rev. **7**(3):1, 1986.
9. Association of State and Territorial Health Officials Foundation: Public health agencies 1980, a report on their expenditures and activities, Pub. No. 61, Washington, DC, 1981, The Association.
10. Association of State and Territorial Health Officials Foundation: Public health agencies 1983, vol. 2, services and activities, Pub. No. 80, Washington, DC, 1985, The Association.
11. Association of State and Territorial Health Officials Foundation: Public health agencies 1983, vol. 4, an inventory of programs and block grants, Pub. No. 82, Washington, DC, 1985, The Association.
12. Burt, B.A.: Financing for dental care services. In Striffler, D.F., Young, W.O., and Burt, B.A., editors: Dentistry, dental practice and the community, ed. 3, Philadelphia, 1983, W.B. Saunders Co.
13. Campbell, E.M., Hayden, C.H., and Van Burskirk, H.: Summaries of recent legislation affecting dentistry, Bethesda, MD, 1968, Public Health Service, Division of Dental Health, p. 29.
14. Clark, J.P. and Goforth, V.: Organizing dental programs for Head Start preschool groups, Washington, DC, U.S. Department of Health, Education and Welfare, Office of Child Development, p. 52.

15. Editorial, J. Public Health Policy **6**(4):435, 1985.
16. Foege, W.: On AMA's interest in public health, Am. Med. News **29**(36):4, 1986.
17. Forward plan for health, F.Y. 1977-1981, DHEW pub. No. (05) 76-50024, Washington, DC, 1975, U.S. Department of Health, Education and Welfare.
18. Gibson, R.M., and Mueller, M.S.: National health expenditures, F.Y. 1976, Soc. Secur. Bull. **40**(3):22, 1977.
19. Greene, J.C.: Federal programs and the profession, J. Am. Dent. Assoc. **92**:689, 1976.
20. Haggerty, R.J., and Darney, P.D.: Maternal and child health services. In Last, J.M., editor: Maxcy-Rosenau public health and preventive medicine, Norwalk, CT, 1986, Appleton-Century-Crofts.
21. Hanlon, J.J., and Pickett, G.E.: Public health administration and practice, ed. 8, St. Louis, 1984, The C.V. Mosby Co.
22. Health Services Administration: The Children and Youth Projects, DHEW Pub. No. (HSM) 72-5006, Washington, DC, 1972, Public Health Service.
23. Health Services Administration: Dental Health Projects for Children, DHEW Pub. No. (HSM) 72-5006, Washington, DC, 1972, Public Health Service.
24. Health Services Administration: The Maternity and Infant Care Projects, DHEW Pub. No. (HSM) 75-5012, Washington, DC, 1975, Public Health Service.
25. Health Services Administration: Promoting community health, DHEW Pub. No. (HSA) 77-5000, Washington, DC, 1976, Public Health Service.
26. Ingle, J., and Blair, P., editors: International dental care delivery systems, Cambridge, MA, 1978, Ballinger Publishing Co., p. 263.
27. Jack, S.S.: Use of dental services: United States, 1983, Medical Benefits, Charlottesville, VA, p. 3, August 31, 1986.
28. Jordheim, A.E.: Welfare kids: outlook bleak, Medical Tribune **27**(27):3, 1986.
29. Knutson, J.W.: What is public health? In Pelton, W.J., and Wisan, J.M., editors: Dentistry in public health, ed. 2, Philadelphia, 1955, W.B. Saunders Co., pp. 1-10.
30. Leske, G.S., and others: Dental public health. In Last, J.M., editor: Maxcy-Rosenau public health and preventive medicine, Norwalk, CT, 1986, Appleton-Century-Crofts.
31. Manpower Analysis Branch, Division of Dentistry: Dental manpower fact sheet, Bethesda, MD, February 1977, Public Health Service, p. 10.
32. Minnesota Department of Health: Services for children with handicaps, SCH-706, Minneapolis, March 1984, The Department.
33. National Caries Program, National Institute of Dental Research: The prevalence of dental caries in United States children, 1979-80. NIH Pub. No. 82-2245, De-

cember 1981, U.S. Department of Health and Human Services.

34. National Center for Health Statistics: Decayed, missing and filled teeth among persons 1-74 years, United States. Pub. No. (PHS) 81-1673, August, 1981, U.S. Department of Health and Human Services.

35. National Health Service Corps rules and regulations, Federal Register 40:34080, 1975.

36. Project Head Start dental services, Washington, DC, U.S. Department of Health, Education and Welfare, Office of Child Development, p. 31.

37. Schoen, M.H., and Freed J.R.: Prevention of dental disease, Annu. Rev. Public Health 2:71, 1981.

38. Services, expenditures, and programs of state and territorial health agencies, 1974, Washington, DC, 1976, Association of State and Territorial Health Officials, Health Program Reporting System.

39. Smith, D.C.: Organization of maternal and child health services. In Wallace, H., and others, editors: Maternal and child health practices, problems, resources, and methods of delivery, Springfield, IL, 1973, Charles C Thomas, Publisher, p. 30.

40. Social and rehabilitative statistics from Medicaid statistics. F.Y. 1976, DHEW Pub. No. (SRS077-03154, Washington, DC, 1977, U.S. Department of Health, Education and Welfare.

41. U.S. Department of Health and Human Services: Head Start program performance standards (45-CFR-1304, DHHS Pub. No. (OHDS) 84-31131), Washington, DC, November 1984.

42. U.S. House of Representatives: Opportunities for success: cost-effective programs for children, staff report of the Select Committee on Children, Youth and Families, Washington, DC., August 1985, U.S. Government Printing Office.

43. Willcocks, A.J.: Dental health and the changing society. In Slack, G.L., editor: Dental public health, Bristol, England, 1981, John Wright & Sons, Ltd.

44. Wilson, F.A., and Neuhauser D.: Health services in the United States, ed. 2, Cambridge, MA, 1985, Ballinger Publishing Co.

45. Wilson, W.A.: The future role of government in dental practice and education, J. Am. Coll. Dent. 40:111, 1973.

46. Winslow, C.E.A.: The untilled field of public health, Mod. Med. 2:183, 1920.

47. World Health Organization, Expert Committee on Dental Health: Organization of dental public health services report, Technical report series no. 298. Geneva, 1965, The Organization, p. 44.

48. Young, W.O.: Dentistry looks toward the twenty-first century. In Brown, W.E., editor: Oral health dentistry and the American public, Norman, OK, 1974, University of Oklahoma Press, p. 3.

CHAPTER 2

Factors Affecting the Practice of Dentistry

As we approach the turn of the century, the role of the dental professional is changing. Some of the changes are a function of advances in technology. Others are the result of increased and improved education, both of patients and dentists. But some are the result of the changes in society and the socio-economic structure of which dentistry is a part. People and systems over which dentists have limited control are affecting the way dentistry is practiced today. The purpose of this chapter is to explore some important issues in dentistry and discuss implications for the profession. The issues selected for discussion are those that most significantly affect the profession, for example, demographics, financial considerations, and the medically compromised patient.

DEMOGRAPHICS

Several factors have been operating concurrently over recent years to change the characteristics of the population that the dental profession serves and the characteristics of the dental profession itself.

The post-World War II baby-boom cohort is choosing to have fewer children than its historical predecessors. Moreover, women who have begun careers or are in the educational process in pursuit of careers are delaying the start of their families so that the average age of the mother among college-educated women has risen to the early thirties. Therefore there are relatively fewer pediatric dental patients. Of those, the incidence and prevalence of dental caries has declined.[5,6,9]

The introduction of fluoride, both topically and in public water supplies, has had the greatest impact on reducing dental caries. During the 1940s conclusive documentation showed that 1.0 part per million of fluoride in drinking water effected a two-thirds reduction in dental caries. In 1946 efficacy of sodium fluoride solution applied topically to the teeth was demonstrated. Use of fluoride rinses, ingested fluoride supplements (in nonfluoridated areas), and fluoridated dentifrices have also been shown to reduce the decay rate. Prevention of dental disease has become the thrust of the profession's goals and objectives. Even so, fluoridation is still a hotly contested issue in some areas. Antifluoridationists campaign vigorously and vociferously to prevent fluoridation of community water supplies. Their attacks are based on political or ideological issues or simply misinformation. Presently about 80 million individuals using public water supplies do not have community fluoridation. Despite the irrefutable evidence about the efficacy of fluoridation, almost 40% of public tap water remains unfluoridated or does not have enough fluoride to combat caries effectively. Dr. Harold Löe, director of the National Institute of Dental Research, attributes this to lack of public funding.[18] Since fluoridation of public water supplies is determined locally and is often determined by referenda, the implementation of this dental public health policy is subject to local political action groups. Misguided antifluoridation activists, some of whom claim that fluoride promotes cancer, sickle cell anemia, and AIDS, have succeeded in persuading local government agencies and voters in many areas to reject fluoridation.

Increased dental health education through school systems and professional offices as well as the generalized increase in nutritional education of the public has also had a positive impact on decreasing dental caries. However, a decrease in dental caries does not necessarily mean a decrease in dental disease or a lessening of demand for dental care. Lower incidence of caries and loss of teeth resulting from caries at a young age means that at adulthood, more teeth have been retained. This fact, taken in conjunction with another demographic trend, the increase in the number of elderly in the population, has created a new pool of dental need.

THE ELDERLY

The over-65 age group is the fastest growing segment of our society. By the end of the century, it is expected that the U.S. population over 65 years of age will increase from the present 11% of the population to 13%, and by the year 2030 will reach 20%. In 1981, according to U.S. census figures, 48.2 million people were in the 55-plus segment of the population. By 2010 the number will soar to 74 million. The population doubled from 1950 to 1980 and will nearly double again by 2030 to 98.6 million people over 55 years of age (Table 2-1).

At a conference on Geriatric Education for Health Professionals in 1985, Dr. Lawrence Kerr, past president of the American Dental Association, discussed the state of oral health of the elderly and identified the following group of dental diseases requiring treatment[19]:
1. Mobile and brittle teeth
2. Periodontal disease
3. Fractured crowns of teeth with sharp edges
4. Recession of gingival tissue
5. Root caries
6. Ill-fitting bridges and dentures, full and partial
7. Malaligned jaws with temporomandibular joint diseases
8. Higher incidence of caries
9. Neglect of oral hygiene
10. Edentulousness
11. Xerostomia—salivary gland impairment
12. Changes in the oral mucosa
13. Tissue changes in the tongue
14. Bone changes
15. Changes in tooth structure

Table 2-1. Elderly population estimate, 1980-2000 (in millions)

Age group	1980	1990	2000	Annual rate of change	
				1980-90	1990-2000
65-69	8,780.8	10,006.3	9,110.2	1.3%	-0.9%
70-74	6,796.7	8,048.0	8,582.8	1.7%	0.6%
75-79	4,792.6	6,223.7	7,242.2	2.6%	1.5%
80-84	2,934.2	4,060.1	4,964.6	3.3%	2.0%
85+	2,239.7	3,460.9	5,136.3	4.4%	4.0%
Total	25,544.1	31,799.1	35,036.1	2.2%	1.0%

From U.S. Bureau of the Census. Population Estimates and Projections, Series P-25, No. 937, 1983.

The impact of this increase in the elderly population on dental practice will be significant. Historically, use of dental services by the elderly has been less than significant. According to a report issued by the American Dental Association in 1983[2]:

Except for children under six years, the percentage of elderly persons who visit a dentist is lowest compared to other age groups. Lower income is a further barrier to receiving care. About one of five among the poorest elderly (under $5000) visit the dentist in a year's time. The percent rises to one-third of the elderly with incomes of $5000 to $10,000; 41 percent in the $10,000 to $15,000; and 48 to 56 percent for the elderly with incomes of $15,000 or more. For those utilizing dental services, number of visits per person is highest in the lowest income group. This indicates the impact of Medicaid and access for the elderly programs, combines with the large amount of care needed by the oldest and poorest, which is being converted to demand.

That existing need will be translated into demand is substantiated by the following information from Robert J. Forbes, a staff member of the American Association of Retired Persons[8]:

Myth 1: Older people have limited needs and limited dollars

In part this is true. People in retirement no longer have children at home or in college, and some economists estimate that because of smaller household size, lower taxes, no regular commuting costs, and limited wardrobe purchases, older households need only 60 to 80 percent of their former income to maintain their lifestyles.

On the other hand research statistics tell us that households headed by persons 55 and over receive about 30 percent of total aggregate income in the United States; own 80 percent of all money currently in savings and loan institutions; and are responsible for 20 percent of all discretionary money spent in the marketplace— nearly double that of households headed by people under 34.

Myth 2: Most older people are in institutions

A 1982 study by the U.S. Census Bureau states that fewer than 5 percent of people 65 and 74, only 1.5 percent are institutionalized. . . . In fact, 70% of all older Americans own their own homes and the majority of mortgages are paid in full.

Myth 3: Most older people are in poor health and inactive.

A recent survey of retirees found that 70 percent stated that they were in good health and were enjoying active lives in their families and communities.

Other supporting information is found in marketing journals. *Madison Avenue* in 1984 published an article called "The Invisible Consumer," which discussed the senior market.[11] The author states that the 1981 household per capita income for those ages 55 to 64 was $9,874, 34% higher than the national average. This age group comprises a third of all buying power in the U.S. marketplace. The author further suggests that those who perceive the elderly as being in their *vital* years or *freedom* years will have more success in reaching them than those who perceive them as the grey market. The suggestion seems appropriate for those in the practice of dentistry as well. (More detailed information on geriatric dentistry can be found in Chapter 5).

Three demographic and epidemiologic trends have been discussed: declining birth rate, declining incidence of caries in children, and the growth of the elderly segment of the population. Issues involving the numbers of dentists and dental auxiliaries will be addressed next.

STATUS OF DENTAL PERSONNEL IN THE UNITED STATES

The educational system for dental professionals has experienced major changes over the past ten years.* First year enrollments in dental schools peaked at 6,301 from 1978-79 but have declined since then. During the period from 1984-85, first year enrollments numbered 5,047 (Table 2-2). Applications to dental schools have decreased dramatically. The declining trend in

---

*For more comprehensive data on the issues discussed here, the reader is referred to the American Dental Association's Council on Dental Education Annual Reports and the Fifth Report to The President and Congress on the Status of Health Personnel in the United States, March, 1986.

applicants since 1975-76, despite a decrease in the number of first year places since 1978-79, has resulted in a steady increase in the applicant/ acceptance ratio. In 1975-76, 37% of all applicants were enrolled; in 1984-85, 78% of all dental applicants were enrolled.

Table 2-2. Number of dental schools, students, and graduates: selected academic years 1950-51 through 1984-85

Academic year	Number of schools	Number of students		Number of graduates
		Total	First year	
1950-51	42	11,891	3,226	2,830
1955-56	43	12,730	3,445	3,038
1960-61	47	13,580	3,616	3,290
1961-62	47	13,513	3,605	3,207
1962-63	48	13,576	3,680	3,233
1963-64	48	13,691	3,770	3,213
1964-65	49	13,876	3,836	3,181
1965-66	49	14,020	3,806	3,198
1966-67	49	14,421	3,942	3,360
1967-68	50	14,955	4,200	3,457
1968-69	52	15,408	4,203	3,433
1969-70	53	16,008	4,355	3,749
1970-71	53	16,553	4,565	3,775
1971-72	52	17,305	4,745	3,961
1972-73	56	18,376	5,337	4,320
1973-74	58	19,369	5,445	4,515
1974-75	58	20,146	5,617	4,969
1975-76	59	20,767	5,763	5,336
1976-77	59	21,013	5,935	5,177
1977-78	59	21,510	5,954	5,324
1978-79	60	22,179	6,301	5,424
1979-80	60	22,482	6,132	5,256
1980-81	60	22,842	6,030	5,550
1981-82	60	22,621	5,855	5,371
1982-83	60	22,235	5,498	5,756
1983-84	60	21,428	5,274	5,337
1984-85	60	20,588	5,047	—*

From American Dental Association, Council on Dental Education. *Dental Students' Register* for each selected academic year from 1950-51 through 1966-67. *Annual Report on Dental Education* for all subsequent academic years.
*Data are not available at this time.

The cost of dental education may be a significant factor in the declining number of dental school applicants. Student indebtedness increased by 58% between 1978 and 1984 (Table 2-3). Factors contributing to this increase include higher cost of living, higher tuition, higher interest rates, and reduced availability of low-cost loans and scholarships.

The total number of dental schools grew from 42 in 1950 to 60 in 1978. As of 1986, there were still 60, but two have announced plans to close (Oral Roberts and Emory University), and the status of at least three more is publicly questioned.

Table 2-3. Average annual cost to public and private dental schools per dental student: academic years 1967-68 through 1983-84

Academic year	All schools	Public schools	Private schools
	(In thousands)		
1967-68	$ 7.3	$ 8.9	$ 5.9
1968-69	8.5	10.1	6.8
1969-70	9.5	11.1	8.0
1970-71	10.3	11.7	8.8
1971-72	12.0	—*	—*
1972-73	13.4	15.9	10.9
1973-74	14.7	17.4	11.7
1974-75	16.4	19.4	13.0
1975-76	17.8	20.7	14.5
1976-77	19.8	23.1	15.9
1977-78	21.2	24.5	17.1
1978-79	22.7	26.2	18.3
1979-80	24.9	28.5	20.3
1980-81	27.9	31.7	23.1
1981-82	30.4	34.6	25.1
1982-83	32.2	36.6	26.8
1983-84	35.4	41.2	28.5

From American Dental Association, Council on Dental Education. *Financial Report, Fiscal Year Ending June 30, 1984; Supplement 4 to the Annual Report on Dental Education 1984-85.* Also prior annual reports.
*Further breakdown of school costs are not available.

The number of women enrolled in first-year dental classes has increased from 2.1% in 1970-71 to 27.1% in 1984-85. Their number as first-year enrollees and graduates is expected to increase through the year 1995 and then level off, although the number of active female dentists is projected to increase through the year 2000.

Of concern to practicing dentists is the number of active dentists per 100,000 total population because this number represents the relative proportion of the dental market each practitioner holds (Table 2-4).

In 1984 there were 58.0 dentists per 100,000 people. Regardless of the methodology used for future projections (that is, low or high), this

Table 2-4. Number of active dentists and dentist-to-population ratios: estimated 1984 and projected for selected years, 1985-2000*

Year and alternative projection	Number of active dentists	Active dentists per 100,000 total population
1984	137,950	58.0
1985	140,770	58.7
Low	140,770	58.7
High	140,770	58.7
1990	150,760	60.1
Low	150,760	60.1
High	151,200	60.3
1995	156,800	60.2
Low	156,500	60.1
High	159,820	61.4
2000	161,180	60.0
Low	158,900	59.1
High	167,020	62.2

From Department of Health and Human Services, Health Resources and Services Administration, Bureau of Health Professions, Division of Associated and Dental Health Professions.
*The basic methodology was used for the projections shown for the years 1985 through 2000; alternative assumptions were used for the low and high projections. Includes dentists in Federal service.

number will remain fairly stable through the year 2000. An interesting and confounding variable may be seen by considering lines 2 and 3 in Table 2-5.

Of dentists who practice 30 or more hours per week, 78.3% are male and 55.6% are female. Of dentists who practice less than 30 hours per week, 10.6% are male and 17.5% are female. It would seem, therefore, that as the number of female dentists increases, although the dentist per 100,000 population ratio may remain stable, the full-time equivalents (FTE) may actually decrease, thereby increasing the relative proportion of the dental market each practitioner holds. It may also be seen that 88.9% of male dentists list private practice as their primary type of dental employment, in contrast to 73% of female dentists. In every other category given in Table 2-5, percent of female dentists is greater than percent of male dentists. This would indicate that female dentists have become proportionately more involved in areas of the dental profession other than private practice.

The numbers of dental auxiliary students and practicing auxiliaries is important to examine because they are critical to the success of any practicing dentist. These will be discussed in Chapter 3.

FINANCIAL CONSIDERATIONS IN THE PRACTICE OF DENTISTRY

Reimbursement for dental services is a major factor affecting the practice of dentistry. Although much of the cost of dental care is out-of-pocket expense for the patient, an increasingly large number of patients have some type of third party payment system in place. Some examples of third party payment systems include private dental insurance, Medicaid, and capitation programs. These programs will be discussed in greater detail in Chapter 6. However, a few salient issues concerning the impact of these programs on the practice of dentistry will be addressed here.

Table 2-5. Primary type of dental employment of active dentists, by sex: December 31, 1984

Primary type of dental employment	All active dentists		Male		Female	
	Number	Percent distribution	Number	Percent distribution	Number	Distribution (%)
All active	137,950	100.0	130,970	100.0	6,980	100.0
Practicing dentist (30 or more hours per week)	106,367	77.1	102,484	78.3	3,883	55.6
Practicing dentist (Less than 30 hours per week)	15,161	11.0	13,942	10.6	1,219	17.5
On faculty or staff of dental school	3,577	2.6	3,210	2.5	367	5.2
Armed Forces dentist	5,200	3.8	4,840	3.7	360	5.2
Other federal dentist	2,000	1.4	1,800	1.4	200	2.9
Dentist in state or local government	1,247	0.9	1,097	0.8	150	2.1
Hospital staff dentist	497	0.3	435	0.3	62	0.9
Intern or resident	2,454	1.8	1,940	1.5	514	7.4
Other student	655	0.5	540	0.4	115	1.6
Staff member of health or dental organization	792	0.6	682	0.5	110	1.6

Estimated by Health Resources and Services Administration, Bureau of Health Professions, Division of Associated and Dental Health Professions, based on data from the American Dental Association, Bureau of Economic and Behavioral Research.

Implicitly and explicitly, the involvement of a third party in the practice of dentistry involves loss of control by the dentist. The communication process is affected in many ways. Purely on a technical basis, the number of communications between the practice and insurance carriers (written, verbal, and occasionally on-site verification) places additional demands on the dentist and staff. Many, if not most, offices have had to employ additional personnel whose primary, if not sole, responsibility is insurance forms and follow-up. Communication between dentist and patient is affected because of the potential for misunderstandings about the role of dental insurance in paying for treatment. Issues of deductibles, copayments, coinsurance, maximum allowances, service benefits, and services excluded from coverage are all areas where reality may differ significantly from patient expectations. The following definitions will help clarify these terms:

Deductible. Amount payable by the insured before insurance benefits start being paid. Can apply per event (such as, hospitalization), period of time (for example, year), or lifetime. May apply to one service (for example, under basic plans) or any combination of covered services (usually under major medical plans).

Copayments. Dollar amount payable by the insured for units of covered services; applies only after any applicable deductible is exhausted and up to any out-of-pocket maximum.

Coinsurance. Percent of charge or allowable charge that the insured must pay; it may apply only after a deductible has been met and may be limited to an out-of-pocket maximum payable by the insured.

Maximum allowances. Highest amounts of insurer liability for covered services. May apply per medical event (such as, hospitalization), period of time (for example, year), or lifetime.

Service benefits. A benefit traditionally associated with Blue Shield plans, under which the provider agrees to accept the payment allowed by the insurer for the covered expense as payment in full.

Services excluded from coverage. Those services or units of service not covered under insurance plan.

In addition, the requirement of prior approval by the insurance carrier for certain types of treatment and/or for treatment above established dollar amounts often introduces a new variable into the treatment planning process, for example, "I'll do it if my insurance company will pay for it." Often approval or denial of proposed treatment can take up to 6 weeks from date of submission to receive, and it is certainly not prudent to begin treatment without both the dentist and patient having a clear understanding of with whom financial responsibility lies and who is responsible for how much. The demand for postoperative radiographs by some third party carriers to affirm treatment and quality may clearly countermand established professional guidelines for minimizing patient exposure to unnecessary radiation.[13]

An example of the locus of control moving from the practitioner to a third party (that is, neither the provider nor the patient) may be seen in the following excerpt from a helpful brochure prepared by the Massachusetts Blue Shield Corporation.[4]

METHODS OF REIMBURSEMENT

Depending on the type of benefit plan your patient has, Blue Shield reimbursement to dentists is made in either of two ways:

- a *"usual and customary" payment plan*—based on a profile of your usual charges and those of dentists throughout the state who participate with Blue Shield
- a *fee schedule payment plan*—based on a set amount established by Blue Shield as well as a co-payment from the patient.

DETERMINING REIMBURSEMENT
Usual and customary

Usual and customary payments to dentists represent the lowest of three amounts:

- your submitted charge for a particular procedure,
- your "usual" charge—based on your individual profile (the Level I allowance), or
- the "customary" charge—based on the statewide maximum allowable charge (the Level II allowance).

Levels I and II are explained below.

Usual and customary plans base payment on either 95 or 100 percent of a usual and customary allowance, depending on the patient's plan. If the patient's plan provides full coverage for a service with no patient co-payment, Blue Shield pays you 95 percent of the usual and customary allowance as payment in full.

If the patient is covered through a co-payment plan, you will receive 100 percent of the usual and customary allowance. Blue Shield pays you a designated percentage of that allowance and the patient pays the balance (the co-payment) up to the allowance, according to the provisions of that patient's plan.

In either case, since payment is based on the usual and customary allowance, the patient is not responsible for the difference between that allowance and your actual charge for the service.

Fee schedule

Fee schedule payments represent the lower of two amounts:

- your submitted charge for a particular procedure, or
- the Blue Shield scheduled fee for that procedure.

Under this plan, the patient is responsible for the difference between your submitted charge and Blue Shield's scheduled amount.

A brief summary of reimbursement is shown in Fig. 2-1.

DETERMINING YOUR PROFILE

Because usual and customary reimbursement amounts are based on Level I (usual) and Level II

(customary) amounts, it is important that you understand how these profiles are developed.

Level I

Your Level I profile is developed from a list of your submitted charges for a particular procedure during a calendar year. Charges are arrayed from low to high and the median of this range of charges becomes your "usual" charge, or individual profile.

Level I Example

Charges reported for performing adult prophylaxis, procedure code 1110, in 1985:

1. $24
2. 24
3. 28⎫ $28 is the median of charges submitted in
4. 28 1985, thus this figure becomes your "usual"
5. 30 profile allowance effective July 1, 1986.

To determine your profile, add the number of charges for a service. When the result is an even number, divide by two and add one. When the result is an odd number, add one and then divide by two. In the example above, the total number of charges is 5. 5 + 1 = 6 divided by 2 = 3.

In the example, the dollar amount that corresponds to the third charge is the median. Therefore, your Level I profile for this procedure is $28.

Your profile is based on claims submitted during the calendar year prior to the year in which a profile update takes place. For example, profiles effective July 1, 1986 are based on charges reported for services rendered in 1985. Please note that July 1986 Level I profiles were developed from 1985 claims submitted to Blue Shield and Dental Service Corporation of Massachusetts. The Dental Service Corporation's data is jointly owned by both corporations.

Blue Shield reviews and updates participating dentists' profiles annually.

At least two charges per service during a calendar year are needed to develop a profile. All reported claims, whether paid or denied, are used in develop-

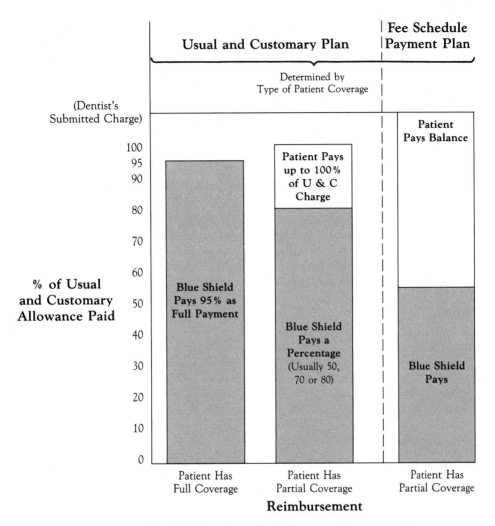

Fig. 2-1. Overview of reimbursement.

ing your profile. Until a profile is developed, reimbursement will be based on the lower of two fees:

- your submitted charge, or
- the statewide maximum allowable charge (Level II).

Level II

Level II allowances are the maximum allowable charges for a service or procedure, based on Level I profiles of all participating dentists throughout the state.

Level II Example

Dentists' Level I Profiles	# of Charges	Cumulative # of Charges
$24	10	10
$25	15	25
$26	25	50
$28	25	75
$29	15	90
$30	10	100

After Level I profiles for a particular service have been developed, they are weighted by the number of times that service was reported. The Level I profiles are arrayed from low to high and the total number of charges is calculated. From this information, Blue Shield is able to determine the 90th percentile, which is designated as the Level II profile for dentists in practice for a year or more, and the 50th percentile, which is designated as the Level II profile for dentists in practice less than a year.

To determine the 90th percentile, multiply the total number of charges by .90 (100 × .90). In this example, the 90th percentile is the 90th charge—$29. Therefore, the Level II profile for this procedure is $29 for dentists who have been in practice for more than a year. For dentists who have been in practice less than a year, the Level II profile is determined by the 50th percentile which, in this example, is the 50th charge—$26.

The Level II profile is particularly important if you do not have a Level I profile for a procedure. In that instance, your submitted charge would be compared to the 90th percentile or the 50th percentile, depending on the length of your practice, and Blue Shield pays the lower of the two amounts.

The following table shows several actual 1986 maximum allowable charges for commonly-performed procedures.

Examples of 1986 Allowances
(For services rendered on or after July 1, 1986)

Procedure Code	Narrative	Level II Allowances
00220	Intraoral periapical—single, first film	$ 10
01220	Topical application of stannous fluoride—one treatment (excluding prophylaxis)	$ 18
02330	Composite resin restoration—one surface	$ 35
03320	Bicuspid root canal, single canal (excludes final restoration)	$325
04910	Preventive periodontal procedures (periodontal prophylaxis)	$ 45

LIMITS ON ANNUAL PROFILE INCREASES

The percentage increase for Level II charges may not exceed the percentage increase in the "Boston Consumer Price Index for Urban Wage Earners and Clerical Workers, All Items Less Medical Care." The percentage increase for Level I charges may also be limited by an amount that varies for each annual update of allowable charges.

Third party payment mechanisms provide a new, sometimes perplexing, sense of accountability for the private dentist. The dentist may submit a treatment plan for what is considered optimum restoration of the patient's dentition to proper form and function. The response from the third party payment group may indicate that less than optimum treatment is covered under the plan. The patient, who often believes that all his/her needs will be covered by the third party, may be frustrated or confused. Three hypothetical examples of the effect of third party payment follow. They serve to illustrate some of the ramifications of third party payment to the patient and the practitioner.

Case study 1. A 19-year-old female suffered traumatic injury to all six maxillary anterior teeth at age 16 years. Treatment at that time included root canal therapy to all involved teeth. Her parents could not afford to restore the teeth then. Since that time, her father died. She is now covered by Medicaid. You examine her and submit a form for pre-authorization requesting posts, cores, and crowns for the six maxillary anterior teeth. The form is returned "Approval denied." A handwritten notation states, "Recommend extracting six maxillary anterior roots and fabricating a removable denture."

Case study 2. A 24-year-old male comes to your office requesting that his wisdom teeth be extracted. He also requests intravenous sedation. He wants to pay for the procedure via the Blue Cross/Blue Shield coverage provided by his employer. Blue Cross/Blue Shield, however, covers only procedures for which the patient must be hospitalized. Therefore a relatively simple procedure, which might have been handled effectively by you in your office, requires you to admit the patient to the hospital. In addition to the fee for your services, the patient (and Blue Cross/Blue Shield) is billed for blood tests, chest x-rays, electrocardiogram, and so on. In addition, a bed that might have been used for a more emergent need has been occupied. (In response to misallocation of hospital beds, many hospitals now provide surgical day-care facilities. In this setting patients are treated in the hospital on an ambulatory basis and go home the same day.)

Case study 3. A 31-year-old female comes to your office with her four children, ages 5 through 12 years. Their dental needs range from simple prophylaxis to routine fillings. No child's needs exceed $50 in cost. All the children are covered by Medicaid. For routine dental care not exceeding $50, no prior approval is necessary. All treatment may be rendered expeditiously and fully. A mother who might otherwise have been unable to provide routine dental care for her children because of financial inability can, with the help of Medicaid coverage, see that their dental needs are met.

Malpractice

The issue of malpractice insurance is one of growing concern to health care providers. Insurance rates have soared nationally, with regional differences driving practitioners to make a choice: (1) to relocate; (2) to become employees of health maintenance organizations (HMOs) where malpractice insurance is paid for by the organization, not the individual; (3) to join the Armed Services, for similar reasons; or (4) to leave the practice of medicine altogether through early retirement or change in careers. In Massachusetts, the rates for private practitioners in general dentistry over the past 3 years were as follows:

1984-85	$368	} 427% increase
1985-86	$1940	
1986-87	$2400	23.7% increase
		plus $50 additional for each dental assistant hygienist employed.

The implications of the increasing cost of malpractice insurance are great for two reasons:

The out-of-pocket expense is large; even though payment may be made in installments, this expenditure is in addition to other personal and professional cost-of-living items such as salaries, rent (office, home), mortgage payments, and so on.

Insurance companies such as Blue Cross/Blue Shield place limits on annual profile increases, which may not exceed either the annual consumer price index increase in a given geographic area or an amount determined as the maximum by Blue Cross/Blue Shield for each annual update of allowable charges, whichever is less. This means that although malpractice rates may increase 50% in a given year, if the consumer price index increases only 5%, the increase cannot be passed along to the consumer. It must, in fact, be absorbed by the practitioner. In medicine, there is precedent for Medicare freezing fees for 2 consecutive years in 1984 and 1985. While other costs of practice and living continued to increase, reimbursement by Medicare remained fixed. Medicare, a federally funded health insurance program for the elderly, does not cover any dental services, not even emergencies or prophylaxis.

Medically compromised patients

The responsibility of the dental professional in management of the medically compromised patient has clearly increased over the years. With medical advances in diagnosis and care of patients with systemic diseases, more patients being treated for one or more medical conditions are currently being seen in dental offices. The discussion of medically compromised patients for the purpose of this chapter will be divided into two groups: systemic diseases and infectious diseases. The purpose of this section is to give the reader an overview of how management of these patients affects the practice of dentistry. For more information on specific disease entities, see references listed at the end of this chapter.

Systemic diseases. Among the systemic diseases frequently seen in dental practice are hypertension, bleeding disorders, diabetes mellitus, and patients with damaged hearts. The best way to identify patients at risk for these problems is by taking an accurate, thorough medical history. A sample of the medical history form currently in use at the Boston University Goldman School of Graduate Dentistry is included as an example (Fig. 2-2). Positive re-

BOSTON UNIVERSITY MEDICAL CENTER
HENRY M. GOLDMAN SCHOOL OF GRADUATE DENTISTRY

MEDICAL HISTORY

Name_____ Record No. _____ Date_____

Address _____ Zip_____

Your Age_____ Height_____ Weight_____ State of Health_____

Physician's Name _____ Phone_____

Physician's Address_____

Date of last physical examination: _____ Reason: _____

In case of EMERGENCY contact: Name _____

　　　Address _____

　　　Relationship _____ Office phone_____ Home phone _____

Please answer the following questions by placing a check (√) in the proper blank. Answer YES if you NOW HAVE or have EVER HAD any of the following. If you are unable to answer the question, please leave the space blank.

	YES	NO		YES	NO		YES	NO
1. Any change in health in last year			16. Any unusual *reaction* to drugs, medications or pills			31. Heart murmur/ Heart surgery		
2. Being treated now by a physician			17. Frequent headaches			32. Chest pain on exertion		
3. Taking any medicines, pills, tonics, drugs regularly			18. Dizziness; light headedness			33. Soaking sweats at night		
4. Major operations, hospitalization, or serious illness			19. Eye or ear trouble			34. Ankles swell		
5. Growth or tumor			20. Stuffy nose; Sinus trouble			35. Appetite changes recently		
6. X-Ray examination			21. Frequent nose bleeds			36. Any foods you cannot eat		
7. Radiation/Therapy			22. Cough, hoarseness or sore throat			37. Difficulty in swallowing		
8. Rheumatic fever			23. Breathe through your mouth			38. Indigestion; Heartburn		
9. Arthritis; Rheumatism			24. Shortness of breath			39. Stomach trouble; ulcers		
10. Jaundice/Hepatitis			25. Asthma, hayfever or allergies			40. Regurgitate; Vomit		
11. Diabetes			26. Itch, rash or swelling of the skin			41. Vomited blood		
12. Tuberculosis			27. Had series of shots or injections			42. Bloody diarrhea		
13. Syphilis; Gonorrhea			28. Cough up blood			43. Black bowel movement		
14. Heart attack; Stroke			29. Smoke now			44. Liver; Gall bladder		
15. Epilepsy			30. Low/High blood pressure			45. More than two drinks of alcohol per day		

Fig. 2-2. Sample medical history form.

	YES	NO		YES	NO		YES	NO
46. Kidney trouble			58. Any blood disease			70. Frequent fractures or dislocations		
47. Painful urination			59. Excess bleeding following a cut			71. Condition requiring cortisone (steroid)		
48. Get up at night to urinate			60. Do you bruise easily			72. History of any disease within your family		
49. Urinate more than six times per day			61. Problems in healing			73. Dry Mouth		
50. Thirsty much of the time			62. Blood transfusion			WOMEN ONLY		
51. Blood/Sugar in urine			63. Treated for nervous or mental disorders			74. Menstrual periods difficult		
52. Gland, goiter, or Thyroid			64. Fainting, seizures or convulsions			75. Any pregnancies; number:		
53. Excessive weight gain or loss in last 6 months			65. Neuritis, neuralgia or numbness			76. Any pregnancy problems		
54. Get tired easily			66. Trembles, uncontrolled shaking or loss of speech			77. Pregnant now; trimester:		
55. Hot weather bother you			67. Any body part paralyzed			78. Menopausal problems		
56. Excessively nervous			68. Growing pains or twitching of limbs			79. Hysterectomy; Ovariectomy		
57. Often cry			69. Painful; swollen joints					

Patient, Parent or Guardian Signature

_____

_____

_____

_____

_____

_____

Report from Physician: Required   Obtained   Requested
                          YES NO   **YES NO**   **YES NO**
                          ☐ ☐   ☐ ☐   ☐ ☐

Student Review: *LIST PERTINENT INFORMATION ON FRONT OF RECORD UNDER MEDICAL ALERT.*

Student Signature: _____ Instructor: _____
                                                 Signature/degree:

Update _____   _____

         _____   _____

Fig. 2-2, cont'd.

sponse to one of the questions requires follow-up by the dentist for clarification. The dentist is not expected to diagnose a medical condition, but familiarity with signs and symptoms of systemic diseases is essential in knowing when to request consultation from the patient's physician in determining what measures are necessary for optimum management of the patient in the dental setting. If it is determined that a medical clearance is appropriate, it should be requested in writing to include in the patient's chart for medicolegal reasons. An example of a medical clearance letter is included for reference (Fig. 2-3).

A medical clearance should be designed for clarity of response and ease of completion on the part of the physician. It is also important to provide space for the physician to print his/her name and phone number should additional information be required. It can be frustrating for the dentist and the patient to receive incomplete information and not have the resources available to be able to follow-up in a timely fashion. It is also important for the dentist to be as specific as possible in communicating to the physician about what dental procedures are expected in the patient's treatment and what medical information is needed in this regard. Finally, note that the patient must sign the medical consultation form authorizing the release of pertinent information to the dentist. It is considered a breach of the patient's right to privacy to divulge such information without the patient's consent, and most physicians will not do so.

Blood pressure should be routinely measured and recorded at the initial visit of all dental patients. Since hypertension is usually asymptomatic in its early stages, an undiagnosed hypertensive patient may schedule an office visit for routine dental care with no knowledge of his/her condition. Although "normal" blood pressure is generally defined as 120/80 mm Hg for adults over 18 years of age, attempts at defining

"high blood pressure" have been less productive and are largely based on empirical evidence.[15] A diastolic measurement of 90 and/or a systolic measurement of 140 are generally considered the upper limits of normal; however, a single high reading, especially in the potentially stressful dental office environment, is not diagnostic. Malamed recommends that blood pressure monitoring be done over several visits in an effort to determine whether elevations persist despite efforts to allay anxiety.[12]

The implications of managing the hypertensive patient in the dental office include the following:

1. The patient's increased sensitivity to vasoconstrictors used in local anesthetics and some retraction cord and hemostatic pellets.

2. In patients who are being treated for hypertension with adrenergic inhibitors, xerostomia and postural hypotension are common side effects. Xerostomia can have ramifications in terms of burning mouth and tongue, root caries, and retention and comfort of prostheses. Postural hypotension must be considered when uprighting patients from a reclining position in the dental chair.

3. Minimizing pain or stress should be a primary concern in managing these patients. Length of appointment, amount and type of treatment rendered, and special efforts in making the patient comfortable should be considered by all office personnel.

Bleeding disorders may be caused by primary disease processes such as hemophilia, thrombocytopenia, or hematologic malignancies. They may also be the result of secondary processes such as anticoagulant therapy or cirrhosis of the liver.[7] History taking is again of paramount importance. Anticipation of bleeding difficulties will enable the dentist to control the situation rather than having the situation control the dentist. With proper preparation, many dental procedures can be performed without untoward sequelae, even in patients with severe bleeding problems. For patients undergoing anticoagulant therapy, the dosage may have to be adjusted for several days before and after the dental visit. It is usually best to try to accomplish as much routine dental work as possible within a given appointment to minimize repeated disruption of the patient's anticoagulant regimen. All adaptions of anticoagulation regimens should be decided in conjunction with the patient's physician.

Implications for management of patients with bleeding disorders in the dental office include the following:

1. Tissues should be as healthy as possible before beginning operative or surgical procedures.
2. Maximize visualization of operative site to minimize tissue trauma.
3. Obtain primary closure of tissue whenever possible and stabilize with sutures.
4. Protect surgical site from trauma.
5. Establish a system for follow-up to ascertain patient status and mechanism for referral if professional support is needed if postoperative hemorrhage occurs.

The dentist and dental hygienist are sometimes able to synthesize individual pieces of data obtained through the medical history to identify patients with undiagnosed diabetes mellitus. Even in the absence of a family history (but certainly in the presence of a hereditary pattern), positive responses to questions regarding frequent urination (polyuria) and having to get up in the middle of the night to urinate (nocturia), feeling thirsty or tired much of the time, and recent history of weight gain or loss should alert the diagnostician to the possibility of diabetes mellitus as an underlying process. Patients in whom diabetes mellitus is suspected should be referred for medical follow-up.

Treatment of a well-controlled diabetic for most routine dental procedures does not vary from treatment of a nondiabetic patient. However, one must be aware of the following implications for management of diabetic dental patients:

1. Appointments should be kept reasonably short and should not interfere with normal meals. Skipping breakfast or lunch can lead to a hypoglycemic state.
2. A liquid containing sugar (juice, soda) should be available in the event hypoglycemia occurs.
3. Local anesthesia may be used in reasonable amounts without concern.
4. Diabetic patients have a greater likelihood of enhanced response to acute infections or of susceptibility to infections because of circulatory compromise. Routine prophylaxis with antibiotics is not indicated; however, active infections should be treated with antibiotics to prevent spread.
5. Diabetic patients may have a slower healing process than nondiabetic patients, so they should be monitored closely following periodontal or oral surgery.

The conditions considered to fall within the category of damaged hearts are congenital heart disease, rheumatic heart disease, and valve prostheses. The primary reason these patients require special consideration in the dental office is the prevention of bacterial endocarditis. Most patients with these conditions are aware of their cardiac state. Since few dentists include auscultation of the heart as part of the initial dental workup, the medical history must be relied upon for the determination of the condition.

Antibiotic prophylaxis should be provided to all patients who give a history of the above conditions, consistent with the currently accepted regimen of the American Heart Association (Table 2-6).

The most frequent issue the practitioner will face in treating patients with damaged hearts is when the dentist requires that the patient take appropriate antibiotics prior to dental treatment

Boston University
Henry M. Goldman
School of Graduate Dentistry
at Boston University Medical Center

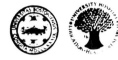

100 East Newton Street
Boston Massachusetts 02118
(617) 638-5129

Paula K. Friedman, D.D.S.
Director
Division of Oral Diagnosis and Radiology

Chart no. _____

To: _____   Date _____

Reason for consultation

_____ States that S/he:

_____ is currently under your care
_____ will seek a consultation at your office
Patient indicates a previous or current history of _____

_____

_____

This patient will require:

_____ Routine dental care (fillings, prosthetics, etc.)
_____ Periodontal treatment (possible surgery,   )
_____ Oral surgery (extraction,   )
_____ Use of local anesthesia with vasoconstrictor, epinephrine _____ /ml)
_____ General anesthesia

Would you please provide:

_____ Brief medical history
_____ List of current medications
_____ Precautions which need to be taken
_____ Prophylactic antibiotherapy/dose
_____ Other(s) _____

Dr. _____   _____
     Division of oral diagnosis and radiology   Patient signature: patient consent to
Report of consultant: release medical information to be sent
_____   directly to BUSGD

Name of responding physician: (please print) _____
Signature of responding physician: _____
Telephone number if we have further questions: _____
                    Thank you.

Fig. 2-3. Sample medical clearance letter.

(This side for Boston University of Graduate Dentistry use only)

Clinical protocol to be followed at BUSGD

Date established _____

_____

_____

_____

_____

_____

_____

_____

_____

_____

_____

Dr. Farid G. Boustany

Note: This clinical protocol should be approved and reviewed
with Dr. F.G. Boustany (Room G104, X5129) prior to the
initiation of any treatment at BUSGD. It will also be discussed
at the treatment planning session.

Fig. 2-3, cont'd.

and the patient responds that they have had dental treatment performed before and never had to take antibiotics. In this situation patient education is of paramount importance. When it is explained that it is in the patient's best interest to protect the heart from any potential effects of dental treatment, most patients readily accept the recommendation. Although it may be tempting to think that if nothing happened to the patient before, nothing will probably happen now, the dentist should be cautioned that once a significant medical (cardiac) history has been elicited, it becomes the dentist's professional responsibility to follow all appropriate precautions. However, the patient cannot be forced to comply. A case study will illustrate the point:

A nurse sought dental care at a major Boston teaching hospital. She reported a history of heart murmur which was found to be of the type that required premedication (that is, not "functional" or benign). She refused to take the recommended antibiotics because she said that on previous occasions when she had done so, she got a severely irritating vaginal candidiasis that took weeks of Mycostatin therapy to clear up. It was felt that because of her profession and level of education, she was competent to make that decision. An entry was made in the chart indicating that the recommendation of antibiotic prophylaxis had been made, the possible adverse effects of lack of prophylaxis explained, and that the patient understood. The nurse signed the entry, it was cosigned by the dentist, and treatment was rendered.

Other prosthetic devices besides heart valves are being placed with more frequency, including artificial knees, toes, hips, and ureters. It is

Table 2-6. Summary of recommended antibiotic regimens for dental/respiratory tract procedures

Standard regimen	
For dental procedures that cause gingival bleeding, and oral/respiratory tract surgery	Penicillin V 2.0 gm orally 1 hour before, then 1.0 gm 6 hours later. For patients unable to take oral medications, 2 million units of aqueous penicillin G intravenously or intramuscularly 30-60 minutes before a procedure and 1 million units 6 hours later may be substituted
Special regimens	
Parenteral regimen for use when maximal protection desired (for example, for patients with prosthetic valves)	Ampicillin 1.0-2.0 gm intramuscularly or intravenously, plus gentamicin 1.5 mg/kg intramuscularly or intravenously, one-half hour before procedure, followed by 1.0 gm oral penicillin V 6 hours later. Alternatively, the parenteral regimen may be repeated once 8 hours later
Oral regimen for penicillin-allergic patients	Erythromycin 1.0 gm orally 1 hour before, then 500 mg 6 hours later
Parenteral regimen for penicillin-allergic patients	Vancomycin 1.0 gm intravenously slowly over 1 hour, starting 1 hour before. No repeat dose is necessary

From J. Am. Dent. Assoc. **110:**99, January 1985. Copyright by the American Dental Association. Reprinted by permission.
Note: Pediatric doses: Ampicillin 50 mg/kg per dose; erythromycin 20 mg/kg for first dose, then 10 mg/kg; gentamicin 2.0 mg/kg per dose; penicillin V full adult dose if greater than 60 lb (27 kg), one-half adult dose if less than 60 lb (27 kg); aqueous penicillin G 50,000 units/kg (25,000 units/kg for follow-up); vancomycin 20 mg/kg per dose. The intervals between doses are the same as for adults. Total doses should not exceed adult doses.

thought that each of these may be the site of a bacterial cluster and resultant bacteremia. Therefore antibiotic prophylaxis is recommended in these instances as well.

Infectious diseases. The oral cavity harbors microorganisms with potential to transmit a wide spectrum of infectious agents. The dental professional is therefore at risk for any orally transmissible disease from the blood and/or saliva of the patients he/she treats.

The three infectious diseases that are currently of greatest concern to the dental professional are hepatitis B, autoimmune deficiency syndrome (AIDS), and herpes, although the list of transmissible diseases is more widely encompassing (see box). Each of these three diseases will be discussed in terms of etiology, tests available for diagnosis, and risk of transmission. Recommendations for prevention of these diseases in dental professionals will follow.

Hepatitis B. The disease is produced by a

TRANSMISSIBLE DISEASES OF CONCERN TO DENTAL PROVIDERS

Hepatitis (types B, A, non-A/non-B)
Acquired Immune Deficiency Syndrome
Syphilis
Gonorrhea
Influenzas
Acute pharyngitis (viral or streptococcal)
Pneumonias
Tuberculosis
Herpes
Chickenpox
Infectious mononucleosis
Rubella
Rubeola
Mumps

From The control of transmissable disease in dental practice: a position paper of the American Association of Public Health Dentistry, J. Pub. Health Dentistry **46**:14, Winter 1986.

virus known as the Dane particle. This intact virion consists of an inner core (HBcAg) and an outer coat (HBsAg). The virus is highly infective. As little as 0.00000001 ml of blood can transmit the disease. Initial symptoms may include vague abdominal discomfort, myalgia, diarrhea, jaundice (30% of cases), lack of appetite, and low-grade fever. *However, approximately 80% of individuals infected with the virus are asymptomatic and unaware that they are infected.* People who are infected with the virus can transmit hepatitis B whether they manifest clinical signs and symptoms or not.

A group of tests have been developed to determine the presence in the blood of hepatitis B antigens and antibodies to those antigens. The presence of hepatitis B core antigen (HBcAg) is associated with active viral infection and infectivity. The hepatitis B surface antigen (HBsAg) appears before acute illness and usually disappears quickly. Anti-hepatitis B core antibody (anti-HBcAb) is not protective, appears early in the illness and decreases in titer in those who become immune. Persistent high titer indicates ongoing infectivity. Hepatitis B surface antibody (HBsAb) does not appear for several months, then rises to a high titer in those who become immune. The e-antigen (HBeAg) is associated with lower risk of chronic liver disease and lower risk of infectivity. Table 2-7 summarizes the way to interpret results of blood tests for hepatitis B.

Fortunately for dental professionals, a vaccine has been developed to immunize recipients against hepatitis B. Three doses are given to confer immunity—an initial dose, followed by a second dose at one month, then a third dose six months after the first. Given dental personnel's high risk of contracting hepatitis B,[3] it is strongly recommended that all dental professionals be immunized. The risks of contracting hepatitis B include not only the morbidity of the acute phase of the disease, but the possible sequelae of chronic carrier state, cirrhosis of the liver, or primary hepatocellular carcinoma.

Table 2-7. Interpretation of results of serological tests for hepatitis B

HBsAg	HBeAg	anti-HBe	anti-HBc		anti-HBs	Interpretation
			IgM	IgG		
+	+	−	−	−	−	Incubation period
+	+	−	+	+	−	Acute Hepatitis B or persistent carrier state
+	+	−	−	+	−	Persistent carrier state
+	−	+	+/−	+	−	Persistent carrier state
−	−	+	+/−	+	+	Convalescence
−	−	−	−	+	+	Recovery
−	−	−	+	−	−	Infection with Hepatitis B virus without detectable HBsAg
−	−	−	−	+	−	Recovery with loss of detectable anti-HBs
−	−	−	−	−	+	Immunization without infection. Repeated exposure to antigen without infection, or recovery from infection with loss of detectable anti-HBc.

Courtesy of Dr. Richard Whitman, Boston University Medical Center, Goldman School of Graduate Dentistry.

Autoimmune deficiency syndrome (AIDS). AIDS is a viral disease that has been identified only recently. The mortality associated with the disease is extremely high; 70% to 80% of AIDS patients with concurrent opportunistic infections died during a 2-year period.[14] The disease is accompanied by weight loss, lymphadenopathy, fatigue, night sweats, loss of appetite, and fever. Groups considered at high risk for AIDS include homosexual men, intravenous drug users, people with a history of multiple transfusions of blood and blood products, and hemophiliacs. The rate of spread of the disease is pandemic; the numbers of those affected are expected to double every 12 months.

There is no specific diagnostic test for AIDS. A screening test (ELISA) has been developed, but the interpretation of the results is equivocal. For example, a positive result could mean any of the following[14]:

1. The person may be protected.
2. The person may be a healthy virus carrier.
3. The person may have AIDS or AIDS-related complex (ARC).
4. The results are a false positive.

Similarly, a negative result could mean any of the following:

1. The person has not been exposed and is not infected.
2. The person may be in the early stages of incubation before the antibody that the test measures has been formed.
3. The person may be an active AIDS victim and is unable to form the antibodies because the functioning of the immune system is diminished.

Also, there is currently no treatment for the AIDS patient other than supportive therapy. Researchers are investigating the use of antiviral agents as well as attempting to develop a vaccine to immunize against this disease.

Herpes. Herpes is included in the discussion of infectious diseases because of its high prevalence (antibodies to herpes simplex virus are present in 95% of the population). The route of transmission is through oral or genital secretions, and transmission may occur both from dental professional to patient and patient to saliva, and herpetic lesions may occur periorally, on fingers (herpetic whitlow), and in the eye. All of these potential sites of infection are high-risk areas for the dental professional as a result of direct contact with saliva (fingers) or splattering formation, erythema, edema, lymphadenopathy, and low-grade fever. The most frequent complication of a herpes simplex infection is recurrence.

Diagnostic testing for herpes simplex may be done with a Tzanck smear, tissue culture, or fluorescent antibody tests.

Treatment of herpes is largely symptomatic, although research on the efficacy of two antiviral agents, acyclovir and idoxuridine, may provide valuable information on their application in recurrent oral herpes simplex infections.

Prevention: infection control

Because treatment of hepatitis B, AIDS, and herpes is symptomatic at best, prevention of the processes is the most important aspect of the discussion of these diseases. Even if a cure were available, protection from the untoward effects and discomfort of each disease would be desirable.

The following recommendations should be used routinely in the care of *all* patients in dental practice to control the spread of infection[16]:

1. Always obtain a complete medical history. Include specific questions about lymphadenopathy, recent weight loss, and infections. Follow-up on all positive responses. Remember that an individual may not be aware of an infective state, so diagnostic acumen may be required.

2. Use protective attire and barrier techniques. To protect yourself and patients, always wear gloves, surgical masks, and protective eyewear. Change gloves between patients so as to minimize the transmission of disease from one patient to another. Cover all surfaces touched by instruments or that may be contaminated by blood or saliva with materials impervious to fluids (plastic, aluminum foil) and discard these after each patient.

3. For routine dental procedures, handwashing with ordinary soap before and after gloving is adequate. It is important to wash hands even when gloves are used because there may be small tears or openings in the gloves that would allow microorganisms to enter.

4. Use disposable needles. Do not recap needles; this will minimize needlestick injuries. Do not purposely bend or break needles. Dispose of them in a special puncture-resistant container after each patient.

5. Decontamination of surfaces should be accomplished through a solution of sodium hypochlorite (household bleach). Dilutions of 1:10 to 1:100 have been shown to be effective. Caution should be used because sodium hypochlorite is corrosive to metals, especially aluminum.

6. All instruments should be scrubbed to remove blood and saliva before sterilization. It is recommended that heavy rubber gloves (household gloves) be worn for this purpose to avoid inadvertent skin punctures.

7. Disinfection or sterilization of instruments should occur at the highest appropriate level for the material in question. Use the autoclave, dry heat, or chemical vapor for metal and heat-stable dental instruments; immersion in boiling water for 10 minutes or an EPA-registered disinfectant/sterilant chemical for the exposure time recommended by the chemical's manufacturer for instruments and materials that cannot be heat sterilized.

8. Dental handpieces pose a particular problem since they cannot be sterilized. They should be thoroughly scrubbed with a detergent and water to remove adherent material and then completely wiped with an absorbent material soaked in an approved germicide that is registered with the EPA as a hospital disinfectant and is mycobactericidal at use/dilution.

These guidelines are meant to provide the reader with an awareness of the precautions that should become a routine part of the daily practice of dentistry.

Variations on these basic precepts may exist within certain school, clinic, or hospital settings. However, common sense and good judgment will help each professional determine the best preventive techniques for each environment.

ENVIRONMENTAL FACTORS

The environment in which dentistry is practiced has changed dramatically over the past decade. Some of the issues effecting that change have already been addressed—demographics, malpractice, educational process, and health status of patients. Other issues that have had a major impact on the professional environment have been prepaid dental care programs, advertising of dental services, emphasis on cosmetic dentistry, and the development of alternative delivery systems for dentistry.

Alternative delivery system is a term that describes the new settings for dental care that have evolved since 1980. Prior to that, the dental office was most likely located over the corner drugstore, in a home-office combination, or perhaps in a professional building. Since 1980, dental offices have appeared in "retail settings"—in shopping malls (within chain stores like Sears or Zayres) and in major downtown business districts as independently standing offices, that is, not part of a dental/medical complex).

The alternative delivery system of dental care has had an interesting history. When alternative delivery systems first developed, dental students were told that the era of the solo practitioner had come to an end, the private practice of dentistry as a cottage industry was a thing of the past, and that the future was "retail dentistry." All dental patients would be given beepers to carry to let them know when the dentist was ready or when their child's treatment had been completed.

They could shop at leisure before and after their appointment in the mall, and parking would never be a problem. Moreover, since these new dental settings all advertised, a price war would erupt, patients would flock to the least expensive dentist, and quality care would become an anachronism.

A few years later, we see that the "retail dentistry" paradigm has indeed contributed to the practice of dentistry, but seemingly not in the way initial predictions foretold. In 1984 Friedman and others[10] conducted a study funded by the American Fund for Dental Health to investigate what effect advertising had on dental consumers. New patients ($N = 3, 287$) in offices that advertised were surveyed for their demographic characteristics and their reasons for having chosen the practice.

Managing a retail dentistry practice is more complex than managing a traditional practice. Since these locations are frequently open up to 14 hours a day (7:00 AM to 9:00 PM) and up to 7 days per week, the issues involved in hiring, training, scheduling, and retention of personnel increase exponentially. Quality control is always a concern in multiperson organizations. Initial capitalization of the operation can exceed $250,000, and monthly overhead is proportionally large. The areas of personnel management, financial management, and organizational administration are ones which the dentist has historically had minimum preparation and experience.

Another alternative delivery system that has been developing is one in which dentistry can be delivered to the patient at home through use of portable dental equipment. These systems have proven especially helpful in providing dental services to frail elderly in their homes, to nursing homes which do not have adequate space for a permanent dental facility, and in rural settings where access to centralized dental care would otherwise be difficult. The systems are flexible, relatively inexpensive, and provide a good alternative to equipping a mobile dental van (which can cost in excess of $80,000). The American Dental Association has prepared information on manufacturers of portable dental equipment.[1]

THE FUTURE

In the past 10 years, significant changes in the style of dental practice have occurred. Fluoridation of water supplies, the increase in number of dental professionals, and dental health education have all had an impact on the incidence of caries. New emphasis is placed on "cosmetic dentistry" in addition to treating dental disease. The biotechnology of dental implants may provide a new dimension to the practice of dentistry. The practice setting is more varied and advertising is now accepted as a normal part of many dental practices. An increasing number of women are entering the profession, and no doubt entering the faculty and administration of many dental schools. It will be interesting to observe how their presence affects the educational process and the practice of dentistry. Our population is aging, and the medical complexity of the patients we treat is increasing. In many ways the practice of dentistry is even more closely linked to the practice of medicine than before. We must be vigilant in our knowledge of medical conditions, pharmacologic agents, and infection control procedures.

As the turn of the century approaches, dental professionals will be challenged by new events, new research, new discoveries. They will have the opportunity, by being better informed and better educated, not only to respond to trends, but to set them.

REFERENCES

1. American Dental Association, Council on Dental Health and Health Planning: Portable dentistry information, Chicago, 1982.
2. American Dental Association, Special Committee on the "Future of Dentistry," Chicago, 1983, p. 717.
3. American Dental Association, Council on Dental Thera-
peutics: Hepatitis B and the dental profession: proceedings of a national symposium, J. Am. Dent. Assoc. **110:**614, April 1985.
4. Blue Shield of Massachusetts, Master Dental™: Facts about reimbursement, Professional Relations, June 1986.
5. Bohannan, H.M.: The impact of decreasing caries prevalence: implications for dental education, J. Dent. Res. **61**, 1982 (special issue).
6. DePaola, P., and others: Changes in caries prevalence of Massachusetts children over 30 years, J. Dent. Res. (Special issue) **60A:**360, 1981 (abstract No. 200).
7. Dugdale, M., and Smith, R.M.: The patient with bleeding problems, Dent. Clin. North Am. (Issue 2)**27:**274, April 1983.
8. Forbes, R.J.: Shattering myths about the mature market, Destinations, April 1985, p. 28. Reprinted by permission of *Destinations* and the American Bus Association.
9. Forsyth Conference on Declining Prevalence of Dental Caries, J. Public Health Dent. **43:**78, Winter 1983.
10. Friedman, P.K., and others: The effect of advertising on the dental consumer, Unpublished data, 1985.
11. Garfield, R.: The invisible consumer, *Madison Avenue*, October 1984, p. 86.
12. Malamed, S.F.: Blood pressure evaluation and the prevention of medical emergencies in dental practice, J. Prev. Dentistry **6:**186, 1980.
13. Manny, E.F., and others: An overview of dental radiology, National Center for Health Care Technology, 1980, p. 23.
14. Massachusetts Department of Public Health: AIDS: updated information for dentists and dental auxiliaries, June 1986, p. 4.
15. Meiller, T.F., and Overholser, C.D.: The patient with increased medical risks. In Baker, W.R., and Cottone, J.A., editor: Dental clinics of North America, Philadelphia, 1983, W.B. Saunders Co., p. 289.
16. Recommended infection control practices for dentistry, Morbid. Mortal. Weekly Rev., vol. 35, April 18, 1986, p. 237.
17. The control of transmissible disease in dental practice: a position paper of the American Association of Public Health Dentistry, J. Pub. Health Dentistry **46:**14, Winter 1986.
18. Tufts University Diet and Nutrition Letter, Vol. 4, October 1986, p. 5.
19. U.S. Department of Health and Human Services, Health Resources and Services Administration: Report on issues and strategies in geriatric education, 1985, p. 28.

CHAPTER 3

Role of Auxiliaries in Dental Care

Demand for dental care and consumer awareness in the area of health services has been steadily increasing. The public is no longer content to view health care as a luxury, available only to those who can pay the rising costs, but rather sees it as a necessary service that should be accessible and affordable to all. Increased demand places a strain on the traditional methods of health care delivery. This is especially true of dentistry, which has largely existed as a private-practice, solo cottage industry. With new emphasis on cost effectiveness and more efficient means of delivery, dentistry has little choice but to respond to the pressure from the public and professional sectors.

Several alternatives to increasing and upgrading the delivery of services have been proposed in recent years. Other professions have delegated services to the various auxiliaries employed in that profession or created new paraprofessionals who can assume duties formerly performed by the highly trained and educated professionals. The federal government provided impetus to this movement in the medical field with the Health Professions Act of 1976. This stimulated the emergence of the physicians' assistant and the nurse practitioner, who were able to provide more extended care yet remained under the supervision of the physician. Furthermore, the Health Professions Educational Assistance Act made a team approach to the delivery of care more feasible through the training and use of new health personnel.

To help the dentist in the delivery of dental care, three types of supportive care providers have evolved: the dental assistant, the dental hygienist, and the dental laboratory technician. Dental assistants and hygienists comprise almost two thirds of the dental workforce. In 1984 the active dental labor pool consisted of 137,950 dentists and 214,100 dental hygienists and assistants (Tables 3-1 and 3-2).

A subcategory of auxiliary is the expanded function dental auxiliary (EFDA), a hygienist or assistant who has completed advanced training beyond the basic professional education. Most EFDAs have been trained through federally funded programs and once trained must work under the supervision of a licensed dentist. Their skills vary according to the program in which they were trained and they are able to utilize their skills according to the state law governing their place of employment.[6]

Dental technicians are generally not considered auxiliaries because their work, in most cases, is performed in a private commercial laboratory rather than in a dental office. They work according to a written prescription or work order from a licensed dentist. Laboratory technicians who are working toward establishing independent professional licensure allowing them to provide care directly to the public are called *denturists*. "Six states allow denturists to provide denture service directly to the public. Maine, Colorado, and Arizona require that the denturist work under the supervision of a dentist. Oregon, Idaho, and Montana denturists can work independently."[20]

The cost and length of training of health professionals are factors that substantiate efforts to

Table 3-1. Estimated number of active dental assistants and number per 100 active dentists: selected years, 1950 to 1984

Year	Number of active assistants	Number per 100 active dentists
1950	55,200	70.0
1960	74,000	82.0
1970	112,000	110.0
1975	134,400	120.0
1977	144,700	123.0
1980	155,500	123.0
1982	161,800	123.0
1984	168,300	122.0

From U.S. Department of Health and Human Services, Public Health Service, Health Resources and Services Administration, Bureau of Health Professions: Fifth report to the President and Congress on the status of health personnel in the United States, Dentistry, March 1986, pp. 5-31.

Table 3-2. Estimated number of active dental hygienists and number per 100 active dentists: selected years, 1950 to 1984

Year	Number of active hygienists	Number per 100 active dentists
1950	3,190	4.0
1960	8,800	9.8
1970	15,100	14.8
1975	26,900	24.0
1977	32,200	27.3
1980	38,400	30.4
1982	43,100	32.6
1984	45,800	33.2

From U.S. Department of Health and Human Services, Public Health Service, Health Resources and Services Administration, Bureau of Health Professions: Fifth report to the President and Congress on the status of health personnel in the United States, Dentistry, March 1986, pp. 5-30.

concentrate on the development of the auxiliary to increase health care services to the public. The average total undergraduate cost (tuition and fees) for all years of dental school is $34,640 for state residents and $44,630 for nonresidents.[20] In comparison, a dental hygiene education costs roughly $4,452, and a dental assisting education costs roughly $1,668.* Educational programs for the dentist take 7 to 8 years as compared to 2 to 4 years of education for the dental hygienist and 2 years or less of education for the assistant.

Dentistry has looked at its resources, the trained auxiliaries, as a viable solution to increased and more efficient delivery of services. How to effectively utilize these auxiliaries has generated considerable conflict and controversy within the dental profession itself and is still far from enjoying a consensus of opinion.

*Average of total costs ꞏ students in district from American Dental Association, Coun̄ ꞏil on Dental Education, Division of Educational Measurements: Annual report on dental auxiliary education, 1985-86.

How can the dental auxiliary be utilized effectively and efficiently to meet the health care needs of the public? Both auxiliaries evolved in response to unmet need in the dental care system and have continued to develop in accordance with need. To understand the issues it is important to review the development of each auxiliary.

DENTAL ASSISTANT

The first dental assistant was hired in 1885 by Dr. C. Edmund Kells of New Orleans. Dr. Kells hired a woman as a "lady in attendance" so that female patients could respectfully come to his office unattended. It was found that these individuals could be enlisted to perform routine dental office chores in the operatory as well as in the business office. Dental assistants continued to serve as office helpers until World War II when there was a crucial shortage of labor to meet the dental care demands of the military service. Thus utilization improved in the armed forces where assistants were trained to work at chairside in an attempt to increase productivity.

Dentists who had trained with assistants retained the concepts of auxiliary utilization on returning to civilian practice.[16]

Dental assisting has experienced a number of significant changes in more recent years. The first was during the 1960s, with the advent of four-handed, sit-down dentistry which necessitated that a dental assistant be actively employed in the delivery of patient care. Operatory design and the use of work simplification principles made for a more efficient method of working. In 1961, the federal government supported a grant program that was designed to train dental students to work using the concept of four-handed dentistry. Since that time other programs have been developed and supported in their attempts to increase the utilization of auxiliaries.

The first organization of dental assistants, The Education and Efficiency Society, was formed in 1921 by Juliette Southard in New York City. Others began to form, and in 1924, the societies met together for the first time on a national level.[16] This organization, the American Dental Assistants' Association (ADAA) remains the recognized professional association of dental assistants. The ADAA met for the first time in conjunction with the American Dental Association in 1924. Since that time, the two organizations, as well as the American Dental Hygienists' Association, continue to meet simultaneously at annual sessions.

The ADAA took as its motto "education, efficiency, loyalty, and service." From its beginning, the organization has worked arduously at developing dental assisting as a competent and acknowledged component of the dental profession and to advocating dental health care for the consumer.

The need for educational guidance was recognized in 1930 when the National Curriculum Committee of the ADAA was formed. This committee consolidated in 1937 with the National Education Committee to become the Education Committee, which initiated a program providing official recognition of educationally qualified dental assistants—a program of individual certification. As a result, the Certification Board was established in 1948 to examine individuals for knowledge and skills in dental assisting. The board was established as an independent corporation since its interests might conflict with those of the ADAA. The two continue to work closely with one another, although each remains autonomous.

Originally there were two routes to becoming certified. One was the *grandmother clause*, which meant that with 10 years of work experience, a dental assistant could become certified on request. The other was completion of a 104-hour course in addition to 2 years of verified work experience. This extension course was the first attempt to standardize the education of dental assistants. The program was developed in cooperation with the Council on Dental Education of the American Dental Association. The courses were at that time the only means of getting a formal education that was approved by the ADAA.

In 1957 the ADA House of Delegates approved the standard for educational regulations of certification of the dental assistant. These regulations established a minimum length of 1 year for a training program that was to be offered in an academic institution. These requirements are now reviewed and established by the Commission on Dental Accreditation, which includes representation from the ADAA. Maintaining and improving the quality of dental auxiliary education are primary aims of the commission. Programs accredited by the commission must be at a postsecondary educational institution. There are presently about 290 accredited programs varying in length from 1 to 2 academic years. Graduates of these programs are eligible to sit for the Dental Assisting National Board Examination (DANBE). Programs offer either a certificate or, in the case of a 2-

year institution, an associate's degree in dental assisting.

At one time it was possible to challenge a seven-course examination that was given as an accredited extension program through the University of North Carolina at Chapel Hill. By successfully challenging these, candidates were considered to have adequately exhibited the competencies necessary to take the certification examination. This route to certification was deleted from the 1982 certification examination application.

In 1978 the Certifying Board of the ADAA (currently DANB) opened the examination for a 3-year period, from 1979 to 1981, to allow anyone with dental experience to take it. The rationale in doing so was to provide a data base reflecting the examination results of students graduating from an accredited program and of those who were trained on the job. It was also stated by the Certifying Board that certification is a credential that indicates a level of knowledge, rather than how that knowledge was attained.

Basic eligibility pathways for the certification examination (CDA) for 1986 are: (1) graduation from a dental assisting or dental hygiene program accredited by the ADA Commission on Dental Accreditation, or (2) high school graduation or equivalent and 2 years of full-time work experience (3,500 hours) as a dental assistant.

A 1986 DANB news release states that nearly 100,000 dental assistants have been awarded the designation Certified Dental Assistant. Specialty certification examinations are also available. They include Certified Oral and Maxillofacial Surgery Assistant (COMSA), Certified Dental Practice Management Assistant (CDPMA), and Certified Orthodontic Assistant (COA).

The Dental Radiation Health and Safety Examination was developed by DANB to enable states to comply with requirements contained in the federal government's Consumer-Patient Radiation Health and Safety Act of 1981, which requires states to institute certification procedures for dental and medical personnel who operate radiographic equipment. This requirement can also be met by passing the basic CDA examination.

There are no baccalaureate programs in dental assisting at this time, although degrees are offered in related areas such as dental auxiliary education, nutrition, management, or health science.

In order for an institution's program to be accredited, the institution must first submit a written document to the Commission on Dental Accreditation; if approved, it will then be subject to an on-site visit from a team of professionals (usually dental assisting educators). Full approval is given for a 10-year period, after which reevaluation is necessary. Although the CDA is not legally recognized in most states, the certificate is currently the only nationally recognized credential available to dental assistants.

The profession of dental assisting has continued to express its goals and objectives through the ADAA. The ultimate goal of the ADAA is to strengthen the association and achieve recognition for the dental assisting profession. Member services and benefits have been revamped and made more responsive to member needs. Health and life insurance plans and a loan program are available.

In 1985 the organization began an intensive marketing program aimed at expanding its market base and making continuing education a viable revenue source. Long-range plans address the need for development, production, and marketing of continuing education products.[10] These activities indicate the Association's current emphasis on education to keep pace with the changing profession.

As the profession of dentistry has changed, so has the role of the dental assistant. Dental assistants are taking a stronger position concerning their rights and responsibilities, and with a workforce of 168,300, that position will not easily be overlooked.

DENTAL HYGIENIST

With the growing demand for increased capacity in the treatment of dental disease, the dental profession in the early 1900s began to seek what Dr. Alfred Fones termed a *subspecialist*, whose primary function would be to serve in the prevention of dental disease. Fones conceptualized this subspeciality as one of training in health care education and oral prophylaxis, completely uninvolved with the treatment of disease. In 1906 he put these ideas into practice by training his assistant to provide these preventive services for his patients.

Subsequently, Dr. Fones developed a course for dental hygienists that stressed the value of oral health care. More specifically, he emphasized health care for children consisting of prophylaxis skills and dental health education programs in the public schools. At its very inception, then, the dental hygiene profession had a bearing on public health dentistry.

Although Dr. Fones is often credited with the development of the first course for dental hygienists and assistants in 1913, the Ohio College of Dental Surgery had developed a program for hygienists and assistants in 1910. However, as a result of strong pressure from the local dentists, the Ohio program was dissolved.

After the third year of his hygiene program, Dr. Fones advocated that the training of dental hygienists be based within recognized education institutions, and in 1915 the Connecticut Dental Practice Act required licensure for dental hygiene. Thus the dental hygiene profession became securely established within the parameters of the dental profession's licensing and educational systems.

Since 1913 the number of dental hygiene programs began to increase slowly, and in the 1940s all programs were required to be 2 or 4 years in length and be based within a college or university. Table 3-3 shows the gradual increase in the number of programs until the 1960s, when the number of programs grew rapidly as the federal government supported the development of allied health programs, and education then shifted from the university to the community college setting. The table also shows that the number of graduates is decreasing in the 1980s. The 1985-86 ADA Annual Report on Dental Auxiliary Education states that there are 198 dental hygiene programs, indicating that two have closed since the 1984-85 report.

By February 1947 the American Dental Association Council on Dental Education developed the Requirements for the Accrediting of a School of Dental Hygiene, and since 1952 accreditation by the American Dental Association Commission on Dental Accreditation Programs has been required for all schools offering programs in dental hygiene.[14]

Today, there are 198 accredited dental hygiene programs that offer a curriculum leading to a 2-year associate's degree or a 4-year baccalaureate degree. In addition, there are opportunities for advanced education. Several institutions have programs especially designed to offer dental hygienists master's degrees with specialized training in public health, education, research, or administration.

Until 1969 dental hygiene was the only dental auxiliary acknowledged in the state dental practice acts. Dental hygiene licensure is required by the state after at least 2 years of training, and the profession is regulated by the state boards of dentistry through examination for licensure and regulation of the delivery of care. The functions that a registered dental hygienist is allowed to perform vary from state to state.

The American Dental Hygienists' Association has been the representative of the registered dental hygienist since 1923, when 46 hygienists met in Cleveland to discuss common professional issues. From this nucleus grew the association, which, as of October 1986, had approximately 30,000 members.

The American Dental Hygienists' Association has taken noteworthy steps toward equipping the hygienist to assume his/her role in dental public health. First the association's Division of Professional Relations created a newsletter in 1978 (entitled *Legislative Bulletin*), designed to increase the practicing hygienist's awareness of legislative activities. This monthly bulletin monitors dental care bills from the time they are introduced in state legislatures and reports the progress of each bill. Second the association's Division of Professional Development is an active resource and advisor to hygienists who, as program planners, are responsible for development, implementation, and evaluation of community programs.

A survey of a cohort of 1,982 dental hygiene

graduates who attended 48 dental hygiene programs in the United States (and included associate and baccalaureate degree programs) indicated that private dental offices, either solo or group practice, were the work sites of approximately 90% of the graduates (Table 3-4).[5] The remaining 10% were occupied in a diverse array of settings such as:

1. *Public:* the United States Public Health Service, the Indian Health Service, neighborhood health centers, Veterans Administration hospitals, state departments of public health, prisons, and diverse rehabilitation institutions
2. *Voluntary:* the American Heart Association, the American Cancer Association, and various other charitable, health-related associations and foundations
3. *Educational:* in teaching capacities in dental hygiene 2-year certificate programs, baccalaureate and master's degree programs, schools of public health, and departments of community dentistry in dental schools

Table 3-3. Dental hygiene programs and numbers of graduates: selected years, 1950-1985

Academic year	Number of programs	Number of graduates
1950-1951	26	632
1955-1956	33	902
1960-1961	37	1,023
1965-1966	56	1,650
1967-1968	67	1,834
1969-1970	100	2,465
1974-1975	160	4,568
1976-1977	179	4,847
1978-1979	196	5,149
1980-1981	200	5,088
1982-1983	202	4,562
1984-1985	200	4,024

From American Dental Association, Council on Dental Education: Dental students' register for each selected academic year from 1950 to 1951 through 1966 to 1967; and annual report on dental auxiliary education for all subsequent academic years.

Table 3-4. Employment site(s) of the cohort of 1982 dental hygiene graduates

Site	Respondents	
	Number	Percent
Solo dental practice	444	64.9%
Group dental practice	182	26.6
Public health clinic	9	1.3
Hospital	2	.3
Health department	3	.4
Dental auxiliary education	3	.4
Dental college	6	.9
Public school	1	.1
Other	34	5.0

From Boyer, E.M.: New dental hygiene graduates: demographic and employment profile, Dent. Hyg. **60**(5):206, 1986.

4. *Special Needs:* the delivery of care to the homebound, hospitalized patients, individuals in nursing homes, day care centers, and elementary and secondary schools.

The reasons that the majority work in private practice are essentially pragmatic. The employment setting has been primarily defined by the needs of the dental profession, and the hygienist will shift from this practice setting when there is an increased demand for his/her skills elsewhere.

FACTORS INFLUENCING DENTAL AUXILIARIES

Both internal and external factors impinge on the dental auxiliary (Fig. 3-1). Internally, the professions of dentistry, dental hygiene, and dental assisting have repeatedly clashed over responsibilities and role delineations. Externally, federal and state governments, as well as consumers, have taken an active role in providing input into dental service delivery, thereby affecting the function of auxiliaries in the provision of dental care.

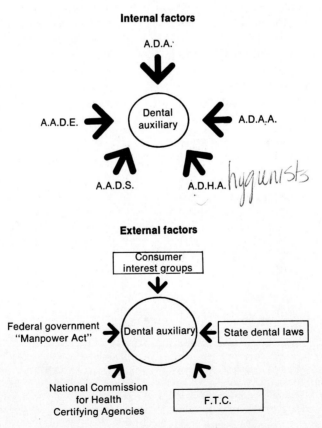

Fig. 3-1. Factors influencing dental auxiliaries.

Internal factors

Within the profession, the issue of auxiliary utilization remains who should provide what service.

A fundamental principle of auxiliary utilization is the realization that the dentist is ultimately responsible for the patient care provided, and furthermore, that there are aspects of a dentist's professional endeavor which should not be delegated to dental auxiliaries since these functions comprise the essence of the practice of dentistry.*

The dental auxiliary has been quick to assume that the dentist is anxious to delegate more repetitive functions to an auxiliary so that he/she may be free to perform more advanced skills. In reality, many dentists may want to hold on to those functions as their primary responsibility.[21] The dentist of the 1980s views what he/she considers the "essence" of the practice of dentistry being taken from him/her by the specialist on one hand and claimed as a responsibility of the expanded duty auxiliary on the other.

The dentist's attitude toward auxiliary utilization has been a vacillating one, and can be reflected by the policies of the American Dental Association (ADA) between 1960 and 1980. The beginning of the 1960s was a time when professional policies, governmental support, and dental education focused efforts on greater utilization of the dental auxiliary. The federal government's funding of Dental Auxiliary Utilization (DAU) Programs in 1961 met with such success in reducing the dentists' chair time that the ADA looked favorably toward research that would study additional methods of auxiliary utilization. In fact, the 1961 House of Delegates of the American Dental Association supported

further research of dental auxiliary utilization and training.

As a result of this philosophy, various experimental programs were conducted across the country at such institutions as the Forsyth Dental Center, U.S. Naval Training Center, University of Alabama, U.S. Division of Indian Health, University of Minnesota, University of North Carolina, University of Maryland, and University of Iowa. These research studies established that utilization of auxiliaries with expanded functions can increase productivity and the quality of care and perhaps, contain the cost of dental care.

In 1969 the need to develop a model dental component for the impending National Health Insurance Program was imminent and prompted the American Dental Association to create a National Health Program Task Force. The Task Force Report supported a program that would experiment with the training and utilization of auxiliaries.

The following year, 1970, the Carnegie Commission Report reinforced the necessity to train auxiliaries by revealing the low level of health in the United States and by predicting a serious shortage of health care labor. The report proposed increasing the number of dentists and physicians being educated and providing funds for training programs that would expand the duties of auxiliaries. In light of these proposals, the ADA 1970 House of Delegates resolved that educational institutions should experiment with alternative methods of dental care delivery utilizing dental hygienists and assistants trained to provide additional functions.

To harness additional support for these programs, the ADA Council on Dental Education established the Inter-Agency Committee on Dental Auxiliaries. The committee was created in order to establish and support educational guidelines for the delegation of expanded functions to the dental auxiliary. This effort combined the leadership and resources of the var-

*Orientation remarks made by L.M. Kennedy, Chairman, Advisory Committee, Workshop on dental auxiliary expanded functions. Sponsored by the American Dental Association, Council on Dental Education, Chicago, March 31, April 1 and 2, 1976.

ious associations that are crucial to the education and regulation of dental auxiliaries. These associations are the American Association of Dental Examiners, the American Association of Dental Schools, the American Dental Hygienists' Association, and the Public Health Service, Division of Dentistry.

The Inter-Agency Committee concluded that more research was necessary to determine which auxiliary should perform what type of expanded function. Again, the necessity for research programs to evaluate efficient utilization of expanded function dental auxiliaries was evident. The committee report concluded that the dental profession was more willing to delegate expanded functions for auxiliaries than the individual state laws allowed.[2]

As the economy worsened in 1972, the attitude welcoming experimentation with expanded function auxiliaries changed. This gradual reduction of support was reflected in the ADA 1973 House of Delegates' resolution that the association stands in opposition to programs that permit a research program using auxiliaries to cut hard or soft tissues.

Finally, in 1975, a resolution was passed by the House of Delegates that stressed "the termination of research in expanded functions and a return to traditional roles and responsibilities of dental auxiliaries."[3] The dental profession's support for so many years in seeking alternative delivery systems by utilizing expanded function auxiliaries was ending, while at the same time the government, through the Federal Health Manpower Legislation (1974), was encouraging dental schools to develop new programs and to remodel present programs to train expanded function auxiliaries. In agreement with the government legislation, the 1975 House of Delegates of the American Association of Dental Schools (AADS) resolved that curriculum in dental hygiene schools should include instruction in all expanded functions, even though the legality of performing such functions varies from state to state. Such a curriculum would provide

future graduates the flexibility to become licensed in any state and to perform the functions legalized within the state. But more importantly, the American Association of Dental School's resolution highlights the professional dichotomy between dental educators and the American Dental Association. By withdrawing support of programs that experiment with the delegation of functions to auxiliaries not legal within the state practice act, dental educators believe that the ADA is restricting academic freedom. During this period, while the ADA and the AADS were making these policy statements, the ADAA and the ADHA were vying with one another and with the ADA for recognition as *the* expanded function dental auxiliary representative.

The authors of a 1979 ADA article reported that all study results showed that properly trained auxiliaries could provide the same quality of care for specific reversible and irreversible procedures as is provided by a dentist.[18] As the research programs proved that auxiliaries could perform expanded functions, the debate grew over *which* auxiliaries should have which expanded functions delegated to them! It was argued that dental assistants should be selected because (1) there are more of them, (2) they are not restricted by licensing requirements, and (3) they command a lower salary than dental hygienists. The proponents for delegating expanded functions to dental hygienists argued that the hygienist (1) has a professional education, (2) is subject to licensure, and (3) is trained as a direct care provider.

The ADHA and the ADAA continue to represent their constituents in the battle over the right to perform various duties. Attempts to bring the dental auxiliaries together through their professional organizations to work on common issues was conceptualized in the form of an annual convention called Partners-In-Progress. However, after 3 years, the meeting was curtailed because of a lack of cooperation between the associations.

While the auxiliaries discuss, debate, and

dream about future roles, the dentist is no longer concerned about whether the auxiliary *is* capable of performing expanded functions, but whether these functions *should be* delegated at all.

The prediction of an increased demand for dental care faded during the 1970s with the postponement of a National Health Insurance Program, a drastic drop in the birthrate, increased water fluoridation, and a sharp setback in the economy. While the dentist became frustrated by his/her decreasing workload, the government was encouraging dental schools to increase the number of students or to develop remote sites for training by funding schools on a capitation basis. Traditionally in favor of these programs, the ADA and the American Association of Dental Examiners no longer supported the capitation program.[22]

As the number of dentists providing care exceeds the demand for care, the question of the delegation of duties becomes a moot point. As the economy worsens, the dentist who finds more free time in his/her work schedule starts to perform the services that he/she used to hire a hygienist to provide.

The years between 1960 and 1980 revealed a reversal in the policies of the ADA, moving from an invitation to experiment with expanded duty dental auxiliaries to a moratorium on research and training in expanded functions and a watchful eye turned toward the number of dentists graduating from the dental schools. During these two decades, the policies of the AADS, ADHA, and ADAA became more supportive toward examining alternative methods of providing dental care and increasing available labor with the hopes of ultimately providing optimal dental health for the public.

In the 1980s there has been a decrease in caries prevalence, and the dentist-to-population ratios have increased from 53.4 per 100,000 in 1980 to 56.3 per 100,000 in 1984.[20] The dental profession is grappling with the issues of an increased supply of dentists and a decrease in the rate of population growth, thereby taking the focus away from expanded utilization of auxiliaries. However, Table 3-5 indicates that a large percentage of dentists still rely on the use of auxiliaries. Dentists as well as hygienists and assistants are seeking alternatives to the narrow practice role of the auxiliary. The office job description may be expanding to include: treatment coordinator,[9] human relations staffer,[11] cost containment advocate,[19] and manager of special patients, as well as general office manager.

From a public health perspective, it is difficult to discuss cutting back on the supply of dental labor, dentist or dental auxiliary, simply because the demand for care is not increasing. The need for greater access to dental care for people not previously receiving care or receiving insufficient care and the underutilization of dental care systems are the real public health issues.

Table 3-5. Percent of independent dentists who employ auxiliaries: selected years 1955-1983

	Percent of dentists employing auxiliaries*		
Year	Dental hygienists	Dental assistants	Any type of auxiliaries†
1955	10.3	70.7	77.1
1961	15.0	76.7	82.6
1967	25.2	86.6	92.4
1972	36.9	90.2	93.6
1979	48.2	87.7	94.5
1981	50.7	87.2	95.5
1983	53.9	88.2	96.4

From American Dental Association, Bureau of Economic and Behavioral Research: The 1984 Survey of Dental Practice; also prior reports of this series.
*Any of these employees may be either full-time or part-time.
†Includes dental laboratory technicians and secretary/receptionists, as well as dental hygienists and dental assistants.

External factors

The external factors that influence dental assisting and dental hygiene have continued to increase both in numbers and intensity. The dental profession has enjoyed relative autonomy until the past few years, when various groups expressed interest in and a desire for input into *all* areas of health care. Dental auxiliaries have become a subject of controversy, caught between the conflicts of different interest groups. The factors that are involved in health care quality, labor, access, and cost are many. The ones that most directly affect the status of dental auxiliaries are federal government, state government, and the current consumer movement.

Federal government

Program funding. The federal government has long played a role in the monitoring of health care delivery. One of its first efforts focused on dentistry was Congressional identification in 1950 of a dental labor shortage and the enactment of legislation dealing with that issue.[13] The major emphasis at that point involved the dental auxiliary in an attempt to increase dental care productivity through greater utilization of auxiliaries. The government began to support the development of programs that would promote the facilitation of auxiliaries in expanding the dental work force capacity. The Dental Auxiliary Utilization program (DAU) was the first of its kind and was instituted in dental schools across the country. The program's primary purpose was to investigate the concept of four-handed dentistry and the feasibility of incorporating this type of delivery system into the practice of dentistry. When the program was proved to be sound and its goals of increasing productivity could in fact be realized, support for the program was gradually increased, until by the early 1970s, virtually every dental school had an operating DAU program.[3]

Two other programs that were sponsored by the federal government were TEAM (Training in Expanded Auxiliary Management) and EFDA (Expanded Function Dental Auxiliary). Federal funding for these programs ended in the early 1980s, and most dental schools discontinued their efforts in this area of education.

Federal Trade Commission. The Federal Trade Commission (FTC) was originally established to monitor any violations of antitrust or fair trade laws. The Magnuson-Moss Act of 1965 gave the commission specific power to set minimum standards of conduct for an industry. This practice is the cause of much debate within the dental profession. The FTC has been conducting investigation into the provision of high-quality dental care at the lowest cost.

The independent practice of auxiliaries has been a major priority for the FTC. The FTC contends that to require dental hygienists to work under the supervision of a dentist unnecessarily limits the public's access to preventive care and may retard competition in the provision of dental services. If the FTC continues in its current path, auxiliaries may be more closely scrutinized to determine their role in providing competent low-cost care.

National Commission for Health Certifying Agencies. This agency was formed in 1976 to establish criteria for professionals working in health areas. The ADAA and the ADHA are represented on the commission, which is involved in setting standards for certifying bodies that attest to the competency of individuals who participate in the health care system.[15] In April 1985, however, DANB relinquished its membership in NCHA because it had not found membership of any direct value in promoting its examination programs and because of the high cost of membership.[7]

The issue of credentialing and/or educational requirements is an ongoing topic of debate and will probably become even more controversial. At a 1984 conference sponsored by the National Commission for Health Certifying Agencies, the ADAA president was informed of a move by the National Association of Health Career Schools to establish a new credentialing mechanism for their program graduates who cannot take the DANB certification examination unless they fulfill a 2-year work requirement. Rather than clarify the role of the dental assistant, a new credential could undermine the recognition of the CDA and legislative advances that have been established.[10]

State government. State governments have more direct control over the function and status of auxiliaries. Through the power vested in it, the state is responsible for the protection and safety of its citizens. Therefore, the state hopes to ensure this protection by enacting laws that will prevent unnecessary harm to the public. Police power gives each state the right to enforce such laws. Thus, state practice acts have evolved that would control the health—as well as other—professions. These practice acts are intended to provide the general public with competent and standardized health care.

State dental practice acts establish minimum qualifications for and delineate the services performed by dental health care providers. In 1915 the state of Connecticut included a definition of dental hygiene in their state practice act. Since that time, every state in the country has written the practice of dental hygiene into its legislation with accompanying qualifications and licensing mechanisms. Despite the fact that dental hygiene statutes may vary from state to state, the educational and licensing requirements are relatively consistent. Dental assisting is not as universally defined, however, and state practice acts can be found that vary from a mere mention of a person labeled *dental assistant* to a person who is mandatorily registered, examined, and defined by statutes. The discrepancies in the boundaries imposed by state practice acts make the role of an assistant arbitrary, vague, and inconsistent.

The State Board of Dental Examiners or Board of Registration, is the appointed group responsible for enforcing a state's dental prac-

tice act. Members of state dental boards have traditionally been the gubernatorial appointments of nominees submitted by the state dental society. A board is theoretically representative of the state, not the profession. There has been increasing impetus to change the composition of boards in many states, to include more representatives of the dental profession as well as lay appointees. It may very well be that the catalyst for more definitive and progressive state practice acts will be in the form of consumer board members rather than the dental profession itself.

State law also involves what is known as *sunset* legislation, which mandates periodic review of such regulating bodies as the professional licensing board. This means that, even if the profession does not raise its own issues concerning the composition and function of state professional boards, they may be raised by the legislature itself. Depending on how states view the dental practice act, states may either give additional opportunities to dental hygienists or end licensing.

Consumerism. As health care costs continue to spiral, the consumer is taking an increasingly active part in finding a means of cost containment. In almost every area of health care, it has been discovered that fuller utilization and delegation of additional functions to ancillary personnel increases service provision. The expansion of dental boards to include consumers lends more clout to the consumer movement. Naturally, the consumer is primarily concerned with making high-quality, low-cost care available to as high a percentage of the population as is feasible. One method that laypersons have found appropriate in providing care on a local level has been the neighborhood health center. Some of these centers have operated successfully, free from professional control. Admittedly, there have been problems encountered when a center operates without adequately trained personnel, but many communities have found their specific needs are best met when representatives of their own neighborhoods make the decisions through the actions of community boards.

Consumers have exercised more control in the delivery of dental care services through payment mechanisms. An increase in availability of care is a direct result of the ever-growing third party payment plan. In this way auxiliaries will be permited a greater role in providing dental care.

PLANNING THE FUTURE ROLE OF THE AUXILIARY

With an increase in third party dental insurance and with the development of more alternatives to the traditional private solo practice setting, the dental auxiliary can be viewed in light of new roles and functions that may have a significant impact on the dental health of the public. In terms of function and capacity, this impact falls into three broad categories: community dental health advocate, educator, and dental care provider.

Community dental health advocate

Certainly the dental auxiliary can and should have significant impact on and influence in the community in terms of promoting effective preventive dental care programs. The objectives of these programs include those aimed at achieving fluoridation, regular home-care procedures, periodic visits to the dentist, an awareness of nutrition as a factor in oral health, and screenings for oral cancer and hypertension.

The dental profession as a whole has made great progress since the time when simply sponsoring an Annual National Children's Dental Health Week was deemed to be a sufficient contribution to the community's dental health. One of the indications of a more comprehensive approach toward improving the dental health of the community is the active role that the dental auxiliary takes in working with dental societies to secure political support for community fluoridation. Public acceptance of water fluoridation

depends in large part on the dissemination of accurate information by committed dental health professionals and consumer groups.

With the signing into law of the National Health Information and Disease Prevention Act in 1977, which encourages the initiation and design of educational programs to help the consumer better understand qualitative health care, the auxiliary acquired another way to serve within the community. Perhaps the most significant recent development in this area has occurred with the appointment of auxiliaries as members of the Boards of Registration in Dentistry in several states. As board members, dental auxiliaries can help to establish rules and regulations that directly affect the delivery of dental care, as well as have a voice on such specific issues as licensure requirements and regulations of quality care (among others), which directly affect public dental health.

In addition to their service on Boards of Registration in Dentistry, trained dental auxiliary personnel are needed to implement programs in public schools and to be administrators within the health components of programs such as Head Start, Health Maintenance Organizations, Health Systems Agencies, and Professional Standards Review Organizations. In the private sector, business concern about the rising cost of dental health care as an employee benefit is increasing, and the era of corporate-sponsored dental clinics and corporate dental health consultants cannot be far off. The dental profession's responsibilities to community needs and its increasing social awareness correspond to the expansion of the auxiliary's role as a community dental health activist.

Educator

The dental hygienist's or dental assistant's responsibility as an educator is well established. Traditionally, a young woman in a white uniform appeared in elementary school classrooms once or twice a year with a picture of Tommy Tooth and Old Mr. Tooth Decay. The presentation included toothbrush instruction, a discussion of the process of tooth decay, and perhaps some reference to certain foods as recommended and certain others as not recommended. Today, with a command of modern educational methods and proven preventive measures, the corresponding presentation would include references to fluoride mouthrise/tablet programs, home-care procedures, periodic dental visits, and more sophisticated nutritional counseling.

Perhaps the most significant trend is away from direct pupil contact and toward teaching and equipping the school nurse, the parent, the teacher of health courses, and even the classroom teacher and principal to convey the dental health message and to act as a dental hygiene model.

In the private practice setting, the auxiliary not only educates the patient about his/her own dental health but also has the opportunity to inform the patient of the issues that are pertinent to the dental health of the community. The interaction between the patient and the auxiliary provides the best opportunity to answer questions and to present facts about such issues as water fluoridation, acceptance of expanded functions for auxiliaries, ionizing radiation, mercury toxicity, and the importance of screening programs for oral cancer and hypertension. When dental public health concerns such as water fluoridation become an issue in the community, the patient has already become an educated consumer and voter. By informing and educating each patient to facts about specific public health problems, the auxiliary can establish a powerful information network and thus effect changes within the community as well as within the individual.

Dental care provider

Rendering of direct dental care to patients falls into three broad categories: primary, secondary, and tertiary. Today the dental auxiliary is taking part in the provision of services that fall

into the first two of these categories, with the possibility of providing care at the tertiary level in the near future. In addition to basic skills in prophylaxis, areas of primary care being provided by the dental hygienist or dental assistant include application of sealants, placement of interceptive orthodontic devices, administration of topical fluorides, and detection of oral cancer and hypertension.

In 1976 the National Preventive Demonstration Program, administered by the American Fund for Dental Health and funded by the Robert Wood Johnson Foundation, was designed to provide preventive and restorative care to all children on a continuous basis. Presently, the program provides school-based preventive services for children, including systemic and topical fluorides, sealants, oral health education, diet regulation, and plaque control. With the advent of these types of programs, expanded duty auxiliaries have been trained to provide these preventive services.

At the secondary level of care, the hygienist and the assistant may perform those expanded duties that are legal within the state in which they practice. As consumer and professional acceptance of the delegation of additional expanded functions to the auxiliary increases, the public should benefit from an increase of available dental services.

Certainly, as the hygienist seeks alternative practice settings from those traditionally under the supervision of the dentist, the public will reap the benefits by receiving increased direct dental care. The concept was pioneered in California by Linda Krol (see Case study, p. 52), who was the first dental hygienist to become an independent contractor. Ms. Krol established a separate office even though her work was under the supervision of a dentist. The alternative practice setting was designed to solve the problems of patient load, insufficient work space, and insufficient dental hygiene personnel.[12]

In other areas, the concept of the traditional private practice setting for the delivery of dental care is being modified to meet the needs of the public. Presently the law and regulations of some states allow hygienists to provide preventive services to patients in schools and institutions who would not normally receive care through the private practice system. This concept of the dental hygienist as a dental care extender is similar to the physician's assistant in medicine.

Case study: an alternative practice setting. A California dental hygienist, Linda Krol, was frustrated because new dental patients had to wait for 10 months, until a hygiene appointment became available, to see her. When office space adjoining her dentist's office became vacant, she discussed with her employer the possibility of her renting the office space and working for herself.

In California, the state dental practice act requires that a dental hygienist perform services and practice only in a dental office or an equivalent facility approved by the Board of Dental Examiners of the state of California. The two dentists by whom she had been employed for 13 years supported her desire to work independently on a professional level and a contract was established between them. Since she planned to see patients of these dentists, the contract was an agreement by both parties stating the responsibilities of each party.

According to the Internal Revenue Service, this agreement designated Linda as an independent contractor. A copy of the contract was sent to the California Board of Dental Examiners for approval to remodel the adjoining office. The board approved the conditions outlined in the contract, contingent on the dentists' providing necessary supervision. Construction of three dental hygiene operatories, a laboratory, an office, and a reception room was completed, and the new office floor plan established the dental hygiene operatories closer to the supervising dentist than had previously been the case.

When Ms. Krol began providing services under the agreement, complaints came from members of the dental profession. Their concerns were that hygiene services were not being provided under the supervision and control of a licensed dentist. Finally, 13 months into her practice, Ms. Krol received a claim from the office of the Attorney General. Ultimately, this claim was settled out of court on the conditions that Ms. Krol put on the door of her reception room the name of each dentist for whom she was contracting services; that 45 days before seeing a patient of a doctor other than the orig-

inally contracted dentists, the name of that dentist must be submitted to the board in writing; and that appropriate supervision and direction of services be maintained by the contracted dentist.*

In July 1986 an amendment to the Colorado Dental Practice Law that allows the independent practice of dental hygiene became effective. The ADA Commission on Dental Accreditation is challenging the amendment, and two patients with heart conditions are also plaintiffs in the case.

According to the amended statute, unsupervised dental hygiene practice includes: scaling, smoothing, and polishing natural and restored tooth surfaces; gingival curettage; topical fluoride application; gathering patient history; oral inspection and dental and periodontal charting; and administering topical anesthesia. The law also allows the hygienist to own the hygiene office and to buy or lease equipment. Since dental hygiene education and accreditation are based on the fact that hygienists are supervised by dentists, the ADA is concerned that hygienists are not prepared to diagnose dental or periodontal disease or to monitor patients who need special care without the supervision of a licensed dentist.[17]

Although there are disputes over the establishment of the hygienist as an independent practitioner, each small advancement provides the consumer with another alternative way of receiving dental care.

Alternative modes for delivering care may be modeled after examples in other professions. In medicine, the Rural Health Clinic Services Act provides financial support for alternative practice settings. This bill sanctions payments by Medicare and Medicaid for care that physician extenders provide in remote health clinics and does not require the presence of a physician. If a similar policy is ever developed for dentistry,

---

*Modified from Mayuga, P.W.: Linda Krol: independent contractor, J. Am. Dent. Hygienists' Assoc. **53**(4):169, 1979.

the dental auxiliary is well equipped to provide the labor.

Eventually, additional practice settings may be established in nursing homes, shopping centers, day-care centers, and other areas where previously the hygienist could not provide services without the dentist.

At the tertiary level the dental auxiliary is a likely provider of services with the expanded functions defined in the area of rehabilitation. The state of Maine has passed a law in support of denturism, and as part of the educational guidelines, the auxiliary must have completed a 2-year educational curriculum and be under the supervision of the dentist. The dental hygienist, who is already regulated in this manner, provides a ready resource for additional training as a denturist.

SUMMARY

Changes in the political, social, and professional climates, affect auxiliaries, forcing more diversified roles. The political climate will play a major part in how involved the auxiliary will become in performing clinical tasks. For example, if Congress passed a National Health Insurance program including dental services, increased demand would dictate an increased need for service providers. The social trend would also promote expanded use of auxiliaries as the consumer insists on reasonably priced dental services. Societal trends have a great influence on where and how money is spent, and in the case of health care, society is no longer taking a passive role. As a result, auxiliaries may readily gain the support of consumer interest groups in promoting their cause.

The professional climate is the one most directly affecting the auxiliaries' role. As the number of dentists increases and the incidence of dental disease decreases, auxiliaries are looking outside the traditional practice setting for jobs. Two nontraditional areas opening up for auxiliaries are marketing and sales in the dental

products industry and dental coverage review analysis in the insurance industry.

Underlying all of these issues is, of course, the economic one. When the economy declines, everyone feels the pinch. Services that are not viewed as "essential," such as dentistry, are historically the first ones sacrificed. Conversely, when the economy is strong, increased emphasis on dental care programs and services reflect prosperity. Dental research, education, and service provision are all dependent on the amount of public money available to support them.

There are interesting times ahead for dental auxiliaries—opportunities for greater involvement and growth at the same time as potential cutbacks in traditional practice opportunities. Auxiliaries will be best served by being articulate and outspoken advocates for themselves and their profession. Perhaps the real challenge and excitement will be in marketing their clinical and communication skills as a unique contribution to the dental profession.

REFERENCES

1. American Dental Association: Interagency committee report, J. Am. Dent. Assoc. **84**:1027, 1972.
2. American Dental Association: Report of the meeting of the House of Delegates, annual session, Chicago, 1975.
3. American Dental Association, Commission on Dental Accreditation: Memorandum, February 1980.
4. American Dental Association, Council on Dental Education, Division of Educational Measurements: Annual report on dental auxiliary education 1985-1986.
5. Boyer, E.M.: Dows Institute for Dental Research, College of Dentistry, University of Iowa, IA: Dent. Hyg. **60**(5):204, 1986.
6. Council of State Governments, National Task Force on State Dental Policies: Manpower utilization, J. Dent. Educ. **43**(11):85, 1979.
7. Dental Assisting National Board, Memorandum, April 1985.
8. Dreyer, R.: RDHs in the dental industry, RDH **6**(5):22, 1986.
9. Feinman, R.A.: An auxiliary for the 1980s—the dental treatment coordinator (abstract) Dent. Econ. **75**(1):70, 1985.
10. Jespersen, K.: President's address, Dent. Assist. **55**(1):37, 1986.

11. MacLeod, A.E.: Independent management consultants, Halifax, Nova Scotia, Canada: Dental assistants and productivity (abstract) Oral Health **74**(10):71, 1984.

12. Mayuga, P.W.: Linda Krol: independent contractor, J. Am. Dent. Hygienists' Assoc. **53**(4):169, 1979.

13. Meskin, L.H.: Focusing on the future: the dental hygienist as an office manager, J. Am. Dent. Hygienists' Assoc. **53**:9, 1979.

14. Motley, W.: Ethics, jurisprudence, and history of the dental hygienist, ed. 2, Philadelphia, 1976, Lea & Febiger.

15. National Commission for Health Certifying Agencies: Bylaws, Article 2, Section 1, 1976.

16. Peterson, S.: The dentist and the assistant, ed. 4, St. Louis, 1977, The C.V. Mosby Co., p. 17.

17. Shanoff, C.: Colorado statute opposed by ADA commission, Dent. Today **5**(7):1, 1986.

18. Sisty, N.L.: Henderson, W.G., and Paule, C.L.: Review of training and evaluation studies in expanded functions for dental auxiliaries, J. Am. Dent. Assoc. **98**:2, 1979.

19. Smith, H.L.: Cost containment in the dental office, Dent. Assist. **55**(2):17, 1986.

20. U.S. Department of Health and Human Services, Public Health Service, Health Resources and Services Administration, Bureau of Health Professions: Fifth report to the President and Congress on the status of health personnel in the United States, Dentistry, March 1986.

21. Waldman, B.H.: Is dentistry's future threatened? Dent. Surv. **51**(11):50, 1975.

22. Woodall, I.R.: Leadership, management, and role delineation: issues for the dental team, St. Louis, 1977, The C.V. Mosby Co.

SOCIAL AND FINANCIAL ASPECTS OF DENTAL CARE

Although dental disease is prevalent in society, not all Americans avail themselves of dental services. There are many barriers to dental care; some relate to education, some to finances, some to cultural habits.

This section begins with an examination of the social aspects of dental disease; that is, the factors that influence people in responding to dental needs and seeking dental care. It is clear that people respond differently to needs. Some people might not perceive a cavity as needing professional care; some might perceive a need for care but place a low priority on the need and thus not seek care unless severe pain occurs; and other people might seek care on a routine basis, without overt symptoms. The multitude of factors that influence these decisions are presented in Chapter 4.

Chapter 5 deals with a specific population group, the elderly, and describes their particular dental needs. The elderly are the fastest growing age group in this country and at present receive less dental care than younger adults. This chapter investigates some of the reasons for the elderly's lower utilization of services and public health programs that might better address their needs.

Chapter 6 discusses the financial aspects of dental care and dental health programs. It describes methods of payment for dental care and the history of third party reimbursement in the United States. It provides detailed information on a variety of reimbursement mechanisms and a case study of how dental insurance premiums are determined.

CHAPTER 4

Social Aspects of Dental Care

The interactions between community dental needs and dental health services are complex and ever-changing. The sociology of dental care is the study of these needs and services. In some cases, the focus is on particular aspects of dental care, such as how people use services or how they interact with dental professionals. In other cases, the concern is with dental care as an aspect of the larger society, such as studies of how organizations representing dental professionals lobby for particular pieces of legislation or studies of the social costs of poor dental health.

In order to conceptualize the range of topics that comprise the sociology of dental care, one should consider the participants involved.[28] At the first level is the individual. One asks how that individual perceives dental care, how a decision is made to seek treatment, and how a dentist is chosen. At the second level, there is the dental care system. One can inquire about how patients and dental practitioners interact and about how their perceptions of each other may influence the outcome of treatment. Another set of questions involves the relationship between the type of dental delivery institutions—private office, group practice, dental school clinic—and the kind of treatment provided. At the third level, there are the organizations that affect the practitioners. These include educational institutions, certifying boards, national organizations representing dental professionals, and local groups, including peer networks. One must ask how these institutions affect the practitioner and, in turn, the patient. What for example, are the beliefs, attitudes, and values that these institu-

tions encourage in their members? At the fourth level, there is the public at large as represented both by government and by consumer groups. The concern is with planning and regulation of the overall system of dental care delivery as well as in maintaining high standards of care at every encounter between a patient and a dental professional. One must ask how the government can affect the distribution of practitioners in the population, the accessibility of care of all in need, and the long-term improvement in oral health. At the fifth level, there is the international community. At this point, one can compare the efficiency and effectiveness of different types of dental care delivery systems and inquire as to how these systems may or may not serve as models for those societies just beginning to provide organized dental services.

The purpose of this chapter is to serve as an introduction to the different areas of the sociology of dental care. A description of the role of government in dental health care, a comparative analysis of dental health systems in different countries, and a discussion of program planning for dental services are found elsewhere in this text, and for this reason, the discussion of these topics is limited.

SOCIAL EPIDEMIOLOGY

Dental disease is not a random event; it is related to biological, genetic, environmental, and social factors. Social epidemiology seeks to explain the interrelationship between these factors and, in particular, to describe how social phenomena affect both the onset and the outcome of disease. A major concern is to identify those factors contributing to dental disease that can be altered or eliminated.

Diet is an example of an important social phenomenon that plays a role in dental disease. More simply, a high intake of sugar, if accompanied by poor oral hygiene, can lead to dental caries. The question asked by epidemiologists is, What conditions affect a person's diet? Does poverty result in an inability to buy nutritious, unsweetened foods? Is the consumption of highly sugared foods a part of some cultures? Is poor nutrition encouraged by the placement of vending machines containing sweets in schools and work areas?

Once identified, the causes of poor nutrition are not always easy to remedy. One must consider the factors involved in a person's diet. Encouraging good nutrition among people who cannot afford to buy wholesome foods will be futile and perhaps alienating to those being given the advice. Taking candy-filled vending machines out of school cafeterias will not solve the problem of poor nutrition, but it will eliminate a source of the problem.

It is important to study the social epidemiology of dental disease in order to identify some of the paths to eliminating the problem. Nevertheless, not all studies result in a discovery of a solution. An example of this is the work by Heifetz and associates comparing the number of carious teeth found in black and white children living in a rural southern community.[12] Black children used to have a lower rate of caries than white children, but this is no longer the case. The authors hypothesize that this change is a result of changes in the diet of black children who, in recent years, have come to consume more sugar and fewer homegrown foods than was previously the case. Indeed, it is suggested that black children have a diet similar to that of white children and therefore, a similar caries problem. Should this hypothesis be confirmed by later studies, the next step would be to find ways of discouraging

sugar consumption in both black and white children, a problem that has plagued dental health advocates for many years. As suggested earlier, dietary habits, like other basic life patterns, are difficult to change.

The connections between behavior and disease may be obvious, as is the case with diet and decay, or they may be difficult to uncover. In either situation, the ability to respond to the problem will depend on the resources of the society and the individuals involved. Social conditions may need to be altered through efforts such as food stamp programs and income supplements. Patients and practitioners may need to improve their communications so that health habits and behavior can be altered to improve oral health status. Chapter 7 provides a closer look at the factors causing ill health, illustrating the complexity of the events leading to the state we call illness.

THE UTILIZATION OF DENTAL HEALTH SERVICES

Those concerned with policy planning and the oganization of dental health delivery systems are often frustrated by the fact that those who may need the most care often receive the least. Attempts at stimulating utilization through health education in the schools and through the media often have disappointing results. What is most apparent is that the use of services is influenced by many factors, only some of which can be altered for better results.

Sociologists studying the utilization of health services have shown that it is directly related to a number of variables. Economic conditions, sociopsychological processes, sociocultural background, and the characteristics of the delivery system all influence utilization. A behavioral model of health services utilization developed by Andersen and Newman can be used to explain all these factors from the perspective of the individual.[2] The factors involved have been broken down into three groups: (1) those that influence the person to use services, called predisposing factors; (2) those that allow those services to be used, called enabling factors; and (3) those that determine how those services should be put to use, called need factors.

Predisposing factors

Predisposing factors are of three types: (1) demographic variables, for example, age and sex; (2) social variables, which give some idea of the status the person holds in society, such as education and occupation; and (3) health beliefs, such as how susceptible to diseases the person believes himself/herself to be or how serious one believes a particular dental condition to be.

Demographic factors. Demographic factors are relatively easy to measure and have been shown to affect utilization. The Health Interview Survey of 1981, for instance, demonstrated that both age and sex influenced utilization of dental services.[25] Women made more visits to dentists than did men, averaging 1.8 visits per year as compared to 1.5. Age had less of an effect, although it was found that those 65 years of age and over made the least number of visits, averaging 1.5 per year. Of the total population, only 50.1% had seen a dentist during the previous year.

Social factors. Social factors such as race, ethnicity, occupation, and level of education have a greater influence on utilization than the demographic factors reviewed above. A study of the National Health Interview Survey of 1981 found that race was a major determinant of utilization.[25] While dental visits for those of all ages and incomes and for both sexes averaged 1.7 per year, for whites the average was 1.8 while for nonwhites it was only 1.1. Ethnicity as well as race is a factor. In a pioneering survey comparing utilization of dental services by Chicanos and whites, Garcia and Juarez found significant differences in utilization, even when other variables such as socioeconomic status held constant.[11] Occupation has been suggested as a factor by Dunning, who argues that if presentability

is an important aspect of an occupation, more dental treatment would be sought than would otherwise be suggested by a person's background.[7]

Health beliefs. Health beliefs are the most difficult of the predisposing factors to assess, as utilization behavior in this case is linked to a constellation of values and ideas. Dworkin and colleagues describe four types of health beliefs: perceived susceptibility to dental disease, perceived seriousness of dental disease, perceived preventability (the degree to which people believe they can promote dental health through brushing and through seeing a dentist), and perceived salience (the degree to which people view dental care as worthwhile).[8] Health beliefs have received some study. Garcia and Juarez hypothesized that Chicano beliefs about dental care are symptom-oriented—that care is sought to relieve pain and other symptoms of ill health—rather than being prevention-oriented.[11] The suggestion is that one's health beliefs are related to one's culture. Milk, in her article, points out some of the ways in which a person's culture influences the seeking of care.[18] She describes some possible aspects of this, such as the value of beauty, the definition of attractive teeth, and the need for immediate gratification (for example, having teeth extracted rather than undergoing long-term restorative work), as being linked in part to a person's cultural identity.

Enabling factors

The most important family resource enabling people to use services is income. Its effect on utilization has been studied extensively and it has been found to be of major impact. Anderson and Newman studied dental service utilization and found that it increased along with family income.[2] They found that the family's perception of its income was also important; that is, the family must not only have the means to pay for care, it must also be aware that it has those means. Socioeconomic status was also pointed out as a factor by Nikias and associates, who compared poverty and nonpoverty groups on their dental status, needs, and practices. They found that those who were poor were less likely to seek care or, more specifically, preventive care.[20]

Community resources that enable a person to utilize services have sometimes been studied in conjunction with income resources. People with low incomes may live in areas with relatively few services available. Even if this is not the case, low-income people may lack resources, such as time and transportation, necessary to utilize available services. In their study of the demand for dental care, Holtmann and Olsen found that both income and waiting time influenced utilization.[13] They suggest that if low-income people are paid hourly wages rather than the weekly salaries paid to higher income groups, the time spent waiting in the dental clinic or office for care can be very costly. They suggest that, in addition to subsidized dental care, low-income people would benefit from practices that use dental assistants to reduce both the cost and the waiting time.

The major community resource is, of course, the dental care provider. One way to measure the availability of dental services is to look at the number of dentists available to serve a given population. In 1984 there was an estimated civilian dental work force of 132,750 with a ratio of 56.3 dentists for 100,000 people as contrasted to 49 dentists to 100,000 people in 1965.[24] The meaning of these figures to a person in search of a dentist is hard to determine. Leverett has suggested there is a maldistribution of dentists who can offer an appointment to a new patient within 1 week of the appointment request.[15] He suggests that much of the demand for dental care is controlled by the profession and that examining such measures as availability of appointments and the number of hours dentists work may yield better information about provider resources.

Need factors

The need factor in utilization is, very simply, the presence of ill health as it is perceived by the individual and as it is assessed by the dental professional. In dental care, the perception of the need for treatment is an important factor that will be discussed in detail in the section on the patient-practitioner relationship. The need for dental care, as judged by the community of dental professionals, is difficult to describe in numbers, but given that many people have never visited a dental professional and that many who have sought care do have extensive dental problems, it can be said that not all dental needs have been met.

The interaction of predisposing, enabling, and need factors

While predisposing, enabling, and need factors have been described separately, it is obvious that they are related. Age for instance, is mentioned as a predisposing factor, and it was stated earlier that those over 65 years of age use services less frequently than younger members of the population. Income, an enabling factor, was also linked to utilization. If a large percentage of the elderly population has a low income, this may account for a low level of dental services' utilization. Health beliefs may also play a role if older people perceive dental care as less of a purchase priority than other possible expenditures. Dental care professionals may find that elderly people need a different type or amount of care than younger people; for instance, they may hesitate to do extensive restorative work. Putting all these variables together, we find that age, a predisposing factor, income, an enabling factor, and need may combine to result in elderly people receiving less care (or a different type of care) than other members of the population.

Increasing utilization

For those concerned with increasing the effective utilization of dental health services, the behavioral model, which looks at how the individual seeks care, may not be the best perspective from which to view dental services. Instead, the factors involved in the utilization of services may be examined with regards to their mutability, that is, the degree to which they can be altered. Using this as a guideline, it becomes obvious that demographic and social factors are largely impossible to change. Similarly, health beliefs, as they affect the predisposition to use services, are difficult to alter. It is largely in the area of community resources that changes can be made. Chapter 9 on program planning discusses the ways in which community resources can be assessed, augmented, changed, and improved.

THE PROFESSION OF DENTISTRY

Dental care is provided by a variety of workers, including dentists, dental hygienists, dental assistants, and dental technicians. The division of labor is made on the basis of education and training as well as by the type of work performed. Furthermore, the division of labor is hierarchical. Dentists are the dominant group, able to supervise the work of all the others.

The dentist as professional

The term *professional* designates the status with which a worker is viewed by society, not the quality of the work performed. One definition of a profession describes it as a *possession* of: (1) a basis of systematic theory, (2) authority recognized by the clientele of the professional, (3) broader community sanction and approval of this authority, (4) a code of ethics regulating relations of professional persons with clients and with colleagues, and (5) a professional culture sustained by formal professional associations.[14] There are two key issues in professional status: one is the use of peer review rather than outside assessment of the work performed, and the second is the accompanying expectation that professionals, if allowed to judge their work, will live up to a code of ethics and deliver the highest quality care at all times.

In terms of dentistry, the meaning of professional status raises several questions. How does professional status affect the quality of care being provided in terms of dentist-patient communication? How does it affect the interactions between the dentist and other dental care providers? And finally, does peer review succeed in maintaining the performance of high-quality care?

Becoming a professional

While a professional status is granted by the society through a formal proceeding, the development of a professional identity is a slow, unregulated process. The environment of the dental school and the role models of older students and professors on the faculty guide the dental student toward the creation of a self-definition as a professional. Studies of dental students have demonstrated that changes in attitudes and values occur in the course of obtaining a professional education. Vinton, in a 4-year study of the impact of learning structures on dental student values, found that students placed less value on learning from and sharing with others, interpersonal communication, and close personal relations with others as their time in school continued.[27] Students instead came to place more interest in their own personal goals and interests. Loupe and associates studied dental students and dentists over a 10-year period and found that the social environment, as well as the nature of the dental practice, affected the development of interpersonal values.[17]

Another inquiry into professionalization might begin by asking, Who is selected to attend dental school? Does the population of dentists reflect the makeup of the overall population with regard to race, sex, class background, and ethnic identity or are dental students coming from only a small segment of the overall population? The answer is obvious; dentists are not representative of the general population, and it is possible that this difference, as well as the assumption of a professional identity, could make dentist-patient communication difficult at times.

While dental schools have tried to correct the racial and sexual balance of their entering classes, they have been only partially successful. Mulvihill found that, while minority enrollment in dental schools began increasing in the early 1970s, the percentage of Black students had begun to level off and even decline by 1975.[19] This trend reversed by 1980 and by 1984 Blacks made up 6.0% of the first-year national enrollment.[24] The high cost of dental school combined with the lack of scholarships were two of the reasons posited for this imbalance. Another consideration must be the way in which minority students are perceived by the dental school faculty and by their fellow student. If they feel unwanted or unwelcome, they may not bother to apply or they may drop out. The issue of perception has been studied with regard to female dental students. Rosenberg and Thompson discovered that among other things, male dental students and faculty members perceived female dental students as both different from the sex role of a woman and different from the professional role of a dentist.[21] The question, How will these perceptions affect the female dental students' professional self-identity? must await a further study. The number of women in dental school has been increasing and it is expected that 22% of the 1986 nationwide graduating class would be female.[1]

If an enhanced professional identity is the outcome of a dental education and practice, how will this affect the dentists' ability to understand patients and auxiliaries who do not share this professional identity? For instance, will dentists feel more at ease speaking in technical language to fellow professionals than in using common language with their patients?

The dentist and the auxiliary

The delivery of dental care often involves a great deal of teamwork between the dentist and the other providers. At the same time that the dentist plays the role of team member, he/she is also team captain directing as well as providing care. The relationship between the dentist and other providers will depend on both law and custom. The law will determine the limits of the activities performed by auxiliaries. Custom will decree what is actually done in the work environment. In some cases, the auxiliaries will have been trained by the dentist; in other cases, they will be graduates of professional programs or will have trained with other providers. Thus, their abilities and their personal relationship with the dentist will dictate their behavior.

A recent study of the Commission on Accreditation of Dental and Dental Auxiliary Education Programs concerning the professional role of the dental hygienist found that hygienists were highly ranked in terms of professional status, but that they were not seen as equal to dentists.[26] Those interviewed found hygienists to be better educated than ever before, but they also suggested that hygienists were "much too aggressive at the national level for their own good." It seems that while the accreditation commissioners endorse the attempts of hygienists to expand their education and ability, they do not accept them as peers. This view is shared by the society at large, as indicated by the law that believes in both dentists and dentistry but only in dental hygiene and not in dental hygienists.

The dentist and the patient

Dentists are trained in special programs, and in their training they inculcate professional values, including respect for fellow members of the occupation. Their work requires them to make and receive referrals from other dentists, which in turn means that they view the work of others as well as having their own work on display. The question that arises is whether they view the work of other professionals with a critical eye and as part of a process of upholding standards, or whether they refrain from making judgments on those with whom they closely identify. More simply stated, does professional identification conflict with the need to protect patients from fellow members of the trade who fail to perform at the highest levels? The 1979 changes in the law, which permitted dentists to advertise, has been viewed by many dentists as another conflict within the profession. Some dentists feel that advertising denigrates the profession in the eyes of the public, whereas other dentists believe that advertising increases access to care for many patients.[4]

The issues of professionalism and dentistry have become more pronounced in recent years. Questions of the effects of training on the dentists' ability to work effectively with patients have inspired new types of training programs, such as externships. The quest for professional status by dental hygienists has led some to seek to expand the scope of their services and their autonomy, raising further questions about what type of practitioners need perform particular aspects of care giving. The answers that emerge will play a large part in determining the future dental care systems.

THE PATIENT-PRACTITIONER RELATIONSHIP

The expectations that patients and practitioners hold regarding the type of care to be given and received is an important area of inquiry. The interest of each participant often varies. Thus, the outcome of any interaction may depend on an informal negotiation process as well as on the provision of actual services. The patient, for instance, may expect to be given "care" as well as a cure for his/her problems. That is, the patient expects the dentist to be concerned with his/her worries, questions, and level of comfort as well as trying to take care of the presenting complaint. The practitioner, on the other hand, may not be fully aware of this need. In another case, the practitioner may expect to have all instructions understood and followed without question. The patient, in turn, may not be able to meet this expectation because of financial limitations and/or an incomplete understanding of the practitioner's request. In some situations, patients who are members of particular social groups may feel that they are being treated with less than total concern, while practitioners may feel that these patients are difficult to communicate with. In sum, the delivery of care involves a social as well as a service relationship.

While practitioners are defined as such through legal statutes and occupational activities, patienthood is an assumed and temporary status. Moreover, the process of becoming a patient is one that is difficult for a practitioner to observe. A patient may arrive at a dental clinic and be asked by the practitioner why he/she delayed so long before seeking care. The patient in this situation may feel that care was sought as soon as the need for it was recognized.[10]

Becoming a patient—two models

Medical sociologists have sought to describe the process by which a person becomes a patient, and its applicability to dental care should be discussed. Suchman has described the process in terms of five stages or decision points through which a person must pass in the process of becoming aware of an illness, seeking care, and recovering.[22] Zola has instead looked for the triggers to action that result in the person coming into actual contact with the health care system.[30] While both of these models were developed in reference to medical illness, their value in analyzing dental patients must be considered.

The model presented by Suchman begins with the symptom experience stage.[22] At this point, the person has the physical experience of ill health, recognizes it as such, and has an accompanying emotional response to the change in health status. The next step is the assumption of the sick role, whereby the person seeks to alleviate the symptoms and to acquire information about the condition that is causing the illness. At this stage a lay referral network, composed of friends and family members, may help guide the person in the decision-making process by recommending remedies and suggesting probable causes of the illness. The third stage involves contact with the health provider. The practitioner, rather than the lay network, is asked to vouch for the legitimacy of the symptoms being experienced. The fourth stage follows quickly when the individual is treated by the health provider and is thus assumed to be a patient. The fifth and final stage occurs when the patient has recovered or has been rehabilitated and exits from the role of patient.

Obviously, the length of time a person remains at any particular stage is a function of both the illness and a personal decision-making process. In the case of dental care, symptoms of ill health such as deterioration of the supporting structures can be ignored far longer than more acute conditions that cause pain or rapid tooth loss. Similarly, at the second stage when the person has begun to think of himself/herself as ill, the treatment may be sought immediately and with the approval of the lay network, or it may be postponed because of financial, emotional, and other barriers to treatment. In each of the stages outlined, decisions regarding the costs and benefits of proceeding to the next stage must be made by the care seeker, and there will be wide variations among individuals possessing the same symptoms.

A second model of patienthood examines the different processes leading to contact with health care professionals. Zola has delineated five triggers to care seeking that may operate independently of one another in some cases and jointly in others, depending on the values, beliefs, and attitudes of the patient.[30] One trigger to care seeking is an interpersonal crisis that causes the person to become aware of the symptoms of ill health and to seek a cure for them. A second trigger is termed *social interference*, meaning

that the symptoms are seen as threatening a continuation or initiation of valued social activities. An example of this may be a person who feels that tooth loss distracts from personal appearance and is limiting social interaction. Another type of trigger is sanctioning, in which the person feels that those having the authority to suggest it encourage the seeking of treatment. A fourth trigger involves the perception that the symptoms are interfering with physical activity. An example of this case would be extensive tooth loss that interferes with eating habits. Last, there is a trigger that involves temporalizing; that is, the person decides to seek care if the symptoms have not abated within a specific period of time. Along with this temporalizing, there can be a kind of self-examination, which involves comparing one's experiences with those of friends and to past symptomatic episodes. An example of this case may be a person who finds that his/her gums are bleeding and decides to seek care if the condition continues for another week.

Both models present the idea that care seeking involves consultation with others, such as friends and family, prior to contact with health professionals. Sociologists have suggested that the way these consultants view health and illness will have a large effect on the individual and that these health beliefs vary among different social groups. As noted in the discussion of utilization of services, age, sex, race, and income do affect the amount of contact a person has with a dentist. Studies have also indicated that ethnicity may play a large part in determining at what point, and for what reason, a person will decide to seek dental care.

Patient-practitioner interaction

Studies of patient-practitioner interaction have depended on the perspective of only one of the participants. For example, Weintein and associates found that the majority of dentists questioned in their study reported getting along with their patients.[29] The authors raised the issue of how this finding would relate to the quality of care. For instance, do dentists provide better services to those who seemed to appreciate it the most? This question can be asked from the patient's perspective. Is the best quality care provided by the most considerate dentists? Trihart's study of underprivileged patients indicates that some feel that empathy is as important as competence and that the experience of pain by these patients is perceived as an indication that the dentist is unqualified.[23] Dummett suggests that some patients may feel uncomfortable with the aseptic cleanliness of a dental clinic and would prefer a more relaxed environment.[6] He also suggests that practitioners may, at times, have difficulty understanding the speech of some patients, a problem that would be magnified among groups of patients for whom English is a second language. A classic study by Frazier and colleagues points out that while providers thought low-income consumers did not value dental care (as compared with other services and goods), in point of fact, dental care was much desired and well regarded by low-income consumers.[9] The variations in patient and practitioner views of dental services uncovered by these studies may indicate only a lack of congruity in the case of low-income patients or perhaps a more generalized problem.

Theories of interaction

Studies of actual practitioner-patient interaction have been limited. Linn examined behavior in two dental clinics and found that most patients obeyed dentists, conformed to their wishes, and rarely made direct requests.[16] Dentists, in turn, remain calm, orderly, and in control of the social reactions that occurred. The question of patient satisfaction with this environment was not explored. Anderson has begun a study of dentist-patient interactions, focusing on negotiation, pain management, and other aspects of the organization of routine interaction in the dentist's office.[3] Completion of the study will

undoubtedly yield new insights into the actual process of giving and receiving dental care as it examines the environment of a private practice dental office in which the bulk of dental care is provided.

To aid in conceptualizing the practitioner-patient relationship, Davis has developed a model of interaction that proposes to delineate patient orientation and practitioner control.[5] Three levels of patient orientation to the environment are posited: hostile, calculative, and positive. Practitioners are seen as able to exercise three types of power: coercive, utilitarian, and normative. Davis suggests that different combinations of patient orientation and practitioner power are present in different treatment settings. Thus, a dental school clinic would be viewed by the patient as a hostile or alienating setting, one in which the practitioner was able to exercise coercive power. Another example might be working-class patients visiting a private practitioner for corrective purposes where they would find an entirely different situation. These patients' orientation would be calculative, that is, neither hostile nor positive, but one in which a negotiation with the practitioner might take place. The practitioner in this situation would have a utilitarian orientation. Recommendations to the patient would be based on the type of care needed and the patient's ability and willingness to pay for such care. Finally, there is a possible situation in which an upper-class patient, making a regular visit to a private practitioner, might have a positive (moral) attitude toward the situation, while the practitioner may be able to exercise a kind of normative power because of the patient's acceptance of the need for care. While this model has yet to be applied on a large scale to a variety of dentist-patient interactions, the issues raised regarding power are important. The obvious implication is that a variety of interactions are possible, and the environment, the practitioner's perspective, and the use of power may affect the patient's view of dental care.

Recently more dental care has begun to be provided in clinics and Health Maintenance Organizations (HMOs) as well as in group practices. In these situations, there is more opportunity for the practitioner to scrutinize and presumably criticize the work of others. However, there is also the possibility that in these settings the dentist will develop closer ties to fellow practitioners—who share the same background, training, and status—than to the patients. That is, dentists will become peer-oriented rather than patient-oriented, because peers, rather than patients, will be influencing the amount of work the practitioner performs. The effect of the practice setting on the quality and quantity of care delivered will be an important area of inquiry as more practitioners enter into group work settings. It has been suggested earlier that some patients feel uncomfortable in clinic settings, perhaps because practitioners in these situations must meet the needs of the bureaucratic organization as well as those of the patient.

Simply stated, hostile, alienating environments might be identified and changed into calculative or positive situations. Practitioners might encourage compliance with dental regimes through appeal to utilitarian or normative beliefs rather than attempting to use coercion. It is possible that by identifying the alternatives, as this model has done, greater understanding of the situation will result.

THE ORGANIZATION OF DENTAL CARE

Studies in the sociology of dental care require knowledge of both practitioners and practice settings. Information ranging from simple demographic data on the number of practitioners and their geographic distribution to the description of the institutional structures in which they practice must be understood prior to any attempt to inquire about the social relations within the dental care delivery system.

The most basic information necessary to the study of dental care is, of course, the number and type of active practitioners. How many practitioners are there, how many are in training, how many are specialists? Armed with this data, we can ask if more or less are needed. Another type of determination can be made by looking at dentist to population ratios within different parts of the United States. Are dentists evenly distributed on a regional basis? Are people in both rural and urban areas able to get care? Are dentists located in areas where they can refer to other health providers and get referrals from them?

Dental care is generally provided in a private office. A dentist may employ one or more auxiliaries to assist in the delivery of care or may share a facility with a fellow practitioner; but to a large degree, dental care is an interaction involving only two people—the patient and the dental professional. The implications of this interaction in terms of the communication that is possible have been discussed earlier. A further question was raised regarding professionalization: How does peer review operate? Do private practitioners have an opportunity to view the work of others, judge it, and try to ensure quality of work performed by all members of the profession?

It is ironic that the practitioner-patient relationship, being at the core of all dental care and the most important field of study within the sociology of dental care, is studied so little. There are theories that are untested and studies that fail to unite the perceptions of both parties. Environments that provide easy access to investigators, such as dental clinics, and patient populations most available to study, such as low income consumers, are overstudied, while the more frequent type of interaction, that which occurs in the private office of a dental practitioner, has been explored very little. Nevertheless, the questions raised by those studies that have been done on how patients and practitioner perceive each other, how social variables affect these perceptions, and how a person decides to seek care offer guidelines to those who will further investigate this area of study.

THE POLITICS OF DENTAL CARE

The increasing involvement of local, state, and federal agencies with the delivery and regulation of dental services has forced providers to develop a political as well as service orientation to their work. The vast array of regulations brought forth with the purpose of ensuring the quality and accessibility of care have been met with various levels of acceptance on both a personal and an organized basis. To study the politics of dental care, one must examine those who are involved, their goals, and the means they use to achieve them.

At the center of the political arena is the consumer. Represented in law, by the government, and, in fact, by many public and private organizations, the consumer is presumably seeking high-quality, affordable, and accessible dental care as well as the promotion of public health in general. To this end, laws will be passed regarding the licensure of dental professionals, the funding of care for the needy, the financial support of dental students, and numerous other provisions will be enacted to protect the public from harm. Consumers may be organized for the purpose of passing particular pieces of legislation, as is the case with those concerned with television advertising of highly sweetened foods. In other instances, the public may be represented by a national organization with broad goals, such as the American Public Health Association.

Providers, like consumers, have an interest in the law. They are represented by professional organizations such as the ADA. Issues of concern to providers include the continuation of self-regulation by means of peer review, protection from competing groups of workers who would seek to provide care, and the securing the favorable reimbursement rates when work is to be paid for by the government.

A third group of participants in the politics of dental care includes institutions with specific interests in dental care delivery. These include dental schools, hospitals, insurance companies,

and foundations. These institutions will, like the consumers and the providers, have their own priorities and goals.

The interaction between consumer groups, provider groups, and related institutions will vary according to the issues involved. A community dental society may work voluntarily with a school district to provide students with dental health information. Consumers and organizations representing dental providers may unite to press for fluoridation of local water supplies or may find themselves on opposing sides of this issue. Dental schools may join the local dental society in requesting higher reimbursement rates for patients being treated under publicly financed programs, and at the same time, these two groups may be in competition to serve these patients.

The role of government in the delivery of dental care, like the types of interactions between consumers, providers, and allied institutions, shows wide variation. At one end of the spectrum is the situation in which the government controls all aspects of care. Such a case would be a military dental facility in which the consumers and the providers are both government employees and where the cost of care is assumed totally by the government. In other cases, the government is involved in dental care only when a crime is being committed. The government need never become involved in the situation of a private dental professional treating a private patient unless malpractice is the result or if the dentist should lack proper credentials. In the majority of situations, however, government involvement is neither absent nor fully mandated. An example would be the cases of dentists who are part of the Medicaid program. These dentists may find that their work, in some cases, is being closely reviewed and that parts of their billing procedures are being monitored. Nevertheless, the government is not the employer of the dentist, for it is the patient who selects the dentist who will provide the treatment.

The only certainty in the area of politics is change. Economic and social conditions change and this results in new programs and laws. Interested parties will encourage or fight their passage and implementation; the community will reap the benefits or suffer the consquences of these efforts.

SUMMARY

This chapter has presented some of the ways in which social scientists study dental care. The questions they ask, though at times similar to those asked by members of the profession, are framed within different sets of assumptions. Looking at dental care from the outside they ask about the interactions that occur, the outcomes that are possible, and ultimately, what they might do to contribute to the improvement of dental health services. Second, they view dental care as a part of the whole social process. They want to know what interactions within the dental environment are similar to others in areas outside of it. For instance, the question of professionalization and how it affects communication is of importance to those doing other types of highly specialized work.

The intent of this chapter has been to provide a framework for studying dental care with a social science perspective. The levels of interaction presented in the opening section might be considered by those who are involved in program planning, the delivery of services, or the regulation of the provision of care, in order to understand the complexity of the social process we call the delivery of dental care.

ACKNOWLEDGMENTS

I express appreciation to Anthony Jong and Madalyn L. Mann for their help with this chapter.

REFERENCES

1. American Dental Association, Council on Dental Education, Annual Report on Dental Education, 1984-85, Chicago.
2. Andersen, R., and Newman, J.F.: Societal and individual determinants of medical care utilization in the United States, Health Society 51(1):95, 1973.
3. Anderson, W.T.: Behavior in painful places: aspects of the dentist-patient encounter, dissertation. Department of Sociology, Boston University, Boston.
4. Darling, J.R., and Bussom, R.S.: A comparative analysis of the attitudes of dentists toward the advertising of their fees and service, J. Dent. Educ. 41(2):59, 1977.
5. Davis, P.: Compliance strategies and the delivery of health care: the case of dentistry, Soc. Sci. Med. 10:(6):327, 1976.
6. Dummett, C.O.: Understanding the underprivileged patient, J. Am. Dent. Assoc. 76(6):1363, 1969.
7. Dunning, J.M.: Dental care for everyone, Cambridge, MA, 1976, Harvard University Press.
8. Dworkin, S.F., Terence, T.P., and Giddon, D.B.: Behavioral science and dental practice, St. Louis, 1978, The C.V. Mosby Co.
9. Frazier, J.P., Jenny, J., and Begramian, R.A.: Patients descriptions of barriers faced and strategies used to obtain dental care, J. Public Health Dent. 34(1):22, 1974.
10. Freed, J.R.: The educational value of a university sponsored community dentistry clinic: a three-year student evaluation, J. Dent. Educ. 40(2):93, 1976.
11. Garcia, J.A., and Juarez, R.Z.: Utilization of dental health services by Chicanos and Anglos, J. Health Soc. Behav. 19:(4):428, 1978.
12. Heifetz, S.B., Horowitz, H.S., and Korts, D.C.: Prevalence of dental caries in white and black children in Nelson County, Virginia, a rural Southern community, J. Public Health Dent. 36(2):79, 1976.
13. Holtman, A.G., and Olsen, E.O., Jr.: The demand for dental care: a study of consumption and household production, J. Hum. Resour. 11(4):546, 1976.
14. Hughes, E.C.: Men and their work, New York, 1958, The Free Press.
15. Leverett, D.H.: A critical examination of the barriers to the receipt of dental care, J. Public Health Dent. 35(1):28, 1975.
16. Linn, E.L.: Role behavior in two dental clinics: a test of Nadel's criteria, Hum. Organization 26(3):141, 1967.
17. Loupe, M.I., Meskin, L.H., and Mast, T.A.: Changes in the values of dental students and dentists over a ten-year period, J. Dent. Educ. 43(3):170, 1979.
18. Milk, H.C.: The dental patients cultural response to the need for dental care, Dent. Clin. North Am. 21(3):595, 1977.

19. Mulvihill, J.E.: Barriers to identification and motivation of minority group members for dentistry, J. Dent. Educ. **40**(3):142, 1976.

20. Nikias, M.K., Fink, R., and Shapiro, S.: Comparisons of poverty and non-poverty groups on dental status, needs, and practices, J. Public Health Dent. **35**(4):237, 1975.

21. Rosenberg, H.M., and Thompson, N.L.: Attitudes toward woman dental students among male dental students and male dental faculty members, J. Dent. Educ. **40**(10):676, 1976.

22. Suchman, E.A.: Stages of illness and medical care. In Gartly, J.E., editor: Patients, physicians, and illness, ed. 2, New York, 1972, The Free Press.

23. Trihart, A.H.: Understanding the underprivileged child: report on an experimental workshop, J. Am. Dent. Assoc. **77**(4):880, 1968.

24. U.S. Department of Health and Human Services, Public Health Service, Bureau of Health Professions, Fifth Report to the President and Congress on the Status of Health Personnel in the United States, March 1986.

25. U.S. Department of Health and Human Services, National Center for Health Statistics, unpublished data from the National Health Interview Survey, 1981.

26. Vanable, E.D.: The professional role of the dental hygienist as viewed by the accreditation commissioners and consultants, J. Dent. Educ. **41**(2):59, 1977.

27. Vinton, J.C.: A four-year longitudinal study of the impact on learning structures on dental student lifestyle values, J. Dent. Educ. **42**(5):251, 1978.

28. Weinstein, P., and others: Dentists perceptions of their patients relationships to quality care, J. Public Health Dent. **38**(1):10, 1978.

29. Wiener, J.M.: Medical sociology: a field definition. Unpublished manuscript.

30. Zola, I.K.: Pathways to the doctor—from person to patient, Soc. Sci. Med. **7**(9):677, 1973.

CHAPTER 5

Geriatric Dental Health

In caring for sick old people we've tended to compare them with healthy young people and see the difference as disease.

John W. Rowe
Director of the Harvard Medical School's Aging Division

Interest in the provision of care for the elderly began in the 1960s when the two federally sponsored health programs, Medicaid and Medicare, underscored the enormous and disproportionate cost of health care services to this group. Since then, both the dental and the medical profession have attempted to develop rational systems for the training of personnel and the establishment of delivery systems that meet the needs of this group. This chapter will consider some of the social issues impacting on the elderly as well as the medical and psychological considerations that affect the practice of dentistry. The elderly are not simply another version of younger individuals who happen to have a greater incidence of disease. They are human beings who have attained a stage of life characterized by unique social and biological conditions.

In part the high cost of care to the elderly is a result of their increase in numbers during the twentieth century. In the early 1900s the ratio of individuals over age 55 to the rest of the population was 1 to 10, and for the over-65 age group it was 1 to 25. By 1984 the age-55-and-over population accounted for 1 in 5 Americans, and the over-65 age group accounted for 1 in 9.[39]

Table 5-1 shows the country's age distribution

in 1984 and provides some basis for assessing the future. The increase in the numbers of elderly is not only a result of increased longevity but also of population spurts caused by periods of increased numbers of births. The data reflect the "baby-boom" generation of those individuals born between 1946 and 1962 and who in 1984 constituted the 20- to 39-year age group. This group will be eligible for Social Security during the early part of the twenty-first century.

In 1984 21% of the U.S. population was over age 55. Approximately 12% of the population was over age 65. This has occurred because of increased longevity, and increase in births after World War I, and a decline in births during the 1960s. All of these factors have contributed to a steep rise in the median age of the U.S. population. In 1970 the median age of the U.S. population was 28, while in 1984 this number has jumped to 31. This last number represented a singularly large increase in U.S. demographic history.[39]

The aging of the U.S. population is changing in other respects as well. Not only is the over-65 population growing, but among the over 65-group it is the older age categories or the over age 75 group that is growing the fastest. For exam-

Table 5-1. Distribution of the population by older age groups, 1984

Age group	Number	Percent
All ages	236,416	100
0-54	186,220	79
55-64	22,210	9
65-74	16,596	7
75-84	8,793	4
85 plus	2,596	1
55 plus	50,195	21
65 plus	27,985	12

From U.S. Senate Special Committee on Aging: America in Transition: an aging society, 1984-85 edition, Washington, DC, 1985, U.S. Government Printing Office.

ple, in 1980 the "young" old group (65-74) outnumbered the older group (75 plus) by a 3 to 2 ratio. In the year 2000 the number of individuals over age 75 will equal the number of individuals between 65 and 74.

As the population ages, the distribution by sex also changes. The elderly population is comprised of many more women than men. According to the 1980 census, at age 65 there were 79.4 men for every 100 women. By age 85 there were only 48.5 men for every 100 women. Of the women over age 65, the majority were widowed (66%) and living alone. Men, on the other hand, are more likely to live with a spouse and about 30% continue to work.[29]

Approximately 20% of those over age 65 spend some time in a nursing home or extended care facility. At any point in time about 5% are institutionalized.[29] Most dependent elderly are cared for by relatives and home health care services provide support for those who live alone and require assistance.

Many of the elderly suffer from chronic disease. About 90% have one chronic disease or more. Although a majority of the elderly remain active, almost 17% are unable to carry on major activities. Chronic ailments and associated limitations contribute to the dependence of the elderly and also have major impacts on treatment modalities, treatment plans, and preventive therapy.[29]

LEVELS OF DEPENDENCE

Most individuals over the age of 65 function without assistance. Many, however, although not institutionalized, have major activity limitations as a result of chronic conditions.[35] Elderly living in the community are categorized according to degrees of dependence. Dependence is defined as the "need for assistance in bathing, dressing, eating or transferring from bed to chair."[32] The functionally dependent are those who are seriously impaired and are unable to maintain themselves. They are either homebound or institutionalized. The frail elderly are those who have chronic debilitating physical, medical, and emotional problems and a loss of their social support systems. They are unable to maintain their independence without help from others. Most of these individuals reside in the community. A small percentage are institutionalized.[15]

The elderly who are admitted to extended care facilities usually suffer from one or more of the following conditions: failing intellectual capacity and inability to make life-choice decisions, physical instability leading to falling episodes; immobility as a result of crippling conditions and incontinence. These individuals have dental treatment needs somewhat different from those of the general elderly population.

A survey of nursing home patients disclosed the following regarding their dental health and dental treatment needs: 70.3% had no natural teeth; 30% had some or all of their natural teeth, and most of these believed that their teeth were in good or fair condition. About half of these patients had been transported to a private office for care and the other half had been treated at the home. Approximately 40% of those with teeth had visited the dentist, whereas only about 19%

of the edentulous patients had gone. This discrepancy in utilization between dentate and edentulous patients mimics the pattern of use among noninstitutionalized dentate and endentulous individuals.[9]

There is a vast gap between the institutionalized patients' perception of their treatment needs and the perception of their needs by professionals. Of those who did not visit a dentist during the past year, examining dentists determined that 82.5% were in need of some type of dental treatment. Of those needing care, 71% could be treated in a dental chair and 18.1% required bedside care. Four percent could not be treated because of a mental or physical condition.

As the elderly population increases, the number of institutionalized patients requiring care will also grow. This group is currently underserved and there is need for dentists and dental hygienists to be trained in the delivery of services to this group.[1]

UTILIZATION OF DENTAL SERVICES

The increase in numbers of elderly and the shifts in social factors have been accompanied by changes in the numbers of individuals over age 65 who visit the dentist. In 1964 about 21% of the individuals over age 65 visited the dentist during the previous year.[3,14] In 1979 this figure had increased to approximately 33%. The increased utilization has generally been attributed to changes in the social, educational, and economic backgrounds of the newer generations of elderly rather than to any significant changes in the delivery system.[14]

Although unmet dental treatment needs have been demonstrated, the elderly visit the dentist less often than any other age group except for the very young. Among the elderly, those without teeth tend to seek care less often than the dentate group. The factors that account for these behaviors are complex.

Investigators describe utilization behavior as a function of socio-economic factors such as income, age, race, and gender.[2,14,20,29] Other findings relate user-behavior to utilization patterns that occur during earlier periods of the individual's life.[41] Although this is not surprising, it is helpful in forecasting this type of behavior in future generations of elderly.

The assessment of treatment needs is a difficult and problematic task. Treatment needs are generally described in terms of professionally established criteria. The elderly, however, have less stringent standards in evaluating their oral health status. Perception of treatment needs impacts on use. In part the perception of need may be influenced by education, but it is likely that there will always be a considerable gap between professional judgment and the perceptions of the potential patient. This phenomenon therefore is an explanation of why there is often a difference between the behavior predicted by the professional and the actual behavior of the potential patient. The elderly also tend to have lower expectations for the outcomes of therapy than do the dental professionals. This is particularly true with respect to periodontal and preventive services and especially among men.[41] This factor of decreased expectations may also account for the significantly lower utilization rates among edentulous and denture-wearing groups.

According to the elderly, the key impediment to seeking service is cost. Most elderly have a fixed income and need to apportion this income among various options. Dental services, according to most polls, do not appear at the top of the priority list. The interpretation of cost as a factor in receiving dental care is confounded by the observation that in countries with publicly funded programs there is not a significant difference in the amount of use by the elderly. Utilization behavior, therefore, is determined by a combination of attitudinal and social factors. Other factors that contribute to low utilization by the elderly are the following: fear of treatment, lack of transportation, lack of mobility by the individual, lack of a regular dentist, illnesses, and some concerns about bothering a busy dentist.

The use of dental services by the elderly is also determined by the education of the dental professionals. Surveys of dental professionals indicate an acceptance of many of the popularly held aging myths as well as lack of geriatric information.[11,21] Surveys of dental education reveal a relative absence of courses to remediate this situation. The lack of geriatric sophistication by dental professionals often results in dental offices that are poorly located or poorly designed for the purpose of accommodating the needs of the elderly. Adequate and nearby parking is often lacking. Ramps to assist those who are handicapped or hallways of sufficient width for the passage of wheelchairs may not be provided.[12] Many professionals feel that the elderly or the chronically ill cause discomfort to the other patients. Treatment of the elderly is perceived as being more difficult and more time consuming than treatment of other groups.

TREATMENT OF THE ELDERLY PATIENT

The aging adult must cope with an increasing number of physical and psychological problems. The average older adult living in the community suffers from three and one half major disabilities; the average institutionalized elderly individual manifests six pathologic conditions.[32]

Aging also implies the modification or loss of cells of various organs of the body. The kidney, for example, over the course of a lifespan loses nephrons. Most organ systems, however, function well with only 15% of their cells intact. The loss of cells does limit the reserve capacity of the involved organ and thereby compromises the ability of the individual to cope with stress. The dental practitioner, therefore, must consider this factor as a component to the office visit.

Symptoms of cognitive impairment occur more frequently in older individuals. These individuals may appear to be suffering from fluctuating levels of awareness, mild confusion, stupor, or delirium. Most of the time these symptoms are caused by malnutrition and anemia, congestive heart failure, infection, drugs, head trauma, alcohol, a cerebrovascular accident, dehydration, responses to surgery, and a host of other conditions. Often the health care practitioner may assume that these symptoms are manifestations of chronic brain syndrome such as Alzheimer's disease. It is important to distinguish among the various causes of brain related symptoms in order that the patient receive the appropriate care.

Aging changes and disease

The interplay of aging changes and disease is of particular importance to the practitioner because it is the distinction between these phenomena that permits accurate diagnosis and appropriate treatment. Physiological changes related to aging influence the presentation of disease, the response to treatment and are associated with the complications that ensue. Generally, there are three related categories that describe the impact of physiological change on disease: (1) those physiological variables that remain constant throughout life; (2) those physiologic changes that increase the likelihood of disease; and (3) those physiological changes that have a direct clinical relationship to the appearance of disease. An example of an incorrectly anticipated aging change is the diagnosis of senile anemia. The blood sera factors such as hematocrit, fasting blood glucose, serum electrolyte concentrations, and blood gas values, in normal aging adults, remain the same. A drop in the hemoglobin value should be evaluated for causative agents and not attributed to the aging process.

The changes that increase the likelihood of disease are generally those that deprive the various organ systems of their physiological reserve because of the loss of cells. The systems affected in this manner include the renal, the pulmonary, the immune functions, and the homeostatic mechanisms. This reduction in reserve contributes to the increased vulnerability of the elderly to disease during acute illness, trauma due to burns, major surgery, and the administration of medications. Visits to the dentist or dental hygienist, of course, are potential sessions of increased stress, and the practitioner must modify the management of the patient accordingly.

The purpose of the discussion on aging in terms of physiological change is to clarify the relationship of the aging process to disease. The aging process may have relatively no impact on the body's physiologic functions or, as in the case of the kidney, the process may compromise some organ systems so as to render them and the individual more vulnerable to stress and to disease. In some cases physiological changes may result in adverse symptoms. Examples of these types of changes include age related menopause, arteriosclerotic changes, and modifications of the lens of the eye. The modifications of the lens have important implications for dentistry. Dentists and dental hygienists have observed the tendency of elderly patients to select denture teeth that are several shades too white. This occurs because of the increased opacity and amber tint of the lens of the eye. The patient sees the recommended denture teeth as being too yellow and therefore aesthetically unacceptable. This is but one example of how the understanding of aging changes is important to appropriate patient management.

The relationship of physiological change as a result of aging and disease, as previously discussed, does not account for all disease related phenomena in the elderly. The complexity of the process is underscored by the following occurrences: first, that several diseases occur less frequently in older adults and, second, some diseases or conditions in the elderly initially have symptoms that are different from those found in younger individuals. The immune mediated diseases such as myasthenia gravis or lupus erythematosus are found infrequently or not at all in older adults. Certain antibody titers are higher in the elderly, and this suggests that older adults have increased resistance to some diseases.

With respect to the altered state of disease presentation, there are two interesting examples. The first is hyperthyroidism, found in younger individuals as an elevator of mood and various functions. In the older adult most functions are depressed by the condition. Patients with acute myocardial infarctions also show different symptoms. The elderly are less likely to manifest chest pain, although they are more likely to experience syncope. Findings such as these suggest that pain in the elderly needs to be evaluated differently than in younger individuals.

Dental disease in the elderly

The major dental diseases, dental caries and periodontal disease, may be approached from two perspectives. First, how does the passage of time affect the oral cavity and presence of disease? And, second, does the aging individual respond differently to the etiological agents of dental disease?

Dental caries is thought of as a disease of youth that stabilizes in the middle twenties. Current information indicates a decrease in caries among 5- to 17-year-olds. These findings suggest that the future generations of middle-aged and elderly individuals will have more teeth and more vulnerable tooth surfaces.

Root caries has been studied for several years, but it is only recently that the root caries index (RCI) has afforded the dental profession a realistic picture of root caries prevalence and location.[25,26,27] The root caries index calculates the presence of root caries in relation to the susceptible surfaces, that is, where gingival recession has taken place. The occurrence of root caries is age related (Fig. 5-1), and its occurrence is related to the number of exposed root surfaces. Mandibular molars are the teeth most often attacked.

Strategies that are effective in the prevention of coronal caries are presumably effective in the prevention of root caries. There is evidence that both systemic and topical fluoride will have the appropriate effect.[18] Antimicrobials are under

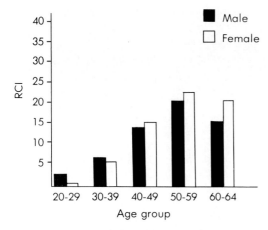

Fig. 5-1. Root caries index (RCI) prevalence rates for males and females by age group. (From Katz, R.V.: Root caries: clinical implications of the current epidemiologic data, Northwest Dent. **60:**308, 1981.)

investigation as caries preventive agents.

Secondary decay is a considerable problem, and some researchers have suggested that restorations with overhanging margins are at increased risk of disease in the elderly. Prevention of these conditions should include the application of fluoride to the potential sites and the elimination of aberrant margins.[30]

Periodontal disease, which is thought to be a disease of middle-aged adults, occurs at an accelerated pace in older adults.[19,30] Related to the occurrence of periodontal disease is the increased rate of plaque accumulation that is observed in the elderly during periods of oral hygiene abstinence. There is also evidence that the appearance of gingivitis is more rapid and that bone loss and the rate of gingival attachment loss is accelerated. Preventive therapy for the elderly needs to be more frequent and more vigorous.

The design of self-administered plaque control programs must include consideration of the inability of many elderly to manipulate conventional self-cleaning devices. This is especially true among victims of stroke, arthritis, or palsy-

like conditions. In some instances, especially among institutionalized elderly, it is necessary for auxiliary personnel to attend to dental hygiene needs. Oral hygiene implements may be modified in order to facilitate use. Modifications or substitutes for the toothbrush include the following: an electric toothbrush; something placed over the handle such as styrofoam ball, a bicycle hand grip or a soft rubber ball; plastic tubing attached to the handle of the toothbrush in order to lengthen the handle; an Ace bandage or aluminum foil wrapped around the toothbrush handle; bending the toothbrush handle; and creating a cuff to fit around the handle. A floss holder may also be valuable (Fig. 5-2).

Oral examinations of older adults should include a thorough examination of anatomical sites that are potential tumor sites. Oral cancer accounts for 5% of cancer in men and 2% of all cancers in women. These lesions are more frequent in older adults. In order to minimize the effect of this disease, the patient should be informed of the hazards of tobacco and alcohol, the need for regular dental checkups, and the need to eliminate tissue irritants.

Discussion of dental treatment

Treatment of institutionalized patients is marked by a dramatic need for oral prophylaxis. Epidemiologists who have attempted to quantify dental disease in this group have commented on the difficulty of clinical examination because of the presence of plaque and debris.[25-27] In addition to preventive services, of those elderly who require services, about 24% need treatment of lesions that are potential sources of pain or infection. Approximately 5% are in need of relief from pain or infection and 84% are in need of treatment of pulpally involved teeth.[9] Nursing home patients, who are on the average older than the elderly who remain in the community, are generally less able to practice personal hygiene and are less able to manipulate dental appliances. Because of this, partial dentures for the handi-

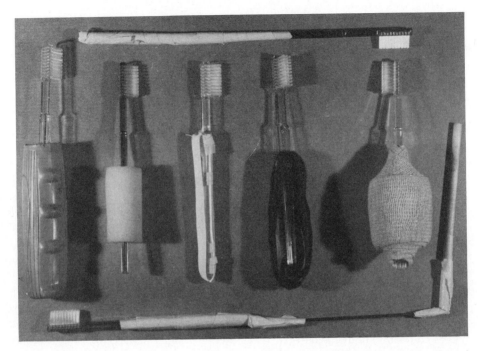

Fig. 5-2. Toothbrush modifications. *Top:* Plastic tubing extension. *Left to right:* Bicycle handle, styrofoam ball, elastic cuff, velcro cuff, ace bandage. *Bottom:* Bent wire extension.

capped elderly are reconstructed with wrought iron clasps in order to facilitate denture removal.

The types of dental services provided to well elderly are described in a program conducted in Minnesota in 1982.[41] The goal of this program was to establish a statewide dental program for the purpose of determining the dental needs of the elderly. In addition to testing the administrative feasibility of a statewide program, the project determined the frequency distribution of types of services. The program was offered to those who were 62 years of age or older and retired. These individuals also need to pass a means test and all services were paid for by the state of Minnesota. Of the 15,000 applications mailed, about 30% were returned (about the same as the national utilization rate among the elderly) and about 40% of these were eligible for services. The mean age of the eligible population was 73.8 years. The services offered were routine examinations, emergency treatment, restorative services, oral surgery, surgical and nonsurgical periodontal treatment, endodontic treatment, and prosthodontic services. A summary of the dental treatment delivered to first year utilizers appears in Table 5-2.

An analysis of the services delivered reveals the following: men were the recipients of more removable prosthodontic and oral surgical services; women received more diagnostic, preventive, and restorative services; provision of diagnostic, preventive, restorative, endodontic, and fixed prosthodontic services declined with the advancing age of the participants; and provision of removable prosthodontic services increased as the average age of recipients in-

Table 5-2. Frequency distribution of utilization by category service

Service	Total claimants %
Diagnostic	80.7
Prophylaxis	56.3
Restorative	55.7
Endodontics (nonsurgical)	6.3
Periodontics (nonsurgical)	8.5
Oral surgery	27.5
Removable prosthodontics	62.2
Fixed prosthodontics	5.1

From Yellowitz, J.A., Katz, R.V., and others: The Minnesota Dental Insurance Program for Senior Citizens: two year results for the utilization of services, JADA **104:**455, 1982. (Copyright by the American Dental Association. Reprinted by permission.)

creased. Although use among the participants declined during the second year, the service distribution profile remained about the same. The results of this project as well as the shifts in the distribution of dental disease among the U.S. population indicate that future generations of elderly will have significant needs for preventive and restorative services. Fewer elderly will require full dentures, and more elderly will be in need of partial denture construction. Therefore as more elderly remain dentulous, it is probable that increased proportions of elderly will seek dental care.

Evaluation of the elderly patient

What is apparent in the provision of care to the elderly is that this is a heterogeneous group both biologically and socially. The over 70 population demonstrates greater variation anatomically, physiologically, and biochemically than any other age category.[33] These differences may be functions of race, sex, geographical location, or socioeconomic factors. The multifarious nature of this segment of the population poses a management challenge to the dental practitioner.

The identification of patient diversity is fur-

ther complicated by factors that impact on the ability of the patient to communicate with the practitioner. Of the population over age 65, approximately 10% suffer from dementia, 22% suffer from impaired hearing, and about 15% have visual handicaps.[32] History taking or interviewing of the elderly often requires increased interview time and dependence on other professionals (the dentist, for example, depends on the patient's physician as well as the dental hygienist). Thus one might conclude that not only is there more information to glean from an interview with an older adult, but that accessing the information is more complex.

Delivery of services to the elderly, more than any other aspect of dental care, requires that the practitioner consider several dimensions of the patient's life. The "dynamics of rational dental care" depicts the relationship of various factors that need to be considered in the development of a treatment plan (Fig. 5-3). Appropriate dental services for the elderly require a comprehensive evaluation of the patient's status.

Medical considerations. The International Classification of Disease published by the World Health Organization lists 120 diseases with oral manifestations.[30] The dental practitioner needs to be aware of these diseases, and medical and dental histories should reflect efforts to identify these conditions.

The most frequent causes of death in the elderly are cardiovascular disease, cancer, and stroke. Recently Alzheimer's disease has been implicated in mortality rates of older adults. Other diseases or conditions that occur frequently in the elderly are thyroid cancer, breast cancer, cervical cancer, occult bleeding, hypertension, postural hypotension, oral disease and its relationship to malnutrition, wax impaction in the ears, auditory or ophthalmic disorders, bowel malfunctions, degrees of urinary incontinence, sleep disturbances, and postural instability, which causes falling.[32]

Concurrent with the presence of disease is the

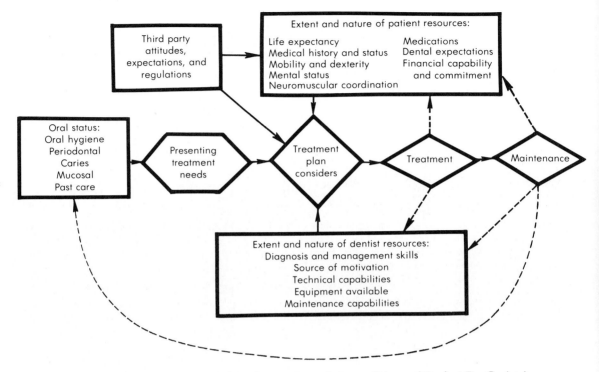

Fig. 5-3. Dynamics of rational dental care. (From Ettinger, R.L., and Beck, J.D.: Geriatric dental curriculum and the needs of the elderly, Spec. Care Dentist. **4:**209, 1984. Copyright by the American Dental Association. Reprinted by permission.)

treatment with pharmacological preparations. The elderly, because of altered metabolic rates, need to have their dosages modified. Patient compliance with drug regimens is an important issue, and many dental practitioners insist that their patients bring their medicines to the office so that a careful drug assessment can be made. The following is a list of drug-related phenomena that are of interest to the dentist or dental hygienist. Table 5-3 cites drug-induced changes in the tissues of the mouth.

1. Antimicrobials are well tolerated but reduced dosages are required.
2. Aspirin and Coumadin may contribute to hemorrhaging.
3. Stomatitis may be related to the administration of dentifrices, mouthwash, denture adhesives, toothache drops, ascorbic acid,

intramuscular gold therapy, antineoplastic agents and folic acid antagonists.
4. Pacemakers may be affected by equipment such as pulptesters and motorized chairs.
5. Long-term administration of phenothiazines may lead to tardive dyskinesia, which is characterized by spastic, uncontrolled movements of the lips and tongue.
6. Several artificial salivas are available. These preparations alleviate some of the symptoms of xerostomia and serve as oral cavity moisteners.

Mental status. Because of the multiplicity of factors that relate to the treatment of the elderly, it is important to evaluate the ability of the patient to communicate and to comply with personal care behavior. The practitioner must determine, either through a psychological evalu-

Table 5-3. Drug-induced changes in tissues of the mouth

Drug	Effect	Drug	Effect
Adrenal hormones		Cyclophosphamide	Stomatitis
Corticosteroids	Oral candidiasis (thrush)	(Cytoxan)	
(general)	Hairy tongue	Folic acid antagonists	Stomatitis
	Oral, laryngeal, and	(e.g. Methotrexate	
Beciomethasone	pharyngeal candidiasis	fluorouracil	Stomatitis
diproprionate		*L*-asparaginase)	
(Vanceril)		Mercaptopurine	Stomatitis
Analgesics		(Purinethol)	
Aspirin	Burns and ulceration of	Plicamycin (Mithracin)	Stomatitis
	oral mucosa	Vinblastine (Velban)	Stomatitis
Oxyphenbutazone	Parotitis	*Gold therapy*	
(Oxalid, Tandearil)		Gold sodium	Somatitis, glossitis
Phenylbutazone	Parotitis	thiomalate	
(Azolid, Butazolidin)		(Myochrysine)	
Antibiotics		Aurothioglucose	
Antibiotics (general)	Oral candidiasis	(Solganal)	
	Hairy tongue	*Heavy metal antagonist*	
Tetracycline	Oral candidiasis	Penicillamine	Taste disturbances
	Hairy tongue	(Cuprimine)	
	Tooth pigmentation	*Heavy metals*	
Erythromycin	Enamel hypoplasia	Lead, bismuth,	Pigmentation of oral
Anticonvulsant		mercury	soft tissues
Phenytoin	Gingival hyperplasia	*Hypotensives*	
Antidepressants		Clonidine	Xerostomia, parotitis
Amitriptyline	Xerostomia	hydrochloride	
(Elavil, Endep)		(Catapres)	
Imipramine	Xerostomia	Reserpine (Serpasil,	Xerostomia
(Tofranil,		Sandril, Reserpoid)	
Norpramin)		*Mouthwashes and gargles*	
Antifungal antibiotic		Hydrogen peroxide	Hairy tongue
Griseofulvin (Fulvicin	Hairy tongue	*Agents*	
U/F, Grisactin		Lithium carbonate	Taste disturbances
Grifulvin V)		(Eskalith, Lithane)	
Antineoplastics			
Adriamycin	Stomatitis		
Bleomycin sulfate	Stomatitis		
(Blenoxane)			

ation or through an interview, the capacity of the individual to respond to treatment. Although instances of senile dementia are rare, they do increase in frequency as the individual ages. The frequency of senile dementia is 2% in those be- tween 60 and 65 years of age, 5% in those over age 65, and between 20% and 30% in those over the age of 85.[16]

The most common type of dementia in the elderly is senile dementia of the Alzheimer type.

This disease is characterized by a gradual deterioration of almost every function of the brain.[7] The patient progresses through a series of behavioral changes and losses. Cognitive skills as well as competency in the life skills decline. There is loss of intellectual prowess and the patient experiences language difficulties, memory loss, concentration difficulties, aberrant emotionality, and altered spatial-motor performance. Verbal and nonverbal communication are affected.

Dental care, even in the early stages of dementia, is generally ignored. This occurs because of the demands on the patient to handle more basic life functions and because of the relative complexity of motion and muscular coordination required in an activity such as toothbrushing. In the early stages of the disease patients require instruction and in the later stages direct intervention by support personnel.[16]

Socioeconomic factors affecting the elderly

The elderly have the lowest median income of any population group. It is conjectured that in order to maintain a constant standard of living, the retired individual must retain an income that is 75% of the preretirement income.[29] In 1980 less than one third of retired persons had income other than Social Security. It is estimated that social security replaced about 45% of preretirement income for couples and only 30% of income for individuals.

The U.S. Social Security program was established in 1935. Twenty-nine other countries, mostly West European, established a social security type of system prior to the United States. All of these countries currently contribute a significantly higher percentage of their national resources to these programs.[5] Although the Reagan administration claimed that the Social Security cost of living adjustments contributed to the federal deficit, this has not been the case. For the period from 1986 to 1990, income generated by the Social Security tax will exceed total expenditures.[31] Since 1974 the economic status of the elderly has stabilized somewhat. This is the result of the cost of living increases that have become an integral part of the system. Despite these adjustments, black elderly women have continued to experience a high rate of poverty (in 1985, 41.7% had incomes below the poverty level). Among all women, 50% had incomes within $800 of the nationally determined poverty level. Among the elderly population, 20% were below or near the poverty line.

Although a key program, Social Security is not the sole source of income for the retired elderly. Private pension plans contribute at an increasing rate, although they are distributed unevenly throughout the population. Existing plans tend to be more prevalent among high-wage and long-term employees. Women have limited coverage when compared to men, and divorced and widowed women have the least coverage.[28]

The utilization of dental services is related to the economic status of the users. Although the Social Security program and private pension plans have contributed to the needs of the elderly, the elderly remain, to some degree, medically and dentally indigent.

Paying for dental care

Direct out-of-pocket payment remains the dominant method of paying for dental services. Since 1954 dental insurance has grown at an accelerating pace. The elderly, however, have been almost untouched by dental insurance programs. This has occurred because most of the insurance plans have been offered to the employed and since 1900 the elderly have declined as a factor in the workforce. In 1980 only 20% of males over the age of 65 were employed.[28] For those elderly who qualify for public assistance and who live in states with dental Medicaid programs there is the possibility of seeking services under this program.

Medicaid, or Title 19 of the Social Security Act, enacted in 1965, provided federal funds to be distributed among the state public assistance programs. The intent of the program was to provide health benefits to the indigent. Eligibility was limited to those eligible for public assistance, and in some states the benefits were extended to those categorized as medically indigent. These were thought to be individuals who could afford to support themselves except for health care. Some services were required under this program, however, dentistry was not one of the services. Where dentistry was included, it was usually underfunded, and where the elderly were included, they accounted for a disproportionate amount of the expenditures for dental care.

Medicare, or Title 18 of the Social Security Act, also enacted in 1965, was a program intended to provide health insurance for those over the age of 65. The program was to pay for hospital and physician services. Dental services, unless provided under special circumstances, were not to be included.

Medicare, under part A, provides for hospital inpatient care, post-hospital extended care, and home health visits by nurses. Part B pays for physician services, outpatient hospital services, and outpatient physical therapy.[6] The patient is responsible for deductibles under part A, and there are premiums and coinsurance provisions under part B. Medicare pays for about 44% of the health care costs of the elderly. Dental care may be provided only under specified conditions of hospitalization; for the most part, this involves oral surgical services. When a dentist provides services that are equivalent to those provided by a physician, such as the treatment of an oral lesion or the treatment of an oral infection (for example, candidiasis), the dentist may bill Medicare. Although this regulation is clearly defined, dentists rarely use it.[10]

Over the past decade there have been initiatives to expand coverage for the elderly. One proposal would have expanded Medicare to cover other outpatient services including dentistry. An auto manufacturer has proposed that upon retirement workers should retain their coverage. Private plans, however, are unlikely to assume programs for the elderly for the following

reasons: (1) the uncertainty of cost as a result of inflation increases the insurer's risk and there is fear of dollar losses; (2) administrative costs are high, especially if only a fraction of the population is involved; (3) current programs, such as Medicaid and Medicare, would undercut the market for these programs; (4) adverse selection, that is, the purchase of insurance by high-risk groups, would drive premiums up and low-income individuals out.[22] Private insurance of any sort for the elderly is unlikely to develop.

Mobile dental care

Dentists have been providing dental services to homebound or institutionalized patients for several years. Recent sensitization of dental students to the existence of dental needs among this population has led to efforts by younger dentists to implement mobile systems. These dentists have seen the treatment of this group as a potential source of income.

Federal and state laws have mandated levels of dental services for institutionalized patients. In 1974 the federal government required that skilled nursing facilities retain an advisory dentist. Medicare funds were made available for reimbursement of authorized dental consultants.[28] They were to be reimbursed for consultation services only. Some states have strengthened the federal statutes by requiring that recently admitted patients receive an oral examination and thereafter be examined at least once each year. The dental consultants supply the following services: provide inservice education for the nursing home staff, devise strategies for oral hygiene programs, recommend policies for emergency care and assist patients who seek dental care. Although these policies have existed for many years, there are no funding mechanisms or enforcement procedures that ensure dental care for nursing home patients.[34]

An anecdotal account of a longstanding (22 years) private mobile dental program reports the need for trained dentists and several support personnel. Although general practitioners provide adequate services to the well elderly, the dependent elderly require specially trained practitioners. The specially designed vehicle transports teams of dental practitioners consisting of one dentist and two dental auxiliaries. Backup personnel include a full-time administrator, a laboratory technician, and a full-time coordinator.[35] Coordination of this project is exceedingly complex. Persons who need to be consulted or informed during the treatment process include: intraoffice personnel, nursing home personnel, the patient, the patient's family, the physician and the physician's staff, government agencies, and third party payers.

The treatment of the older adult is a time-consuming process. The complexity of the operation is not limited to medical and dental considerations but extends into social, economic, and management areas. Treatment of the elderly requires consultation at all levels and the team approach, involving several disciplines, in order to provide the necessary support. Although dental hygiene education has only recently begun to increase the sophistication of its geriatric curriculum, dental hygienists are well educated to contribute to the care of institutionalized patients as well as the older adult who seeks care in a private practice.[8]

Special roles for the dental hygienist. Institutionalized patients tend to suffer from poor oral hygiene. This condition relates to the aging process and to the infirmities that afflict these individuals. Nursing home personnel, from nurses to nurses' aides, are assigned to assist with the personal oral hygiene of their patients. Generally, nondental personnel are not capable of mounting an effective oral hygiene program. Dental hygienists are the ideal professionals to be program planners, program initiators and implementers, and health educators and practitioners. A dental program in a nursing home consists of four major components: (1) a preventive program (2) a treatment program (3) an administrative procedure for coping with emergencies and (4) program coordination.

The preventive program begins with periodic oral examinations. These examinations require a tongue blade survey. Their purpose is to determine the general state of oral health, the presence of pathological conditions, the state of patient oral comfort, and the degree of personal hygiene achieved by the patient. When necessary the patient may be referred to a dentist. Phase two of the preventive program should include a review of the oral health of the edentulous patients. The oral cavity should be surveyed for oral pathological states and denture sores. All dentures must be labeled in order to avoid the commonplace loss of dentures. Phase three should include the implementation of personal care strategies. This involves patient education but also inservice education for the nursing home staff. The staff should be taught to construct the adaptive devices that enable the patients to care for themselves.

Treatment that requires the services of a dentist is generally achieved by taking the patient to a practitioner in the community. Since this effort is often of great inconvenience and expense to the patient, other delivery systems are being explored. The role of the nursing home dental auxiliary is to confirm the need for a dentist and wherever possible identify situations that may be remedied by the dentist visiting the nursing home. A reline of an old denture, for example, may be handled through a brief visit by the dentist of the institution.

Dental emergencies arise because of toothaches or postoperative bleeding after dental extractions. The dental hygienist may be able to minister to some instances of bleeding but, more importantly, will be able to identify situations that require the services of a dentist.

The administrator of the dental program has two major functions: first, to coordinate all personnel who are involved in the oral health care of the elderly; and second, to attend to the massive, bureaucratic paperwork that accompanies all institutional care. The most important paper management challenge is proposed by the patient chart. The chart contains information that includes the following: a list of the various ailments, a list of drugs being taken by the patient, and a description of orthopedic appliances (for example, hip implants require that the patient receive antibiotic therapy prior to dental extractions). Other paper transactions include the third party forms that need to be processed and the written referrals that need to be formulated.[17]

The need for dental personnel in nursing homes is well documented. The accompanying boxes list the tasks of dental hygienists according to the views of older adults and of dental hygienists themselves.

The portable delivery of dental services, especially to institutions that are domiciliary for groups of elderly, has some cost containment and convenience advantages. This system simplifies the procedure for obtaining care for dependent individuals. Because of the dental hygienist's training, he/she would be invaluable asset for such a program. The functions of the hygienist would be divided into two phases: first, those performed prior to the arrival of the service delivery team, and, second, those provided as a member of the visiting team. During the first phase the dental hygienist screens patients in order to identify those with oral disease and to determine the order of treatment. Coordination and administrative tasks are accomplished. A health history is compiled from information provided by the patient and from available sources. Financial arrangements are negotiated and the sources of payments are determined. Potential payers aside from the patient are the family, Medicaid, and Medicare. During phase two, that is, after the arrival of the team that includes a dentist and perhaps one other auxiliary, the hygienist provides clinical hygiene services.[13]

Private practice

Dental patients over the age of 65 represent one fourth of all dental patients.[34] The proportion of elderly who seek dental care promises to grow. More practice time will be dedicated to care to the elderly, and since care to the older adult is

---

TASKS FOR THE DENTAL HYGIENIST, IDENTIFIED BY OLDER ADULTS (IN ORDER OF IMPORTANCE)

Non-Institutionalized

1. Teach how to keep one's breath fresh
2. Discuss nutritional needs
3. Teach how to care for false teeth
4. Teach how to brush and floss
5. Teach how to retain one's teeth
6. Teaching of preventive dentistry
7. Check dentures for proper fit
8. Perform oral examinations
9. Clean teeth

From Marinelli, R.D.: Oral health care for the elderly patient: the role of dental hygienists, Dent. Hygiene **57**:10, 1983. (Copyright by the American Dental Association. Reprinted by permission.)

TASKS FOR THE DENTAL HYGIENIST IN THE TREATMENT OF THE ELDERLY PATIENT, IDENTIFIED BY DENTAL HYGIENISTS (IN ORDER OF IMPORTANCE)

1. Patient education
2. Oral examination
3. Perform oral prophylaxis
4. Teach oral examinations to staff
5. In-service training
6. Humanistic oral care
7. Nutrition counseling
8. Radiographic survey
9. Institutional oral screening
10. Bedside prophylaxis

From Marinelli, R.D.: Oral health care for the elderly patient: the role of dental hygienists, Dent. Hygiene **57**:10, 1983. (Copyright by the American Dental Association. Reprinted by permission.)

more time consuming, the dentist will need to organize personnel in order to optimize the patient visit. One potential strategy is to use auxiliaries who are trained in geriatric dentistry. These auxiliaries would conduct health interviews and preliminary examinations. Medications would be reviewed, perhaps with the assistance of a computerized summary of medications and their actions. Performance of these tasks during the intake process would free the dentist to concentrate his/her efforts on diagnosis, treatment planning, and the delivery of services.

An auxiliary involved as described in oral health assessment and interviewing and review of pharmacological and medical histories of the elderly suggests the need for dental personnel with additional training. A dental hygienist trained to assess the health status of elderly dental patients would save the dentist time and ultimately contribute to the quality of services provided. The accompanying box lists some suggestions for treating the handicapped and the elderly.

The clinical treatment of the geriatric patient requires a philosophy of care that emphasizes humanism and directs the practitioner to adjust the style of practice to accomodate the needs of the elderly. The practitioner must develop a "sensitivity to the patient's and family's legitimate goals and objectives and to the legal and other requirements of practice in the long-term care system, the acute care hospital, and the patient's home."[4]

The provision of dental care to the elderly patient is basically the same as the care provided to other segments of the population, "yet the effects of aging on normal laboratory values, clinical presentation, and complexities of care management—plus the present reimbursement morass—clearly indicate that this is a different mode of practice."[4] As these factors become more clear, the dental profession will recognize that geriatric dentistry is "not just special, it is different."[4]

SOME RECOMMENDATIONS FOR TREATMENT OF THE HANDICAPPED AND THE ELDERLY IN PRIVATE PRACTICE

1. There must be special emphasis on history taking, including a review of the patient's drug regimen and history of cardiovascular disease.
2. Patient must be questioned regarding episodes of syncope, especially upon awakening or sitting up.
3. Background noise should be minimized during interview sessions.
4. Avoid supine positions and bring dental chair to the vertical slowly.
5. Appointments should be arranged to meet the needs of the patients:
   Cardiac and kidney disease patients are better seen in the A.M.
   Arthritic patients are better seen in P.M.

From Ettinger, R.L., Beck, J.D., and Glenn, R.E.: Eliminating office architectural barriers to dental care of the elderly and handicapped, JADA **98**:398, 1979. (Copyright by the American Dental Association. Reprinted by permission.)

REFERENCES

1. ADA Council on Dental Health and Health Planning: Oral health care in the long-term care facility, Chicago, 1983.
2. Antezak, A.A., and Branch, L.G.: Perceived barriers to the use of dental services by the elderly, Gerodontics **1**:194, 1985.
3. Beck, J.D.: Dentists and the elderly: attitude and behaviors. In Chauncey, H.H., and others, editor: Clinical geriatric dentistry: biomedical and psychosocial aspects, Chicago, 1985, American Dental Association.
4. Blandford, G.: Is geriatric clinical practice different? Center on Aging **2**:1, 1986
5. Butler, R.N.: Why survive? Being old in America, New York, 1975, Harper & Row, Publishers, Inc.
6. Butler, R.N.: An overview of research on aging and the status of gerontology, Milbank Memorial Fund Quarterly–Health and Society **61**:351, 1983.
7. Cohen, D., Kennedy, G., and Eisdorfer, C.: Phases of change in the patient with Alzheimer's dementia: a con-

ceptual dimension for defining health care management, J. Am. Geriatr. Soc. **32**:11, 1984.

8. Cohen, L., Labelle, A., and Singer, J.: Educational preparation of hygienists working with special populations in non-traditional settings, J.Dent. Educ. **49**:592, 1985.

9. Council on Dental Health and Health Planning: Oral health status of Vermont nursing home residents, J. Am. Dent. Assoc. **104**:68, 1982.

10. Doctor, don't cheat yourself! (editorial), J. Am. Soc. Geriatr. Dent. **3**:1, 1985.

11. Ettinger, R.L., Beck, J.D., and Glenn, R.E.: Some considerations in teaching geriatric dentistry, J. Am. Soc. Geriatr. Dent. **13**:7, 1978.

12. Ettinger, R.L., Beck, J.D., and Glenn, R.E.: Eliminating office architectural barriers to dental care of the elderly and handicapped, J. Am. Dent. Assoc. **98**:398, 1979.

13. Ettinger, R.L., Beck, J.D., and Willard, D.H.: The role of a mobile dental unit program in geriatric education and dental care delivery, Paper presented at the American Dental Association Conference on Oral Health Care Needs of the Elderly, Chicago, November 19-20, 1980.

14. Ettinger, R.L., and Beck, J.D.: The new elderly: what can the dental profession expect? Spec. Care Dentist **2**:62, 1982.

15. Ettinger, R.L., and Beck, J.D.: Geriatric dental curriculum and the needs of the elderly, Spec. Care Dentist **4**:207, 1984.

16. Finkel, S.: Senile dementia and dental care. In Chauncey, H.H., and others, editor: clinical geriatric dentistry: biomedical and psychosocial aspects, Chicago, 1985, American Dental Association.

17. Fahs, D.E.: Accessible dental care in an extended care facility, J. Geriatr. Nurs. **7**:21, 1981.

18. Forsyth Dental Center: Symposium on root surface caries, Boston, 1985.

19. Gibson, W.A.: Age, caries, and periodontal disease. In Chauncey, H.H., and others, editor: Clinical geriatric dentistry: biomedical and psychosocial aspects, Chicago, 1985, American Dental Association.

20. Gift, H.C.: The elderly population oral health status and utilization of dental services, J. Am. Soc. Geriatr. Dent. **13**:9, 1978.

21. Gluck, G.M., and Lakin, L.B.: Determination of common myths among dental students and dental school faculty, Unpublished data, 1985.

22. Gluck, G.M., Lakin, L.B., and Nezu, A.: The aging population and the private practitioner, J. Dent. Pract. Admin. **3**:31, 1986.

23. Jacobs, L.: The geriatric patient, Dialog., **14**:10, 1983.

24. Kamen, S.: Introduction to geriatric dentistry, Lecture at St. Joseph's Hospital, Paterson, NJ, 1984.

25. Katz, R.V.: Assessing root caries in populations: the evolution of the root caries index, J. Public Health Dent. **40**:7, 1980.

26. Katz, R.V.: Root caries: clinical implications of the current epidemiologic data, Northwest Dent. **60**:306, 1981.

27. Katz, R.V., and others: Prevalence and intraoral distribution of root caries in an adult population, Caries Res. **6**:265, 1982.

28. Kingson, E.R., and Scheffler, R.M.: Aging: issues and economic trends, Inquiry **18**:197, 1981.

29. Kiyak, H.A.: Psychosocial factors and dental needs of the elderly, Paper presented at the American Dental Association Conference on Oral Health Care Needs of the Elderly, Chicago, November 19-20, 1980.

30. Mandel, I.: Preventive dentistry for the elderly, Spec. Care Dentist **3**:157, 1983.

31. Pollack, R.F.: A wrong way to see the aged, New York Times, March 14, 1985.

32. Rowe, J.W.: Health care of the elderly, New Engl. J. Med. **312**:827, 1985.

33. Rozovski, S.J.: Nutrition and aging. In Winick, M., editor: Nutrition in the 20th century, New York, 1984, John Wiley & Sons, Inc.

34. Shaver, R.O.: Dentistry for the homebound, institutionalized and elderly, Lakewood, Colorado, 1982, Portable Dentistry Publishers.

35. Sinykin, S.: Meeting the patient's needs, Paper presented at Symposium on Clinical Geriatric Dentistry, June 3, 1983.

36. Starr, P.: The social transformation of American medicine, New York, 1982, Basic Books, Inc., Publishers.

37. Tryon, A.: Organization and methods of delivering geriatric oral health care. In Chauncey, H.H., and others, editor: Clinical geriatric dentistry: biomedical and psychosocial aspects, Chicago, 1985, American Dental Association.

38. United States Public Health Service: National interview survey, 1981.

39. U.S. Senate Special Committee on Aging: America in transition: an aging society, 1984-85 edition, Washington, D.C., 1985, U.S. Government Printing Office.

40. Wescott, W.B.: Current and future considerations for a geriatric population, J. Prosthet. Dent. **49**:113, 1983.

41. Yellowitz, J.A., and others: The Minnesota dental insurance program for senior citizens: two year results for the utilization of dental services, J. Am. Dent. Assoc. **104**:453, 1982.

CHAPTER 6

Financing Dental Care

The dental care delivery sector of the U.S. economy is currently in the process of diversification and organizational restructuring. There are market forces affecting dentistry in today's economy that reflect trends that are shaping all health care delivery in the United States. One such development is the change of payment from a purely private out-of-pocket transaction between dentist and patient into a layered group financing of dental care through various types of third parties. This segmentation of payment is a relatively recent phenomenon, recent at least when compared to the growth of hospitalization insurance that has its roots in the 1920s and 1930s. The economic consequences of this trend are just beginning to be felt in dentistry, but have been at work in medical care for the past three decades.

There are other trends with economic consequences that are unique to dentistry. One is the dramatic decline in dental caries in the United States, which has implications for the future of dental care delivery in terms of both the demand and the supply of dental services in the marketplace.

MARKET FORCES—THE DEMAND SIDE

The major forces today in dental care demand can be summarized by two words: *insurance* and *caries*, more specifically the increase of insurance and the decline of dental caries. It is important to note that the 1970s was the decade of dental insurance. In fact in one review it is reported that during one 6-year period (1970-

1976) private sector dental insurance grew 500%, from 4.8 to 23.1 million persons covered. Dental insurance payments by all insurers in 1981 were approximately $5.811 billion or 34% of all dental health care expenses. There are projections that this dollar figure will rise to $14.38 billion by 1990.

Dental insurance is currently considered one of the most desirable employee benefits available. It is estimated that approximately one out of every three Americans is covered by some type of dental insurance plan. In the past 10 years there has been a tremendous growth of such programs. In 1965 there were 2 million Americans covered by Dental insurance, while 148 million had medical insurance coverage. It is expected that by 1990 there will be 120 million beneficiaries of dental plans.

Much of the early growth of dental prepayment was the result of collective bargaining agreements. Unions such as the United Auto Workers, United Steel Workers of America, the International Brotherhood of Electrical Workers of America, the Communications Workers of America, and the Railroad Workers initiated dental benefits in some of the nation's largest industries.

Today employers with fewer than 10 employees are purchasing dental plans. There are about 200 carriers in the prepayment field currently, and, in 1982 their payments accounted for one third of the $19.5 billion spent on dental services. They can be categorized in the following way.

Plan	Beneficiaries (millions)
Commercial insurance companies	77.3 million
Dental service corporations	15.6
Blue Cross/Blue Shield	12.1
Other independent plans	6.0

These estimates are from Health Care Financing Administration, Health Insurance Association of America, Delta Dental Plan Association, and Blue Cross/Blue Shield Associations.*

Unions and large corporations account for many individuals eligible for dental plans.

Organization	Beneficiaries
United Auto Workers	3.00 million
United Steel Workers	.75
International Brotherhood—Electrical	3.00
Railroad union	1.50
Letter carriers	.30
Union Carbide	.20
E.I. Dupont—DeNumors Inc.	.30
Eastman-Kodak	.20
Westinghouse	.12
General Electric	.75
United Mine Workers	.50
Major oil companies	.65

The influx of third party dollars in the marketplace can act as a stimulus to increase the consumption of dental care. With dental care insurance subsidizing the market price for dental services, the consumer demand function will tend to seek a new equilibrium with the market supply function. This is based on the assumption that a reduction in price to the consumer will increase the demand for services.

The more dramatic result of growth of dental insurance is that payment for dental care is consolidating through control of administrators of employee benefit packages. Private industry— management and labor—will play a multidi-

mensional, complex role in health care.

As a consumer of health care whose potential influence derives in part from the massive numbers of workers, industry will become more intimately involved in finding equitable ways to allocate limited resources and improve the quality of the dental care delivery system.

A dramatic decrease in the incidence of dental caries is a countervailing force in the marketplace that might result in a reduction in the use of dental services. Whereas most studies before 1977 showed an average incidence rate of two new cavities per child per year, recent investigations no longer support these data. The 1983 National Preventive Dentistry Demonstration Program, funded by the Robert Wood Johnson Foundation, indicated significant findings of less decay than previously reported. This 4-year national study evaluated preventive dental procedures throughout the United States, starting in the fall of 1977. Results showed that the longstanding pattern of two new cavities per child per year was no longer true.

In December 1981 the National Institute for Dental Research pointed to this lower caries incidence rate. Their study showed tooth decay in children ages 5 to 17 had dropped about 33% from rates reported in Health Examination Surveys of 1963–1965 and 1966–1970. In the early 1970s only 28% of children ages 5 to 17 were caries-free; yet by 1981 the number had increased to 37%. Over the last 30 years caries reduction as great as 60% has been observed.

Comparisons of decayed, missing, and filled surfaces (DMFS) data from four national surveys conducted between 1961 and 1980 in the United States also indicate a substantial decrease in dental caries prevalence and an increase in the number of caries-free children ages 5 to 17 during the last decade. In fact a substantial proportion of children have no caries at all, although 20% of children account for 60% of all decay. Available literature indicates that this overall decline in dental caries is most likely

*Data for listings shown above and below are from the American Dental Association, Council on Dental Care Programs, 1985.

the result of the increased use of fluoride supplements and fluoridated water supplies.

However, a reduction in dental caries has also been observed in nonfluoridated areas. A country-wide survey conducted in 1970 showed a definite improvement in the dental health of patients regardless of fluoride in their water supply. A 1979 study reported a 17.5% reduction in decay in the nonfluoridated water system of Columbus, Ohio. This statistic can most likely be attributed to the use of fluoridated water in processed foods and beverages.

The trend of caries reduction in nonfluoridated areas has also been noted in Massachusetts. Data collected between 1958 and 1978 in some Dedham and Norwood neighborhood schools seem to follow national patterns, though community and school water fluoridation was not a factor during this study period. In both towns there was a marked reduction in the number of decayed and filled surfaces, as well as surfaces both decayed and filled.

In 1951 the average 16-year-old in the United States had 15 teeth affected by decay with 2 extractions. In 1981 the average is 8 affected teeth with virtually no extractions.

The issue, then, is how does the reduction of dental caries translate into changes in demand for dental services? This type of data is usually difficult to obtain and often must be inferred, but the Massachusetts Department of Public Welfare has recently published a study investigating the prepaid method of financing dental care for the Aid to Families with Dependent Children (AFDC) population. It documented a dramatic 6-year reduction in dental claims experience for the AFDC population, primarily for services to treat the effects of dental caries (Table 6-1). As Table 6-1 points out, the Department of Public Welfare experienced a 33% average reduction in the number of restorative services claims submitted for the AFDC population. Despite the fact that welfare patients have traditionally been considered in a high-need

group, this and other studies indicate as significant a decrease in dental caries as that observed in the general population.

Dental practice revenue has traditionally been generated by treating the effects of dental caries. A 1977 review of dental care expenditures is presented in Table 6-2. Data for 1977 are shown as a reflection of the income distribution for the typical general dental practice just prior to the observation by epidemiologists of a pronounced decrease in dental caries among children. As Table 6-2 points out, in 1977 operative and endodontic procedures, services to treat the effect of dental caries, accounted for 34.2% of general practice revenue. Generally fixed prosthetic services are also rendered to treat the effect of dental caries. Therefore a very conservative conclusion is that over 50% of the income of a general dental practice in 1977 was earned from the treatment of dental caries.

Market forces interplay

In the dental care delivery sector of the U.S. economy there are two trends, one in the direction of increased use of dental services and the

Table 6-1. Massachusetts AFDC recipients dental service claims count per 100 patients for 1977 and 1982

Service type	1977	1982	Decline %
1 Surface amalgam	100	43	38
2 Surface amalgam	91	27	30
3 Surface amalgam	56	16	28
Composite restoration	54	20	35
AVERAGE 33%			

From Boffa, J., Medalia, D., and Charette, J.: Dental prepaid capitation pilot study —final report, HCFA Contract No. 11-P-973881, Aug. 1984.

other toward a net reduction in utilization. Although the trends seem to be polar opposites, in reality, future demand for services is not all that easy to predict. The trend in dental caries reduction indicates that in another 10 to 20 years the present population of relatively caries-free children will be adult consumers of dental care. Traditional dental practices centering on the treatment of disease will have to face adjustments in finances and focus.

Changes in dental materials technology has led to the ability to offer an increased range of preventive and cosmetic services. As private practitioners adjust to falling volume in their main service line, they will tend to compensate by raising fees, extending the service line, and/or increasing patient volume.

The office of the future may require a different mix of personnel. The dominant providers may be hygienists and other auxiliaries providing preventive and educational services rather than dentists offering highly skilled restorative services. The primary role of the dentist will be as diagnostician, coordinator of care, and provider of the more complex procedures involving both the hard and soft tissues of the oral cavity.

Does this mean there will be less of a demand for dentists in the future? A decrease will primarily depend on overall shifts in consumer demand for dental services. At present most surveys indicate that only 50% of the U.S. population will visit a dentist in any given year with approximately 30% seeking regular care. If the overall impact of dental insurance is to increase the regular consumption of dental care from, for example, 30% to 70% of the population, then the general effect, even when taking into account caries reduction, may be a dramatic increase in dental care demand.

Unfortunately, most of the available actuarial analysis performed for dental insurers in both the public and private sector concludes that the percentage of eligible persons actually seeking care is consistent with overall national statistics. Dental insurance help seems to expand the purchasing power of those individuals who are already predisposed to seek dental care. It has not yet significantly altered the behavior of a large segment of the population that for reasons often having to do with aversive consequences decides not to seek regular care. Some such consequences may be treatments to reduce pain and/or infection or injection of local anesthetic to allow cutting of hard and soft tissues.

A recent economic review by Cohen and Roesler tends to substantiate the view that price does not in itself regulate the demand for dental services. They found a highly variable price elasticity of demand for dental services. Price elasticity is an economic measure calculated by dividing percent change in demand for a product or service by the percent change in its price. Price elasticity measures the sensitivity of demand for a product or service to fluctuations in price. The review states that the demand for dental services by children was price elastic, but for adults, the price was inelastic. Income was found to be a more consistent predictor of utilization of dental services. The factor the authors

Table 6-2. Percent and expenditures by dental service type for general practice in U.S. in 1977

Service	Expenditure %	$ millions
Fixed prosthetics	34.51	3,458
Operative	27.85	2,791
Removable prosthetics	9.63	965
Diagnostic	8.25	826
Preventive	7.67	769
Endodontics	6.35	636
Surgery	3.89	390
Orthodontics	1.07	107
Periodontics	.78	78
TOTALS	100.00	10,020

From Douglass, C.W., and Day, J.M.: Cost and payment of dental services in the U.S., J. Dent. Educ. **43:**7, 1979.

did not consider in this review is price elasticity given the impact of caries reduction.

Perhaps in the future a synergism will develop between caries reduction and increase in dental care insurance coverages. If a positive feeling of well-being can replace the association of aversive experiences, a larger portion of the population will seek dental care on a regular basis. The net impact of reduction of aversive treatments and the increase in purchasing power may lead to increased dental care demand resulting in higher patient volume.

Dental insurance may also provide the impetus in extending the service line in dental care utilization. In traditional or preinsurance private practice, fees could more accurately be described as true market prices or an equilibrium price between market supply and demand functions. It was not that long ago that dentists would provide a free examination as a "loss leader" so that monetary issues would not interfere in establishing good communication with the patient. Once patient rapport was established and a total treatment plan accepted, certain service lines such as dentures would be a "net gain," which would compensate the dentist for the "loss leader" examination. Most dentists realized that the most important aspect of initial patient contact was to establish rapport and confidence that would eventually lead to patient acceptance of treatment options. The unfortunate consequence of this pricing and consumption pattern was the traditional fee schedule's emphasis on the dentist's role as provider of tangible services such as fillings, dentures, and crowns rather than as diagnostician.

Dental insurance should influence this traditional utilization pattern and revenue service mix. With the advent of partial or full coverage for diagnostic service there should be an observable yet gradual increase in the percent of dental practice revenue derived from these services. In addition, most dental plans largely, if not fully, cover preventive services; therefore with the decline of dental caries, a larger percentage of practice revenue should also be derived from preventive services.

Is there any evidence for such revenue shifts? Analysis of the claims and patient copayment experience for six separate union management benefit trust funds involving approximately 110,000 eligible enrollees throughout the Commonwealth of Massachusetts indicates that there is sufficient evidence. Table 6-3 compares the 1977 percent expenditures derived from Table 6-2 with the 1986 percent expenditure as derived from the union claims data for general practitioners.*

Although such comparisons are open to charges that the populations are not comparable, the union data reflect the consumption pattern of a professional, skilled and unskilled labor pool of an industrial Northeast state. The enrollment base of 110,000 individuals ensures that it is unlikely that the consumption pattern observed is grossly atypical or subject to adverse selection.

As Table 6-3 points out, according to the 1986 data, diagnostic and preventive services represent an 8.1% increase as compared to the 1977 percent of revenue. On the other hand, operative and fixed prosthodontic services indicate a decline of 12.1% for the general practitioner. The other interesting and not unexpected observation is that in 1977 periodontics was almost a negligible 0.8% of total revenue. The 1986 combined union trust fund data indicate that periodontic services now represent a more respectable 8.1% of total private practitioner revenue. A reasonable conclusion derived from Table 6-3 is that there is evidence that the countervailing forces of caries reduction and increased dental insurance do appear to have an impact on the service mix of consumer demand.

---

*Claims analysis provided by the author, September 1986.

Table 6-3. Percent expenditure by dental service type comparing 1977 U.S. data with 1986 Massachusetts union data

Service type	% 1977	% 1986	Net change
Diagnostic	8.2	12.9	+4.7
Preventive	7.7	11.1	+3.4
Operative	27.9	22.6	−5.3
Fixed prosthetics	34.5	27.7	−6.8
Removable prosthetics	9.6	6.9	−2.7
Endodontics	6.9	7.5	+0.6
Periodontics	0.8	8.1	+7.3
Surgery	3.9	2.1	−1.8
Orthodontics	1.1	1.1	0

From Douglass, C.W., and Day, J.M.: Cost and payment of dental services in the U.S., J. Dent. Educ. **43:**7, 1979.

MARKET FORCES—THE SUPPLY SIDE
Background

As previously discussed, the economics of health care delivery have evolved from a system of private transactions between physician and patient to one involving various third parties. This development certainly will have its impact on the demand side or consumption of dental services, but what was unforeseen was its impact on the supply of dental services, more specifically the organization and structure of the financing and delivery of dental services.

The growth of insurance is not the only major force to shape and foster changes in dental care delivery. The other factor is the 1976 Supreme Court decision maintaining that state organized restrictions on advertising by professions is a violation of the First Amendment.

Dentistry, along with other similar professions, maintains that the doctor/patient relationship is sacrosanct and because of this is separate from other types of economic activity. What is evolving is not a repudiation of this concept but a clearer definition of the doctor/patient relationship that is consistent with economic reality and constitutional law.

When the payment of services was primarily a private transaction between physician and patient, all aspects of the therapy environment were private in nature. In today's economy dental care payments are becoming benefits derived from an employer. In reality they have become another factor in computing labor costs for the production of goods and services in the U.S. economy. It is unrealistic to believe that industry, both labor and management, will not attempt to use its scarce resources to maximize benefits for its workers. If this requires a more active role in the payment and delivery of dental services, this will be pursued. The U.S. economy is now facing aggressive worldwide competition, and it is inevitable that all costs of the factors of production will be periodically reviewed. If, for example, a particular industry finds that by maintaining its own health clinics it can reduce labor costs by a certain amount, the economic choice is clear. Maximize production efficiency so prices are competitive.

Of course, what is evolving is not as simple as industry starting clinics and hiring doctors but payment reimbursement by various types of third parties representing a range of financial arrangements between industry and the health care sector. It should be added that the union or company clinic is an option that some industries have pursued, but the main thrust is not to get involved in the delivery of services but to negotiate an acceptable financing structure. Some of the new third parties in health care are health maintenance organizations (HMOs) and their dental counterpart, the prepaid group dental practice. In this particular arrangement the provider of services and insurer of care are the same organization.

This and other types of arrangements will increase competition in the third party marketplace. It is in essence this competition between traditional insurance companies and other third party arrangements that will encourage efficiency in the health care delivery system.

In order to flourish these newer organizations must be free to develop marketing strategies to both penetrate the existing dental prepayment market and to attract persons now without coverage. However, there has been a good deal of professional resistance to the idea of marketing health services. Until 1976 most state court decisions upheld states' rights to inhibit advertising for professional services. For example, in two court decisions, *People v. Duben* (10 N.E. 2nd 809 Ill.229) and *Cherry v. Board of Regents of the State of New York* (44 N.E. 2d 405 N.Y. 148) the Supreme court stated and reaffirmed the states' right to limit advertising by physicians and dentists. With this legal precedent most professional organizations, including dentistry, traditionally restricted professionals from using various forms of advertising.

With the evolution of new third parties who may advertise for plan members, the question that would naturally have arisen concerns the ethics of physicians and dentists who are employed by or contract with organizations who in turn advertise on their behalf. This would have been an area of new litigation, but the Supreme Court in 1976 made this a moot issue. The U.S. Supreme Court decided a case on appeal from the Supreme Court of Arizona, *John R. Bates and Van O'Steen Appellants v. The State Bar of Arizona* (76-316 4873,4896); it upheld the right of attorneys to advertise their fees for certain services. The state's rule prohibiting this was found to be in violation of the First Amendment. The Court considered six arguments for restricting price advertising: (1) the adverse effect on professionalism, (2) the inherently misleading nature of attorney advertising, (3) the adverse effect on the administration of justice, (4) the undesirable economic effects of advertising, (5) the adverse effect of advertising on the quality

of service, and (6) the difficulties of enforcements. The Court was not persuaded that any of them was an acceptable reason to inhibit an attorney's First Amendment right to announce to the public his/her prices for basic services. However, the Court did not hold that advertising by attorneys may not be regulated in any way.

Given these economic and legal trends, the practitioner/patient relationship should and must be properly defined so that professionalism and quality of care are fostered. How a particular patient seeks and pays for service from a particular health care provider does not affect the ethical responsibility of that provider. Salaried dentists should maintain the same level of professionalism as those who work in the more traditional private practice setting. It is the role of the dental schools and professional organizations to clearly define and promulgate the concept of professional responsibility.

Supply side restructuring. There are several options available to industry relating to the administrative and provider reimbursement structure for various health care benefits including dentistry. Outlined in this chapter will be organizational arrangements defined in a broad generic sense. It is beyond the scope of this discussion to analyze the finer details of specific organizations.

There are choices industry can and will make concerning the financial management structure of health care benefits. At present there are three possible basic organizational arrangements:

1. Indemnification of dental benefits through an insurance carrier.
2. Self-indemnification and self-administration of the benefit.
3. Self-indemnification but with use of a third party to administer benefit.

Insurance option. In order to establish the proper framework for analysis, a few basic concepts should be discussed. As the list above points out, insuring involves several choices, including to indemnify annual benefit costs through an insurance carrier.

In the attempt to explore the underwriting of health care programs such as dental care through an insurance carrier, there should be a clear idea of the potential benefits to industry and how they can be achieved. A simpleminded idea of "let the insurance company handle everything" may in fact, in the long run, turn out to be more costly to industry.

The use of an insurance carrier to indemnify or protect against possible damage or losses, is at best a short-term risk-ameliorating option. In the long run the insurance company passes all costs on to its customers, in this case, industry. However, there are certain advantages. This type of indemnification makes annual budgeting for benefits much more predictable and efficient, and the technical expertise of insurance underwriters and actuaries can be useful in analyzing program economic impacts. The insurance company also takes on the more burdensome operational tasks such as claims processing, thus freeing management talent to concentrate on long-term strategic planning.

Undeniably the growth of dental prepayment has been marked by an increasing role of the traditional insurance company in the financing of dental services. The insurance company maintains the appropriate administrative talent and resources to maintain large-scale benefits administration. Certainly for particular industries this option makes the most sense and currently most dental benefits are administered under this arrangement.

Self-indemnification and self-administration. Another approach to benefits administration is to self-insure and self-administer the benefit. Usually what is established is a union-management trust fund that pays for care directly rather than paying premiums to an insurance company. In a true self-administered benefit, the trust fund handles all aspects of benefit program administration. There are two main advantages to this approach. The trust fund has complete control of the benefit program from policy initiation to policy implementation and can invest earmarked benefit dollars to expand the resource base or dollars available for future benefits.

If this type of administrative structure is totally maintained by a particular company or union, the cash flow from benefit dollars will remain in its bank accounts until needed to pay for services and will not automatically be sent to the insurance company in regular premium installments. However, as pointed out previously, there is a price to be paid in maintaining this level of control. Industry's management talent must be responsible not only for long-term policy planning and analysis, but also for large-scale day-to-day operational activities. It is this latter responsibility that in reality inhibits policy reformulation and creativity. Once a large-scale initiative has been completed, for example, when a computer data base management system is set up, it becomes very difficult to quickly change direction and consider new economic and benefit policy directions.

Role of the TPA. In the private sector a new type of administrative structure has evolved. Known as third party administrator (TPA), it attempts to bridge the gap between indemnifying and administering through an insurance carrier and self-indemnification and self-administration. This option has the advantage that ultimate budgetary control is in the hands of those who pay for the services. In the private sector this means that if a company self-indemnifies but contracts with a TPA for claims processing and other program management activities, the money budgeted for health care is still in the control of the company for its own cash flow until services are rendered and claims must be paid. The advantage to industry is that the tedious aspect of program management is contracted out, but the analytical and long-term policy tasks remain the provenance of industry benefit administrators.

PROVIDER REIMBURSEMENT STRUCTURE
Medical economics and insurance

The economics of provider reimbursement will play a large part in the final direction relating to dental benefit structure. Once again, we must look to the concept of insurance and what it means for ambulatory care programs such as dental care.

The development of benefit packages and premium calculations for prepaid dental care programs differs greatly from similar work for insurance-type programs. The standard definition of an *insurable risk* contains three essential elements: (1) the loss or incident occurs infrequently, such as a flood; (2) the potential loss is very great, for example, destruction of home by fire; and (3) any single individual cannot affect the risk or frequency of the event in the community. Hospitalization is an insurable risk and meets these three criteria. However, expenditure for dental care, and for that matter most ambulatory care, is not an insurable risk. Dental disease is common. Dental care is not expensive, at least not when compared to the cost of hospitalization, and individuals generally know what their level of need is. This last point is the reason dental care plans cannot be marketed on an individual basis in the private sector. Adverse selection would result from all those persons with heavy accumulated dental needs joining the plan and those who have maintained their oral health not joining. This type of adverse selection would eliminate any element of cost-sharing and force premiums up to an unmarketable level and cause closure of the prepaid plan.

Prepaid dental care plans are essentially a budgeting type of arrangement in which predictible expenditures are planned where groups are large enough. The real economic dilemma occurs when providers, who have considerable leverage over utilization, have no economic incentive to initiate courses of treatment consistent with budgeted premium dollars. With traditional private sector insurance the role of the third party is to assume risk for dental claims, while the role of the consumer and the provider is to maximize benefits derived from the plan.

Changes in the marketplace

The introduction of the concept of risk-sharing in prepaid programs is a product of the past decade. In its purest form the insurers of care and the providers of services fuse into one umbrella organization. This is the HMO concept in which the provider is also given an incentive to initiate courses of treatment consistent with premium dollars.

Are these same forces at work in the dental care marketplace as in the HMO movement for medical care? According to an American Dental Association conference, this seems to be the case. Around the country, indemnity dental insurance plans are beginning to lose ground to capitation and other provider-type arrangements as large insurers speculate that the market is on the brink of some major shifts. The nature of the more common arrangements are outlined below:

1. Fee-for-service (FFS): Open panel
2. Fee-for-service: Participating provider (no provider restriction)
3. Fee-for-service: IPA/PPO model (selected provider participation)
4. Capitation: staff model groups
5. Capitation: IPA model

Range of choices

Fee-for-service options
Fee-for-service: open panel. This is the structure of the typical indemnity commercial insurance plan. The basic contractual arrangement is

between the insurance company and the insured, whereby the insurance company indemnifies for losses from dental claims as outlined in the policy's list of coverages. The policy holder is free to select the dentist of his/her choice and can either pay the dentist directly for services rendered and later collect from the insurance company or assign such payments directly to the dentist. The insurance company in turn reimburses for care based on a table of allowances or usual and customary fees up to the nintieth percentile. The dentist is free to collect from the patient any differences between his/her own fee and that allowed under the terms of the insurance policy.

Fee-for-service: participating provider (no provider restriction). This is the structure of the typical professionally sponsored insurance plan, such as the Blue Cross/Blue Shield and Delta plans. The basic contractual arrangement is between the insurance underwriter and the provider of services, in this case the dentist. This type of coverage is usually termed *service benefits*, in contrast to the *indemnity benefits* of the previous commercial insurance structure. With Delta plan as a typical example, the provider submits his/her fee schedule with the carrier and cannot charge the patient more than the agreed-upon fees. The ability of becoming a participating provider usually entails the signing of a provider agreement with the insurance carrier, locking the provider into an agreed upon fee schedule that the provider submits. This agreement has caused much controversy because most providers (both dentists and physicians) want the ability to bill patients directly for the difference when their fees exceed the fee schedule of the service benefit contract. "Balance billing" has been the topic of much litigation and legislation.

At the present time a large percentage of providers have become participating providers, usually with the insurance carriers reducing the reimbursable fee by 5% because of guaranteed payment. This has given the Blue Cross/Blue Shield and the Delta plans some leverage in the marketplace, but the commercial carriers have countered this economic advantage by offering a more varied product line and packaging it with other types of insurance.

Fee-for-service: IPA/PPO model. Recently, preferred provider organizations (PPO) or Independent Practice Association (IPA) networks have been observed in the marketplace. These organizations are participating-provider service-benefit insurance arrangements, but with the clear intention of negotiating a reduced fee with the providers. In order to entice providers to reduce their fees as much as 15%-20%, the concept of a closed panel is introduced. This means that only a few offices will be selected to participate in any given geographic area, thereby guaranteeing each office a greater volume of patients than would otherwise be obtainable.

FEE-FOR-SERVICE SPECTRUM. In the spectrum of fee-for-service options noted above, if cost containment becomes of greater importance, the most likely solution is to contain, if not reduce, reimbursable fees. There is simplicity and ease in using this approach. Essentially, the problem is tackled by modifying the structure established long ago with a considerable amount of accumulated experience and professional acceptance in the marketplace today.

However, modifying the structure in this way leaves fee-for-service intact and the concept of risk sharing is not used. I have found that providers in the closed panel PPO arrangement will keep to contracutal fee arrangements, but they are not deterred from trying to expand their service options with the patient or increase fees for non-covered or partially covered services. Once again, the third party is at risk, and the provider and patient have an economic incentive to maximize benefits, in this case dollars from the program.

Risk-sharing options. Dental capitation programs have grown in popularity over the past two decades. Most of the major dental insurers, including companies such as Prudential and

Connecticut General, have established capitation programs. These companies would not have ventured into this area of the marketplace if they did not feel it was in their best interests to do so.

The essential feature of capitation is that the provider receives a predetermined fixed revenue and must budget his/her time accordingly. The typical industry standard for rate setting is to budget according to the cost of delivering dental services in the typical office. Fees do not play a role in the pricing mechanism.

Given that a fixed cost–based payment will be received, the provision of preventive and maintenance services is preferable to the more complex rehabilitation services that are usually associated with higher fees in the marketplace. One of the main advantages is that each dentist can base his/her own treatment assessment on his/her own diagnosis, and a prior authorization/review by an insurance carrier consultant becomes superfluous.

The main criticism of this approach is that the provider will not have an incentive to perform needed dental work and may in fact collect the capitation payments without delivering the services. However, with adequate monitoring and utilization review, most providers will follow accepted treatment standards. As with any system of reimbursement, there will be a small percentage who will abuse the system for personal gain.

Capitation: staff model groups. Prepaid capitation group practice is the HMO concept as applied to the delivery of dental services. In one setting the patient can receive all of his/her required dental services. The economic incentive of this concept is to improve the oral health status of the enrolled population, and the patient has the advantage of one-stop shopping for dental care.

Although this option is enticing, there is a problem in the widespread application of this approach. Approximately 88% of the delivery of dental services is by solo practitioners. Large multispecialty groups are not the mainstay of dental care delivery; however, with the growth of retail-based dental centers, this is rapidly changing. From the perspective of benefits administrators, there are dental care delivery units that do have the potential for this type of arrangement such as the growing number of group practice outlets in various shopping malls.

Capitation: IPA model. The independent practitioner association model (IPA) has the advantage of fitting the benefits of risk sharing of capitation with the dental care delivery system as it presently exists. At first glance it seems a perfect match, however, it does introduce a few problems. How does one handle the issue of specialist services? Should capitation payments go to the general practitioners who in turn pay the specialists? Should the specialists be capitated directly, or should they be kept on a closely monitored fee-for-service system? In the private sector there are several variations of this arrangement and each more or less seems to work as intended.

CONCLUSION

In this chapter we discussed the factors that have led to changes in dental care delivery and the economics of dental care. We are currently in a period of transition during which alternative modes of delivery of services and financing of these services will evolve. We have also discussed the potential impact of caries reduction in dental care delivery.

The reduction of dental caries and the role of fluorides have been well documented by the dental profession. The first step in its understanding occurred in 1902, when Frederic S. McKay gave systematic attention to the mottling he found in his patients. The unfolding of the fluoride story is a classic case study in chronic disease epidemiology. The dental profession can point with pride to its role in significantly preventing a disease that a few years ago was considered ubiquitous and its treatment an almost insurmountable task.

In this decade dental care delivery is also influenced by the unfolding of historical events that at first appear to have no bearing on current dental practice. The growth of fringe benefits is one such factor. Fringe benefits developed during World War II when the federal government prohibited nearly all wage increases. War industries attracted workers by offering benefits in addition to wages. For example, many employers paid part of the cost of food served in their cafeterias. Later companies offered medical insurance, life insurance, and accident and disability insurance. Since then, fringe benefits have grown in importance. Labor and management have introduced new benefits, including dental care and stock purchase plans. Unions often accept fringe benefits instead of higher wage because most benefits are not subject to income tax.

Dental professionals must and will adapt to this changing environment. Our responsibilities will not diminish; instead we must remain involved to ensure the highest standards of care and professionalism to the consuming public.

Case study. A.B.C. Insurance Company dental plan

In this case study we will examine the financial planning that must be developed in order for a dental insurance program to be financially viable. If the Board of Directors of the A.B.C. Insurance Company feel it is time to enter the dental insurance market, they must conduct two key sets of analysis to help them through their strategic planning phase. One piece of analysis will be provided by the company's actuaries to properly price the cost of dental insurance and the other by the company's market analysts. In the presentation of this case study we will first outline the basic tools of the actuary and later show how the marketing analyst will use input from the actuary to measure possible cash flows, given different market penetration rates.

ACTUARIAL ANALYTICAL TOOLS. The actuary of an insurance company has the primary responsibility for the financial soundness of its insurance operations. The business of insurance is underwriting risks at proper rates. The basic actuarial function is calculating insurance risks and rates. It is the starting point to determine the prices to be charged for contractual agreements.

TERMINOLOGY. There are times when semantics may be responsible for confusion on the part of those not familiar with rate-making principles and techniques. For instance, the terms *rate* and *premium* are often used interchangeably. Actually a rate is the price an insurance organization charges for each unit of risk it assumes. In dental expense coverage the unit of risk is the individual. The rate is usually expressed in terms of price per policy holder or employee member of a plan. Another term commonly used for unit of risk is *eligible*, and it is not unusual to see insurance rates expressed as price per eligible per month. When there are significant differences in the chance of loss among various units of risk, such units may be subcategorized within a given group with a separate rate being calculated for the various categories. In the determination of dental insurance rates the proper assessment of rates for significant subcategories is of utmost importance. One basic breakdown of rate calculation is for adults versus children. Dental care costs for adults are generally much higher than for children. Another significant subcategory is the breakdown of rate calculation for (1) *rehabilitation patients*, those who seek only episodic care for specific current problems when a backlog of unmet needs are cared for; and (2) *maintenance patients*, those who seek regular care. It has been repeatedly shown that patients who seek regular preventive and early maintenance care generate fewer claims in both volume and dollar amount than those who only seek care when a problem arises.

A premium, in the technical sense, is derived by multiplying the rate for a given category of risks by the number of risk units. Thus the premium is the total cost for a group of risks, whereas the rate is the unit cost. It should be noted that a low rate implies low anticipated claims per insured under the policy, whereas a low premium can result from either low anticipated claims or a small number of insureds, or both. Therefore one firm may have a lower premium for its dental expense coverage than another firm for one of several reasons, including such factors as having a smaller number of employees, less liberal benefits in the coverage, better health among those covered, or lower charges by dentists.

The term *pure premium* is often used to describe that portion of the total premium, or total rate, that is required for the payment of claims. The *gross premium* is the total premium and thus includes the pure premium and amounts to cover an insurance corporation's administrative expenses and reserve requirements.

BASIC ILLUSTRATION OF A RATE CALCULATION. The cost of dental coverage exclusive of overhead expenses and reserves is determined by the amount paid with respect to each service multiplied by the number of times each of the various services is rendered. The rate per subscriber, also known as the *pure premium,* is ascertained by dividing the total anticipated cost (or, in some instances, the actual cost) for the particular category of subscribers by the number of subscribers. For the purpose of this section it will be assumed that the factors that enter into the rate are known. The figures are for illustrative purposes only; the codes, fees, and cost determenents are for calculation by the hypothetical A.B.C. Insurance Co.

Table 6-4 is an illustration of a worksheet section of a cost calculation for operative procedures under a dental care program. Columns 1 and 2 are respectively the code numbers and the corresponding designations of the procedures. The next two columns, 3 and 4, are the cost determinants. Column 3 is a fee schedule of the amounts the A.B.C. Company will pay with respect to each particular procedure. Column 4 figures are assumed annual frequencies of each service, that is, the number of times each service is expected to be rendered per year to a group of people, in this particular example 1,000 enrolled eligible rehabilitative adults. Obviously, the cost calculation considers only those services included in the particular coverage. Multiplying the fee for each procedure by the number of its occasions, column 3 times column 4, gives the net annual cost, column 5, of each procedure for the 1,000 eligible adults. The total of column 5, $56,000, divided by 1,000, the number of eligibles in the group, gives an average annual net cost of $56.00 for each eligible. This figure reflects the cost only for operative dental procedures. The monthly net cost per eligible is $4.67, one twelfth of $56.00. The $4.67 net monthly cost is called the monthly *pure premium,* that is, the part of the premium that is expected to be pooled for the payment of claims.

Table 6-4. Illustrative pure premium calculation for operative procedures (rehabilitation adults)

(1) Case	(2) Procedure	(3) Fee schedule	(4) Procedures per year per 1,000 eligible rehabilitation adults	(5) Annual net cost
210	Amalgam restorations			
211	One surface	$30	600	$18,000
212	Two surface	$40	700	28,000
213	Three surface	$50	200	10,000
Net cost per 1,000 rehabilitative adults				$56,000
Net cost per adult per year				56.00
Net cost per adult per month (pure premium)				4.67

Table 6-5. Illustrative monthly pure premium for various types of dental services

Code	Procedure category	Adult rehabilitation	Adult maintenance	Child rehabilitation	Child maintenance
000	Diagnostic	$1.50	$ .88	$ .47	$ .26
100	Preventive	2.10	1.02	.65	.37
200	Operative	4.67	2.41	1.42	.80
300-900	Other	6.30	3.29	1.96	1.10
	Pure premium all procedures	14.57	7.60	4.50	2.53

Similar calculations must be carried through for all categories of procedures covered under a dental care program. Illustrative components of pure premiums of a comprehensive program for all eligible adults and their children in a group would appear as shown in Table 6-5.

The monthly premium to be paid per employee is the pure premium cost for the type of coverage provided plus the pro rata costs of operating the dental insurance plan and certain contingency factors. A plan's operational and contingency cost usually is expressed as a percentage of the rate. If, for instance, these costs have been calculated to be 15% of the final rate, the final rate is obtained by multiplying the pure premium by 1.15. Table 6-6 illustrates the results of this procedure. Table 6-7 shows an anticipated mix of eligibles and the consequent monthly rate that should be quoted to pay for dental claims and also cover the A.B.C. Insurance Company's operating costs.

MARKET POTENTIAL ANALYSIS. Though the actuaries of an insurance company may be able to calculate a sound rate for dental care coverages, program success is by no means ensured. As with any other business enterprise, the directors of A.B.C. Insurance Company must fully assess if a dental insurance plan is marketable. This is the analysis the marketing department must conduct. The marketing department must determine who will purchase A.B.C.'s product line and whether the anticipated level of demand is sufficient to invest in a new A.B.C. Company line of insurance.

There are many different types of market research studies that market analysis can use to answer the previous question. A common approach is to conduct analysis of focus groups to determine market potential. A focus group is a small group of potential customers who are asked to participate in a special study to determine their opinions regarding the product or service being analyzed. The analysts of the A.B.C. Insurance Co. could ask benefits managers from several of their existing clients to participate in such a study.

The focus group analysis could revolve around showing benefit managers various possible dental benefit coverages and soliciting comments both on an open-end basis and/or using a more structured response. This analysis is very useful in helping A.B.C. analysts more clearly define the nature of their new product line consistent with both the needs and desires of their potential customers.

Focus group analysis is very useful in deriving a qualitative sense of marketability. Financial feasibility

Table 6-6. Illustrative gross premium figures for all services and classes of insured

Class	Monthly pure premium	Operational cost (15% of rate)	Final monthly rate
Adult (rehabilitation)	$14.57	$2.19	$16.76
Adult (maintenance)	7.60	1.14	8.74
Child (rehabilitation)	4.50	.68	5.18
Child (maintenance)	2.53	.38	2.91

Table 6-7. Composite rate calculation

Class	%	Gross premium per class	Component monthly total
Adult: rehabilitation	50	$16.76	$ 8.38
Adult: maintenance	20	8.74	1.75
Child: rehabilitation	15	5.18	.78
Child: maintenance	15	2.91	.44
	100		Composite rate per eligible = $11.35

would require a more quantitative analytical approach. Once the initial focus group analysis is completed, a telephone or questionnaire survey could be conducted using appropriate statistical sampling techniques. This should help analysts derive a quantitative sense of marketability.

MARKET POTENTIAL CASH FLOW. After the actuaries and market analysis have completed their analysis, a report must be written and submitted to the board of directors. The report must be concise, to the point, and by all means focus on potential profits and/or losses. The most graphic way to display marketability is to present a cash flow projection of anticipated dental plan performance. Tables 6-8 and 6-9 outline such a projection. Table 6-4 indicated summary statistics that both the actuaries and market analysts have developed. The plan actuarial statistics section of Table 6-8 are derived from Tables 6-4 through 6-7 already presented. The rate is the $11.35 gross premium per eligible per month that is essentially the market price for services.

Though we have said that administrative charges are an add-on of 15% to the pure premium, most loading factors are usually regulated by various state insurance laws. However, the start-up of a new venture does entail start-up costs that are incurred prior to significant market penetration and consequent revenue generation. The plan enrollment projection section of Table 6-8 outlines a reasonable growth of new members to a dental insurance plan. However, administrative costs do not increase at a smooth rate. Certain fixed costs and semivariable costs such as salaries are incurred right away in order to properly administer the plan. It is crucial to examine investment in a new product over time.

Table 6-9 provides us with such a cash flow projection that would tell the directors when they can expect a return on their investment in dental insurance. Of course the directors should not be satisfied with just one projection. They probably will and should demand to see many cash flow projections. "Worst case" scenario and "best case" scenario should also be ex-

amined to get a full range of possibilities. Only then would the directors be able to properly judge the economic consequences of their decisions.

In the final analysis the decision will only be as good as the information supplied to the decision makers. Fancy graphics and computer simulations will never replace competent analysts who do their homework. Table 6-9 will be the strategic planner's tool to make long-term organizational decisions, but the detail work must be completed first by competent actuary and market specialists.

Table 6-8. Dental insurance plan cashflow—market analysis

Plan enrollment per month	
Enrollment per month 1-6 =	50.0
Enrollment per month 7-12 =	100.0
Enrollment per month 13-18 =	150.0
Enrollment per month 19-24 =	200.0
Enrollment per month 25-30 =	250.0
Enrollment per month 31-36 =	300.0
Plan monthly budget	
Admin. budget month 1-6 =	2000.00
Admin. budget month 7-13 =	2500.00
Admin. budget month 13-18 =	3500.00
Admin. budget month 19-24 =	5000.00
Admin. budget month 25-30 =	6500.00
Admin. budget month 31-36 =	8500.00
Plan actuarial statistics	
Proportion rehabilitation =	0.65
Proportion adult =	0.70
Cost per rehab. adult =	174.84
Cost per rehab. child =	54.00
Cost per maint. adult =	91.20
Cost per maint. child =	30.36
Monthly rate =	11.35

Table 6-9. Dental insurance plan cashflow—market analysis

Month	Total members	Direct care costs	Monthly total cost	Monthly revenue	Monthly net income	Total cash flow	YTD cash flow
1	50	481.72	2481.72	567.50	-1914.22	-1914.22	-1914.22
2	99	955.42	2955.42	1125.54	-1829.88	-3744.10	-3744.10
3	148	1421.22	3421.22	1674.28	-1746.94	-5491.04	-5491.04
4	195	1879.26	3879.26	2213.88	-1665.38	-7156.43	-7156.43
5	242	2329.66	4329.66	2744.48	-1585.18	-8741.61	-8741.61
6	288	2772.56	4772.56	3266.24	-1506.32	-10247.93	-10247.03
7	383	3689.80	6189.80	4346.80	-1843.00	-12090.94	-12090.94
8	477	4591.76	7091.76	5409.35	-1682.40	-13773.34	-13773.34
9	569	5478.68	7978.68	6454.20	-1524.48	-15297.81	-15297.81
10	659	6350.82	8850.82	7481.63	-1369.19	-16667.00	-16667.00
11	748	7208.42	9708.42	8491.93	-1216.48	-17883.48	-17883.48
12	836	8051.73	10551.73	9485.40	-1066.33	-18949.81	-18949.81
13	972	7395.90	10720.90	11029.81	308.91	-18640.90	308.91
14	1106	8414.23	11739.23	12548.48	809.26	-17831.64	1118.17
15	1237	9415.58	12740.58	14041.84	1301.26	-16530.38	2419.43
16	1367	10400.24	13725.24	15510.31	1785.07	-14745.32	4204.49
17	1494	11368.50	14693.50	16954.31	2260.81	-12484.51	6465.30
18	1619	12320.61	15645.61	18374.23	2728.62	-9755.89	9193.92
19	1792	13637.39	18387.39	20338.00	1950.61	-7805.28	11144.53
20	1962	14932.22	19682.22	22269.03	2586.81	-5218.47	13731.34
21	2129	16205.47	20955.47	24167.88	3212.41	-2006.06	16943.75
22	2294	17457.50	22207.50	26035.08	3827.58	1821.53	20771.34
23	2456	18688.66	23438.66	27871.16	4432.50	6254.03	25203.84
24	2615	19899.30	24649.30	29676.64	5027.34	11281.38	30231.19
25	2821	26038.00	31888.00	32019.53	131.53	11412.91	131.53
26	3024	27911.47	44761.47	34323.37	561.91	11974.82	693.44
27	3224	29753.70	35603.70	36588.82	985.11	12959.93	1678.55
28	3420	31565.24	37415.24	38816.50	1401.26	14361.19	3079.82
29	3613	33346.58	39196.58	41007.06	1810.48	16171.67	4890.30
30	3803	35098.24	40948.24	43161.11	2212.88	18384.55	7103.17
31	4039	37282.18	44932.18	45846.76	914.58	19299.13	8017.75
32	4272	39429.73	47079.73	48487.65	1407.92	20707.05	9425.67
33	4501	41541.48	49191.48	51084.52	1893.04	22600.09	11318.71
34	4762	43618.04	51268.04	53638.11	2370.07	24970.16	13688.78
35	4947	45659.99	53309.99	56149.14	2839.15	27809.15	16527.94
36	5165	47667.90	55317.90	58618.32	3300.42	31109.73	19828.36

BIBLIOGRAPHY

American Dental Association, Council on Dental Care Programs, March 1984.

Boffa, J., Medalia, D., and Charette, J.: Dental prepaid capitation pilot study—final report, HCFA Contract No. 11-P-973881, Aug. 1984.

Burnelle, J., and Carlos, J.: Changes in the prevalence of dental caries in U.S. school children, 1961-1980, J. Dent. Res. **61**(special issue), (Nov. 1982), p. 1347.

Cohen, D.M., and Roesler, T.W.: The effect of dental insurance and patient income level on the utilization of dental services and implications for future growth in dentistry, J. Dent. Prac. Admin. **3:**4, Oct.-Dec. 1986.

Douglass, Chester, W., and Day, J.M.: Cost and payment of dental services in the U.S., J. Dent. Educ. **43:**7, 1979.

Eilers, R.D.: Actuarial services for a dental service corporation, U.S. Department of Health, Education and Welfare, Public Health Service, 1967.

Glass, R.: Secular changes in caries prevalence in two Massachusetts towns, Caries Res. **15:**448, 1981.

Leverett, P.: Fluorides and the changing prevalence of dental caries, Science **217**, July 1982.

Moen, B., and Poetsch, V.: Survey of dental services rendered 1969: more preventive less tooth repair, Bureau of Economic Research and Statistics, J. Am. Dent. Assoc. **81:**25, July 1970.

Praiss, I.L., and others: Changing patterns and implication for cost and quality of dental care, Inquiry **16:**131, Summer 1979.

Weisfeld, R.: National preventive dentistry demonstration program, The Robert Wood Johnson Demonstration Program, Special Report, No. 2, 1983.

SECTION THREE

DENTAL DISEASE—PREVALENCE AND PREVENTION

The prevention of disease of the oral cavity requires a multifaceted approach. It behooves the dental professional to understand the etiology and the prevalence of the disease, as well as specific means for preventing it.

Chapter 7 introduces the concept of the study of dental disease by systematic observation of population groups. The science of epidemiology paved the way for the discovery of fluoride as a caries preventive agent; it allows us to describe the effects of caries and periodontal disease in the population of the United States through the use of indices of disease.

Chapter 8, on the prevention of dental disease, defines prevention and systematically reviews the current approaches to prevention for individuals and groups. A variety of programs such as fluoride mouthrinses, school water fluoridation, and occlusal sealants are described in detail. The cost-effectiveness of these preventive measures is compared and recommendations for particular approaches are given.

CHAPTER 7

Epidemiology of Dental Disease

What does epidemiology mean to the average dental health professional in America today? To one, it means relating the findings of studies read in scientific journals to what he/she observes in his/her private practice. To another, it means noting changes in caries rates among young patients after the introduction of fluoride in the community water supply. To yet another, who has a highly developed preventive program, it indicates success through a reduction in dental disease among those who adhere to their prescribed home-care regimen.

Epidemiology is a science to which the general practitioner, the specialist, the researcher, and academician alike can relate. The term itself is derived from the Greek *epidemios*, meaning prevalent. Epidemiology is the study of the distribution and determinants of disease. Its primary tool is the systematic observation of human beings as they relate to their environment. Through the brief scenario of modern dentistry, epidemiological studies have played a leading role. Were it not for the astute observations and accurate recording of findings by dentists in Colorado and other parts of the United States, the correlation between mottled enamel and reduced caries incidence might never have been made and the value of fluoride in caries prevention might never have been discovered.

Epidemiology is more than observation and deduction. Although it is a young science, it is firmly founded in medicine, biology, statistics, and the social sciences. More recently, the advances in computer science have enhanced the capabilities of epidemiology.

Dentistry is one branch of medicine to which epidemiological methods are readily adaptable. The oral cavity is continually exposed to a variety of environmental factors that affect its state of health. The quantification of many of these factors and their correlation with the state of oral health in many instances is reasonably straightforward, for example, frequency of sugar consumption and increase in plaque production. In others, suspected causative agents might be more difficult to define, as is the case with aphthous ulcers. Dental epidemiology provides a framework within which we can scrutinize our data to determine whether our theories of cause and effect are valid.

Dental epidemiology is useful in determining the needs of populations. Dental diseases vary greatly from country to country; indeed, from community to community. Epidemiology is used to delineate disease patterns in communities. This is of value to dentists involved in program planning for dental care delivery. A single survey might disclose that a certain neighborhood is populated by an equal distribution of older adults and young children. The caries rates of the young are low relative to similar neighborhoods because the water in the community was fluoridated 15 years ago. The survey also shows that a large number of the elderly are affected by root surface caries of periodontal disease or are fully or partially edentulous, without adequate dental services. The program planner may weigh all the findings of the study and decide that rather than a dental health education program for local school children, what is needed most by this population is a program for low-cost dentures and dental treatment for the elderly.

Other policy decisions can be aided by epidemiological studies. If limited resources are made available to a city to provide dental treatment for children, a decision maker has a number of options. He/she may decide to earmark the funds for a program of comprehensive dental care for children of low-income families who are not eligible for Medicaid. If a survey of the oral health status of the city school children is available, and it shows that a high caries rate exists among the children in all socioeconomic strata, this information may alter his/her determination of need. Alternative programs that would affect the entire school population may appear to be a more equitable use of public funds.

THE SCIENCE OF EPIDEMIOLOGY

Epidemiology as a science is organized into three distinct divisions: descriptive, analytical, and experimental. Each branch employs specific methods and measurements and evaluates the disease status of a population from different perspectives. Any or all may be of value to the health professional, depending on the population and investigation at hand.

Descriptive epidemiology is used to aid in the conceptualization and quantification of the disease status of the community. The major parameters of interest in descriptive epidemiology are incidence and prevalence. These terms are used to describe the extent to which the problem under inquiry exists in the population.

Incidence is the number of cases that will occur within a population during a specified time period. Incidence is usually expressed as a rate, that is, cases per population per time. It is the result of the force operating on a population over time. For example, the annual death rate in a community is the result of the force of morbidity on the population of that community during the year. Let us say that 60 people in a city of 300,000

died of oral cancer during the year 1986. We could then express the rate of death caused by oral cancer in this population as 60 deaths per 300,000 persons per year.

Now, think of the population as individuals all contributing 1 year of life to a communal concept of living known as person-years. Together, these people in 1986 have accumulated 300,000 person-years. We can now express the death rate caused by oral cancer as 60 deaths per 300,000 person years. We can further compress this expression of morbidity and express it using exponential notation as the rate of 20 deaths per 10^5 person-years. This is a general form in which incidence rates are expressed: $I_R = $ cases/person-time. The range for incidence rates is from zero to infinity.

Prevalence is the term used to indicate what proportion of a given population is affected by a condition at a given point of time. It is expressed as a percentage of the population, and its range is 0% to 100%.

If we examined 1,000 school children in September 1986 and found that 200 had gingivitis, we could say that the prevalence of gingivitis in this population in September 1986 was 20%. The general expression for prevalence is $p = \frac{\text{Cases}}{\text{Population}} \times 100\%$. Most dental surveys, such as decayed, missing, filled (DMF) counts, measure the prevalence of dental disease in populations.

The distinction that must be drawn between incidence and prevalence is one of time. An incidence rate is the expression of an instantaneous force; it is not a period or point in time. Prevalence is an expression of a point estimate. At a given point in time, Y number of individuals have a disease. We do not know when the disease first came into being, but we do know that at the time of examination, a specific percentage of the population showed signs of having the disease. These cases are the prevalent cases. Their ratio to the total population expressed as a percentage is termed *prevalence*.

Say we re-examined our school children in October 1986 and found 16 new cases of gingivitis. We now know that operating under the force we call *incidence*, etiological factors have produced 16 incident cases of gingivitis in 1 month's time. If we consider that each of the previously unaffected 800 children contributed 1 month to the communal concept of person-time, we can compute our incidence rate of 16 cases per 800 person-months. We can further compress this idea by converting this to an annual figure:

$$\frac{16 \text{ cases}}{800 \text{ person-months}} \times \frac{12 \text{ months}}{\text{year}} = \frac{0.24 \text{ cases}}{\text{person-year}}$$

If our originally affected 200 students still had gingivitis at the October examination, we could compute our prevalence for October as:

$$p = \frac{216 \text{ cases}}{1,000 \text{ students}} \times 100\% = 21.6\%$$

Analytical epidemiology is most often used in studies to determine the etiology of a disease. With analytical epidemiology a researcher may attempt to establish that a causal relationship exists between a factor and a disease. In epidemiology causative agents may be considered alone or together with other agents to be necessary or sufficient to cause a disease. A necessary cause is one that must be sustained in order for a person to get the disease. A sufficient cause is one that is sustained and may cause the disease. There may be more than one necessary or sufficient cause for a disease.

Fig. 7-1 illustrates a hypothetical causal theory for periodontal disease. There are two sufficient causes under this theory: sufficient cause 1 accounts for 75% of the cases examined, and sufficient cause 2 gives rise to the remaining

25% of the cases. Factor A is a necessary cause of periodontal disease for both sufficient causes 1 and 2 under this theory. If factor A is not present, the disease will not occur. The presence of factor A alone, however, will not result in the disease state. Factor A, therefore, is a necessary cause but not a sufficient cause.

The remaining factors B, C, and D act together with A to form sufficient causes 1 and 2. Factors B, C, and D, taken individually, are not necessary causes since if any one of them is blocked, the disease can still occur. Separately or together, factors B, C, and D do not constitute a sufficient cause.

The concepts of necessary and sufficient causes are important to a researcher trying to determine the etiological basis for a disease. If a factor is necessary, and blocking this factor results in 100% of the disease prevented, this is important information. If the factor is probably necessary but not sufficient, the researcher

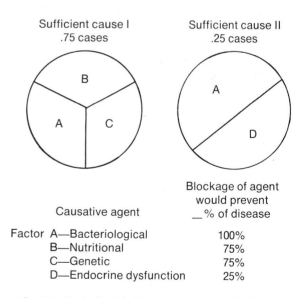

Factor	Causative agent	Blockage of agent would prevent _% of disease
A	Bacteriological	100%
B	Nutritional	75%
C	Genetic	75%
D	Endocrine dysfunction	25%

Fig. 7-1. Periodontal disease—causation in hypothetical population.

must look further to unravel the causal web and discover the relationships between all causal factors.

In analytical epidemiology there are several types of studies that are commonly used by researchers to determine the etiology of a disease. Three common study designs are prospective cohort studies, case control studies, and retrospective follow-up studies. Each type has its own strengths and limitations and is suited for specific kinds of research problems.

The prospective cohort study, commonly referred to simply as a cohort study, is the closest to experimental epidemiology. This study is conducted on a general population that is followed through time to see which members develop the disease or diseases in question. Once this subpopulation is established, the various exposure factors that affected this group are evaluated. This type of study can generate a hypothesis, since multiple endpoints are examined.

Prospective cohort studies allow an investigator to examine a larger number of hypotheses at one time. The temporal sequence of cause and effect may be clearly seen in a prospective study. A major disadvantage of this type of study is that time must elapse for data to be generated, and often subjects drop out of the study along the way for various reasons. A prospective cohort study is a very expensive one since it must be conducted over a fairly long period of time, and the population must be large enough to ensure adequate sample size after attrition.

A case control study is conducted using a population that has a disease and a matching population that does not. Such a study asks the question, What has been the exposure of the disease group? In this study a researcher thinks back from effect to cause. Case control studies are especially good for diseases with long induction periods, since a full picture of the etiology may be obtained. A researcher conducting a case control study uses questionnaires and medical histories to review past events and exposures. This type of study is usually relatively inexpensive and requires a fairly short period of time to obtain results. Matching of cases and controls according to factors that may have influenced the course of disease development, for example, race, age, and sex, is important in ensuring the validity of a study.

A retrospective follow-up study is used to evaluate the effect that a specific exposure has had on a population. It is commonly used in the area of occupational health hazards. This study starts with an exposure in time past and evaluates the histories of those exposed through to time present. An example of this type of research might be a study of dental assistants who were employed in Anytown, U.S.A., during the period 1940 to 1945 and who were exposed to significant quantities of mercury by mixing amalgam with mortar and pestle. If one could identify this group adequately and follow the health histories of this group through to 1985, various patterns of diseases related to this occupational hazard might emerge. Retrospective follow-up studies are relatively easy and inexpensive, provided that a select exposure group is available and that the follow-up data can be obtained.

Experimental epidemiology is used primarily in intervention studies. Once the etiology of a disease has been established, the researcher may wish to determine the effectiveness of a program of prevention or therapy. One method of doing so is by selecting an experimental population that corresponds to the general population for which the program has been designed. The researcher may then divide the experimental population into two groups, a study group that will receive the preventive or therapeutic treatment and a control group that will not. The researcher must take measures to ensure that these groups are as nearly identical as possible in composition to ensure that the trial will be valid. Measurement of disease incidence in both groups before and after treatment and careful analysis of results provide the researcher with information about the effectiveness of the proposed program. He/she may then extrapolate this information to apply to the general population.

INDICES IN DENTAL EPIDEMIOLOGY

Researchers in dental epidemiology have found that in order for their observations to be readily quantified, analyzed, and understood, they must be collected and arranged in an orderly manner according to carefully defined criteria and conditions. For this purpose various indices in dental epidemiology have been developed, including those in the areas of caries, periodontal disease, and orthodontics. A dental index is objective mathematical description of a diagnosis based on carefully determined criteria under specified conditions. In theory an index should be reproducible.

In dentistry the most widely used and best developed in terms of methods and interpretation are the caries indices. The decayed, missing, filled index is commonly used to measure surfaces (DMFS) affected by dental caries or number of affected teeth (DMFT) in adult populations. In primary dentitions the index usually employed is decayed, extracted, filled surfaces (defs) or teeth (deft).

The criteria on which a DMF index is based may vary from study to study, and these must be considered when analyzing data and comparing results of independent investigations. Variations may be found in definitions of what constitutes a carious lesion, the number of teeth at risk, and so on. The definition must be clear as to what is considered to constitute a filling, and what is a missing tooth. Differences such as 28 teeth at risk rather than 32 will yield considerable disparity in results and thus make comparisons difficult.

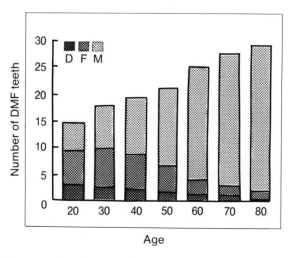

Fig. 7-2. Example illustrates how bar graphs can be used to show breakdown of DMF components. (From National Center for Health Statistics: Selected dental findings in adults by age, race, and sex: United States, 1960-1962, PHS Pub. No. 1000, Series 11, No. 7. Washington, DC, 1965, U.S. Government Printing Office.)

The conditions under which the examination is conducted are also of major importance when evaluating study results. For example, if identical surveys are conducted, data will vary greatly if one uses bitewing radiographs and the other does not.

DMF counts provide us with a broad overview of caries activity in a population. More specific information about the population may be garnered by examining the individual components of the index. Fig. 7-2 illustrates the use of a graph to display the breakdown of DMF components. The total DMF count of a poor urban population may be identical to one of an affluent suburban population, and yet the oral health status of the groups will probably be dissimilar.

For many purposes, such as determining population needs, DMF data may be utilized to yield more informative data. An example of this is the unmet restorative treatment needs (UTN) index,[3] which analyzes the needs of the population as follows:

$$UTN = \frac{\text{Mean number of decayed teeth}}{\text{Mean numbers of decayed teeth and filled teeth}} \times 100$$

This simple, yet elegant mathematical manipulation provides us with information about this population that may be readily comprehended by professionals and laypersons alike.

Indices may be used to compare oral health status of populations following intervention or treatment. An example of this is a study of the effect of water fluoridation on school children in Providence, Rhode Island. The water supply of the city was fluoridated in August 1952. In 1953 baseline data were gathered by Clune.[2] A 1972-1973 study was done by Yacovone and Parente

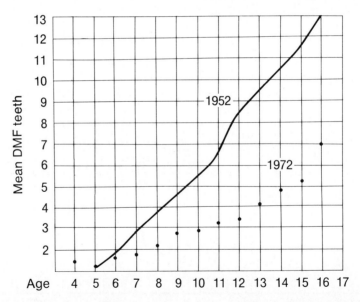

Fig. 7-3. Mean DMF permanent teeth in 1952 (before exposure to fluoridated water) and in 1972 (after 20 years exposure to fluoridated water). Graph depicts reduction in age-specific DMFT attributable to water fluoridation. (From Yacovone, J.A., and Parente, A.M.: Twenty years of community water fluoridation: the prevalence of dental caries among Providence, Rhode Island school children, J. Rhode Island State Dent. Soc. 7:3, 1974.)

using the same techniques and a comparable school-aged population.[10] A reduction of 68% of DMFT was found. Table 7-1 and Fig. 7-3 illustrate how data from such a study may be presented in table or graph form to effectively dramatize the results.

An assessment that is often used to evaluate the need for, or success in, oral hygiene and health education is the measure of oral cleanliness. One popular index for this program is the Oral Hygiene Index Simplified (OHI-S) of Greene and Vermillion.[4] This index sets forth a simple method for quantifying the amount of plaque and calculus in its two components, the Debris Index and the Calculus Index. These components are added to obtain a single score. This simplified index is based on the six surfaces scored from four posterior and two anterior teeth. Its well-defined criteria for both tooth selection and scoring make it an index that can be determined fairly rapidly and consistently. These qualities make the OHI-S a good index for a survey of a large population.

The Personal Hygiene Performance Index (PHP) of Podshadley and Haley, as modified by Martens and Meskin (PHP-M)[7] (Fig. 7-4), is an index that is designed to be repeated following patient oral hygiene education. It may be used to both document and assist in motivating changes in oral health habits. For this purpose teeth selected for scoring are recorded and used at subsequent examinations. Each of six selected teeth are divided into five areas, labeled a, b, c, d, and e on both facial and lingual surfaces. Presence of plaque in lettered areas is noted on the record, and 1 point is given for each area of plaque. The range of scores is from 0 (best) to 60 (worst). In Fig. 7-5, this index has been used to score the patient before and after oral hygiene instruction and at the follow-up visit.

The recorded information from the examination gives us information as to the total amount of plaque present, as well as which areas in the mouth and which surfaces of the teeth are not adequately cleansed. This can be compiled for all individuals and may be used to analyze and eval-

Table 7-1. Caries prevalence in permanent teeth before and after 20 years of fluoridation according to sex

	Male		Female		Both	
	1952-1953	1972-1973	1952-1953	1972-1973	1952-1953	1972-1973
Number of children	4,448	2,092	4,405	2,690	8,853	5,592
Caries	11,789*	1,991	12,250	2,037	24,039	4,028
	(2.65)†	(0.69)	(2.78)	(0.76)	(2.72)	(0.72)
Missing	3,177	217	3,317	201	6,494	418
	(0.71)	(0.07)	(0.75)	(0.07)	(0.73)	(0.07)
Filled	6,588	2,156	7,968	2,515	14,556	4,671
	(1.48)	(0.74)	(1.81)	(0.93)	(1.64)	(0.84)
Total DMF‡	21,554	4,364	23,535	4,753	45,089	9,117
% Reduction	69.1		66.9		68.0	

From Yacavone, J.A., and Parente, A.M.: Twenty years of community water fluoridation: the prevalence of dental caries among Povidence, Rhode Island school children, J. Rhode Island State Dent. Soc. 7:3, 1974.
*Total number of teeth.
†Mean score.
‡DMF data shows success of water fluoridation program in Providence, Rhode Island.

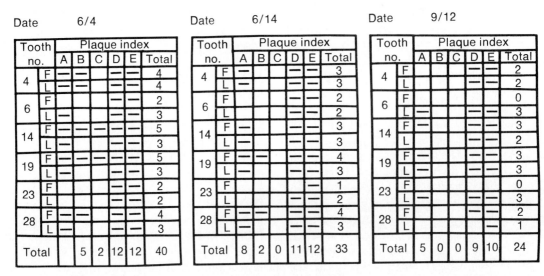

Date   6/4

Tooth no.		A	B	C	D	E	Total
4	F	—	—		—	—	4
	L	—	—		—	—	4
6	F				—	—	2
	L	—			—	—	3
14	F	—	—	—	—	—	5
	L	—			—	—	3
19	F	—	—	—	—	—	5
	L	—			—	—	3
23	F				—	—	2
	L				—	—	2
28	F	—	—		—	—	4
	L	—			—	—	3
Total		9	5	2	12	12	40

Remarks: Pretreatment examination

Date   6/14

Tooth no.		A	B	C	D	E	Total
4	F	—			—	—	3
	L	—			—	—	3
6	F				—	—	2
	L				—	—	2
14	F	—			—	—	3
	L	—			—	—	3
19	F	—	—		—	—	4
	L	—			—	—	3
23	F					—	1
	L				—	—	2
28	F	—	—		—	—	4
	L	—			—	—	3
Total		8	2	0	11	12	33

Remarks: Brushed as usual; home-care instruction given in brushing and flossing

Date   9/12

Tooth no.		A	B	C	D	E	Total
4	F				—	—	2
	L				—	—	2
6	F						0
	L	—			—	—	3
14	F	—			—	—	3
	L				—	—	2
19	F	—			—	—	3
	L	—			—	—	3
23	F						0
	L	—			—	—	3
28	F				—	—	2
	L					—	1
Total		5	0	0	9	10	24

Remarks: Scored prior to treatment—reviewed flossing technique

Fig. 7-4. Use of modified Podshadley method to evaluate oral hygiene performance.

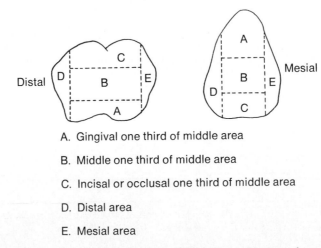

A. Gingival one third of middle area

B. Middle one third of middle area

C. Incisal or occlusal one third of middle area

D. Distal area

E. Mesial area

Fig. 7-5. Plaque scoring—the PHP method, modified. (From Martens, L., and Meskin, L.: An innovative technique for assessing oral hygiene, J. Dent. Child. **39:**12, 1972.)

uate the effectiveness of home-care methods that are being used in the program.

Repetition of this index measures change in individual behavior. In a large population the information is an indication of the amount of change in individual behavior rather than just a change in behavior of the total population. The range of change in individual performance may be used to estimate success and set goals for later in the program or in future programs.

Information about periodontal disease can also be gathered and quantified by means of a widely used index, Russell's Periodontal Index (PI)[9], or a modification of it. Russell's index assigns a numerical score to each tooth standing in the mouth and then takes an average of these values for a PI score. The range of the Russell score is from 0 (no inflammation or disease evident) to 8 (advanced destruction with loss of masticatory function), as indicated in Table 7-2. Although the criteria for the Russell examination are fairly well delineated, because of the nature of periodontal diagnostics, evaluation may be subjective. Reproducibility of scores may be more difficult for this periodontal index than for others.

As knowledge in dentistry advances, our ways of looking at dental disease change, and so must our ways of measuring the disease experience of our population. In recent years periodontists have shifted their focus of concern from pocket depth to attachment levels. Instead of using simple measurement of pocket depth as the indicator of periodontal health and disease, the loss of periodontal attachment is estimated by using a fixed point on the tooth. It is now thought that this gives a broader picture of the extent of periodontal disease. The National Institute for Dental Research sponsored a nationwide study in 1985-1986 called the National Survey of Adult Dental Health.[8] For this study an index was devised to record the loss of attachment. For this index the cervico-enamel junction (CEJ) is used as a reference point. Two

measurements are taken, the distance in millimeters from the CEJ to the free gingival margin (FGM), and from the FGM to the base of the pocket. The difference between the two measurements is *the loss of attachment,* thus:

FGM/CEJ − FGM/Pocket = Loss of attachment.

Other reasons why new indices may be developed include population shifts and changes

Table 7-2. Russell's method for scoring periodontal disease*

Russell score	Criteria for field studies
0 Negative	There is neither obvious inflammation in the gingival epithelium nor loss of function due to destruction of supporting tissues.
1 Mild gingivitis	There is an obvious area of inflammation in the free gingiva, but this area does not circumscribe the tooth.
2 Gingivitis	Inflammation completely circumscribes the tooth, but there is no apparent break in the epithelial attachment.
6 Gingivitis with pocket formation	The epithelial attachment has been broken and there is a pocket (not merely a deepened gingival crevice due to swelling in the free gingiva). There is no interference with normal masticatory function, the tooth is firm in its socket and has not drifted.
8 Advanced destruction with loss of masticatory function	The tooth may be loose, may have drifted; may sound dull on percussion with a metallic instrument or may be depressible in its socket.

From Russell, A.L.: A system of classification and scoring for prevalence surveys of periodontal disease, J. Dent. Res. **35:**350, 1956.
*When in doubt about a given score, the lesser score is assigned.

in disease experience. The fastest growing segment of our population today is our geriatric population. Because of better dental care, older patients in the United States today are far more likely to keep their teeth throughout their lives than previous generations. This demographic shift and concomitant change in health care have increased the likelihood that we will see older adults who have root caries. In order to better understand the etiology of root caries, it is necessary to study populations to determine who is at risk for root caries and to begin to formulate intervention strategies.

The Root Caries Index (RCI) is one that attempts to deal with assessing the extent of root caries experience within the context of individual risk for the disease.[6] Katz reasoned that only root surfaces that are exposed to the oral environment are at risk to develop root caries. Those root surfaces where gingival recession has not occurred cannot develop root caries and therefore should not be considered in assessing the attack rate of root caries. The Root Caries Index records these data as follows:

$$\frac{(R\text{-}D) + (R\text{-}F)}{(R\text{-}D) + (R\text{-}F) + (R\text{-}N)} \times 100 = RCI$$

where: R-D = Root surface with decay
R-F = Root surface which is filled
R-N = Sound root surface.

This index has been further refined by others to include a classification for recording root caries recurrent around a restoration.[5]

One important way of compensating for the subjectivity of diagnosis is the use of a single examiner or a limited number of examiners who have been calibrated. Calibration is a method of bringing the examiners to a unified diagnostic technique and product. This may be accomplished through examination of sample cases and careful definition of diagnostic criteria until diagnoses concur. Examiners should be checked and recalibrated periodically during a study to ensure uniformity of diagnostic technique.

Many other indices have been developed and are used in the literature. The selection of an index is largely determined by the research at hand. What should a dental health professional look for when selecting an index for his/her research?

The researcher should choose an index that addresses the specific information in which he/she is interested. For example, a PI is not a good measure for evaluation of the effects of a home-care regimen. A simpler index, such as OHI-S or PHP-M, would be more appropriate. The index should be suitable for the population. An index that uses key teeth to measure periodontal health or half-arch techniques to assess caries experience may be fine in young adult populations. In children with mixed dentitions and in geriatric populations, however, we may find that key teeth may be missing or that the attack rate of caries may be different in right versus left arch. In choosing an index we must be careful that it will provide valid estimates of disease in the population.

The data should be relatively easy to gather. A caries index requiring bitewing radiographs may be difficult to carry out in a population of rural Arkansas school children. The resultant data base may not be worth the added cost of radiographs. A mirror and explorer determination may yield information that gives an adequate indication of the caries activity in that population. Once gathered, the data should be easy to interpret. The simpler the calculations and presentation, the wider the audience on which the study can impact.

Reproducibility and reliability of data are important. Uncalibrated examiners and poorly defined examination criteria can undermine an otherwise good project.

A final consideration is the current literature. Often a study is to be compared to existing work in other populations or to baseline data gathered by another agency. If this is anticipated and comparable criteria are established, data manipulation may be kept to a minimum and validity of the comparison is enhanced.

EPIDEMIOLOGY AND THE ETIOLOGY OF DENTAL CARIES

With current scientific knowledge of the causation of dental diseases, why epidemiological surveys? Certainly needs determination is one reason, and program planning and evaluation another. The etiology of a dental disease may be so complex that the combination of factors contributing to the cause may vary greatly between populations. Thus the intervention methods well suited for one population may be totally inappropriate for another.

The etiological factors that contribute to any disease are usually divided into three categories: host, agent, and environmental factors. All factors must be present to be sufficient cause for the disease. Table 7-3 illustrates the factors usually recognized as causative in two types of dental caries.

Intervention and removal of any necessary factor may prevent all or part of the disease. Examination of a population should include an assessment of host, agent, and environmental factors that may be used to limit the disease.

A study done in Baja, Hungary, provides an interesting example of how environmental factors can influence the outcome of a disease. In 1955 baseline data were collected in kindergarten children, ages 3 to 6 years, consisting of DMFT counts stratified according to age at last birthday. In order to assess the results of improved vitamin D prophylaxis that occurred after this time, a second age-specific DMFT was done in the kindergartens in Baja in 1975.[1] Analysis of the data revealed an increase of 10.9% frequency of caries (number of children affected by caries). Intensity of caries experience (mean number of carious lesions per child) increased by 43.5%. Examiners then had to look for factors that might have brought about this unanticipated increase in dental caries. One factor that researchers discussed was the rise in annual sugar consumption from 24.4 kg per person to 37.5 kg per person. Analysis of contributing factors in a case such as this can lead to a shifting of priorities in program planning.

Worldwide, variations in host, agent, and environmental factors interact to produce a variety of dental diseases at varying rates and intensities. Cultural, genetic, geographic, and other factors all contribute to these variations. An understanding of these factors is essential if prevention and intervention are to be successful. Local customs, values, dietary habits, and hygiene differ throughout the world. Radical changes in these patterns are not achievable, even if desirable.

THE FUTURE OF DENTAL EPIDEMIOLOGY

There will be those who say that enough holes have been counted in teeth, enough plaque disclosed, and enough pockets probed; that it is

Table 7-3. Etiological factors contributing to dental caries

Disease entity	Host factors	Agent factors	Environment factors
Dental caries	Morphology (pits, fissures) Arch form (irregularities)	*Streptococcus mutans* Plaque	Nutrition Oral hygiene Fluoride
Root caries	Decreased salivary flow Gingival recession	*Actinomyces viscosus*	Nutrition Oral hygiene Toothbrush abrasion

time to get on with some good laboratory research to prevent and cure dental disease. Epidemiology provides us with data analysis, which can support and supplement biomedical research. Who is to say, after all, that the world's population is not our global laboratory?

REFERENCES

1. Bruszt, P., and others: Caries prevalence of preschool children in Baja, Hungary in 1955 and 1975, Health Serv. Rep. **87**(5):456, 1972.
2. Clune, T.W.: Prevalence of dental caries on primary and permanent teeth: a study of 8,853 school children, Rhode Island Med. J. **36**:653, 1954.
3. Gluck, G.M., and others: Dental health of Puerto Rican migrant workers, Health Serv. Rep. **87**(5):456, 1972.
4. Greene, J.C., and Vermillion, J.R.: The simplified oral hygiene index, J. Am. Dent. Assoc. **68**:7, 1964.
5. Heifetz, S.B., and others: National survey of adult dental health: diagnostic criteria for root caries, Unpublished working paper, National Institute for Dental Research, 1985.
6. Katz, R.V.: Assessing root caries in populations: the evolution of the root caries index, J. Pub. Health Dent. **40**:7, 1980.
7. Martens, L.V., and Meskin, L.H.: An innovative technique for assessing oral hygiene, J. Dent. Children **39**:12, 1972.
8. Morrison, E.C., and others: National survey of adult dental health: NIDR periodontal destruction assessment, Unpublished working paper, National Institute for Dental Research, 1985.
9. Russell, A.L.: A system of classification and scoring for prevalence surveys of periodontal disease, J. Dent. Res. **35**:350, 1956.
10. Yacavone, J.A., and Parente, A.M.: Twenty years of community water fluoridation: the prevalence of dental caries among Providence, Rhode Island, school children, J. Rhode Island State Dent. Soc. **7**:3, 1974.

CHAPTER 8

Prevention of Dental Disease

Prevention of disease is a prime objective of public health work, and one where team work is most often of great advantage.

James M. Dunning

Dentistry has traditionally functioned within the private setting, the one-on-one treatment of the patient by the dental professional. In this century, however, scientific research, technological advances, and a better understanding of the disease process have contributed to dentistry's emergence from a purely reparative art toward a preventive-oriented science. This emergence encompasses both a greater variety of practice settings and a greater reliance on auxiliary personnel to assist in the provision of services. Significant contributions to the promotion and protection of the public's oral health can now be accomplished by concurrent and cooperative efforts by the dental professional, the individual, and the community. The purpose of this chapter is to provide the future dental professionals— that is, de. *ists, dental hygienists and dental assistants, expanded-function dental auxiliaries, and dental technicians—with highlights and a brief overview of current preventive concepts and their application.

PREVENTIVE DENTISTRY DEFINED

In its broadest sense, preventive dentistry is all of dentistry and encompasses those practices by individuals and communities that affect oral health status. In this regard, preventive dentistry has been conceptualized in a number of ways. These include a sequence of levels of pre-

vention, a set of priorities, a taxonomy, and a category of services (Table 8-1).[27,64,65,66] The student should be familiar with these concepts and terms since they are used throughout the dental literature. Each of these concepts commonly looks at preventive dentistry in relation to the oral health/disease continuum. A basic division is made between the prepathogenesis and the pathogenesis stages of the disease. Major emphasis is logically placed on those services aimed at the time before the origination and development of the disease, the prepathogenesis stage.

Services directed toward the prepathogenesis stage are referred to as primary preventive services, services that prevent the initiation of disease. They are designated as services that provide health promotion and specific protection. Health promotion activities, such as providing instruction in proper plaque removal or daily toothbrushing and flossing, are designed to promote general optimum health, in this case periodontal health. Specific protection activities include services that are designed to protect against disease agents by decreasing the susceptibility of the host or by establishing barriers against agents in the environment. The ingestion of optimally fluoridated water and the application of pit and fissure sealants provide specific protection against caries.

Services directed toward the initial stages of

117

Gurlcidos4Le4Hart.....

Table 8-1. Prevention concepts and health/disease continuum

Levels of prevention	Primary	Secondary	Tertiary
Prevention concepts			
Priorities of prevention	Prevention of disease initiation	Prevention of disease progression and recurrence	Prevention of loss of function
Taxonomy of prevention	Prepathosis	Intervention	Replacement
Preventive services	Health promotion Specific protection	Early diagnosis and prompt treatment	Disability limitation Rehabilitation
Health/disease continuum	Prepathogenesis	Pathogenesis	

Modified from Dunning, J.M.: Principles of dental public health, ed. 4, Cambridge, MA, 1986, Harvard University Press; Leavell, H.R., and Clark, E.G.: Preventive medicine for the doctor in his community, ed. 3, New York, 1965, McGraw-Hill Book Co.; Lutz, B.L.: Preventive dentistry: proposal for definition of terms, J. Dent. Educ. **37:**24, 1973; and Mandel, I.: What is preventive dentistry? J. Prev. Dent. **1:**25, 1974.

disease pathogenesis are referred to as secondary preventive services, that is, those that intervene or prevent the progression and recurrence of disease. They are designated as activities that are aimed at the early diagnosis and prompt treatment of disease in order to prevent sequelae. For example, the prompt treatment of a small carious lesion will result in the prevention of extended loss of tooth structure.

Finally, services directed toward the end results of disease pathogenesis are referred to as tertiary preventive or replacement services, those that prevent loss of function. These activities provide disability limitation and rehabilitation. Prosthetic appliances and implants are included in this category.

This global perspective of preventive dentistry is based on the premise that every oral health activity implemented by the individual, the community, and/or the dental professional is targeted toward the prevention of some aspect of the health/disease continuum. This logic entails the anticipation of disease initiation and its progression or recurrence if appropriate activities are not implemented. Priority is given first to primary preventive services, followed by secondary, and then tertiary services. It is this rea-

soning and this methodical selection of priorities and implementation of health-specific and disease-specific measures that emerge from this definition of preventive dentistry.

PREVENTIVE DENTISTRY SERVICES

A multitude of preventive dentistry services that can be applied to all levels of prevention are presented in Tables 8-2 through 8-5. Services targeted toward dental caries, periodontal diseases, oral cancer, orofacial defects, malocclusion, and accidents are listed. These tables demonstrate the intricacies of the strategies that need to be taken to prevent these categories of oral diseases and disorders.

Singular efforts by the dental professional, the individual, or the community are not sufficient to attain and maintain optimum oral health because of the complexity of disease etiology. A hypothetical example related to the specific oral disease of dental caries would be an individual who practices excellent oral hygiene, has resided from birth in a community that has optimally fluoridated water, and yet who might develop dental caries on the occlusal surfaces of his/her teeth. In this example these occlusal lesions can be prevented by application of dental sealants. In

Table 8-2. Dental caries: individual, community, and dental professional preventive dentistry services

Levels of prevention	Primary		Secondary	Tertiary	
Preventive services	Health promotion	Specific protection	Early diagnosis and prompt treatment	Disability limitation	Rehabilitation
Services provided by the individual	Diet planning; demand for preventive services; periodic visits to the dental office	Appropriate use of fluoride Ingestion of sufficient fluoridated water The appropriate use of fluoride prescriptions The use of a fluoride dentifrice Oral hygiene practices	Self-examination and referral; utilization of dental services	Utilization of dental services	Utilization of dental services
Services provided by the community	Dental health education programs; promotion of research efforts; lobby efforts	Community or school water fluoridation; school fluoride mouthrinse program; school fluoride tablet program; school sealant program	Periodic screening and referral; provision of dental services	Provision of dental services	Provision of dental services
Services provided by the dental professional	Patient education; plaque control program; diet counseling; recall reinforcement; dental caries activity tests	Topical application of fluoride; fluoride supplement/rinse prescription; pit and fissure sealants	Complete exam; prompt treatment of incipient lesions; preventive resin restorations; simple restorative dentistry; pulp capping	Complex restorative dentistry; pulpotomy; root canal therapy; extractions	Removable and fixed prosthodontics; minor tooth movement; implants

Modified from Dunning, J.M.: Principles of dental public health, ed. 4, Cambridge, MA, 1986, Harvard University Press; and Mandel, I.: What is preventive dentistry? J. Prev. Dent. 1:25, 1974.

Table 8-3. Periodontal diseases: individual, community, and dental professional preventive dentistry services

Levels of prevention	Primary		Secondary	Tertiary	
Preventive	Health promotion	Specific protection	Early diagnosis and prompt treatment	Disability limitation	Rehabilitation
Services provided by the individual	Periodic visits to dental office; demand for preventive services	Oral hygiene practices	Self-examination and referral; utilization of dental services	Utilization of dental services	Utilization of dental services
Services provided by the community	Dental health education programs; promotion of research efforts; provision of oral hygiene aids; lobby efforts	Supervised school brushing programs	Periodic screening and referral; provision of dental services	Provision of dental services	Provision of dental services
Services provided by the dental professional	Patient education; plaque control program; recall reinforcement	Correction of tooth malalignment; prophylaxis	Complete examination; scaling and curettage; corrective, restorative, and occlusal services	Deep curettage; root planing; splinting; periodontal surgery; selective extractions	Removable fixed prosthodontics; minor tooth movement

Modified from Dunning, J.M.: Principles of dental public health, ed. 4, Cambridge, MA, 1986, Harvard University Press; and Mandel, I.: What is preventive dentistry? J. Prev. Dent. 1:25, 1974.

Table 8-4. Oral cancer: individual, community, and dental professional preventive dentistry services

Preventive services	Primary		Secondary	Tertiary	
Preventive services	Health promotion	Specific protection	Early diagnosis and prompt treatment	Disability limitation	Rehabilitation
Services provided by the individual	Periodic visits to dental office; demand for preventive services	Avoidance of known irritants	Self-examination and referral; utilization of dental services	Utilization of dental services	Utilization of dental services
Services provided by the community	Dental health education programs; promotion of research efforts; lobby efforts		Periodic screening and referral; provision of dental services	Provision of dental services	Provision of dental services
Services provided by the dental professional	Patient education	Removal of known irritants in oral cavity	Complete examination; biopsy; oral cytology; complete excision	Chemotherapy; radiation therapy; surgery	Maxillofacial and removable prosthodontics; plastic surgery; speech therapy; counseling

Modified from Dunning, J.M.: Principles of dental public health, ed. 4, Cambridge, MA, 1986, Harvard University Press; and Mandel, I.: What is preventive dentistry? J. Prev. Dent. **1:**25, 1974.

Table 8-5. Orofacial defects, malocclusion, accidents: individual, community, and dental professional preventive dentistry services

Levels of prevention	Primary		Secondary		Tertiary
Preventive services	Health promotion	Specific protection	Early diagnosis and prompt treatment	Disability limitation	Rehabilitation
Services provided by the individual		Use of protective devices; habit control	Utilization of dental services	Utilization of dental services	Utilization of dental services
Services provided by the community	Dental health education programs; promotion of protective garb; lobby efforts	Mouthguard program; safety of children's toys; safety of school buildings and playgrounds	Provision of dental services	Provision of dental services	Provision of dental services
Services provided by the dental professional	Patient education	Caries control; space maintainers; genetic counseling; prenatal care; parental counseling	Minor orthodontics	Major orthodontics; surgery	Maxillofacial fixed/removable prosthodontics; plastic surgery; speech therapy; counseling

Modified from Dunning, J.M.: Principles of dental public health, ed. 4, Cambridge, MA, 1986, Harvard University Press; and Mandel, I.: What is preventive dentistry? J. Prev. Dent. 1:25, 1974.

addition, coordinated, cooperative, and concurrent efforts by all three parties are needed to prevent those categories of oral diseases and disorders for which prevention therapies are known. For example, cooperative efforts aimed only at preventing dental caries and periodontal disease may result in the neglect of other categories of oral disease and disorders. The individual and community are then at risk of developing these unprevented diseases.

A survey of Tables 8-2 through 8-5 shows that most of the individual, community, and professional cooperative efforts are available at the primary prevention level. Beyond that level, the dental professional plays a greater role. At the secondary prevention level, the individual can use existing dental services and the community can fund the provision of dental services. Of course, oral diseases and disorders are rarely present at only the prepathogenesis or only the pathogenesis stage. For example, frequently two or more oral diseases may be present and at different stages on the health/disease continuum. An individual may have numerous carious lesions but not periodontal disease, or an individual may have periodontal disease in one quadrant or the oral cavity but not in any of the others. In both cases, primary, secondary, and/or tertiary preventive dental services are needed, and cooperative efforts are still required to attain oral health.

A multitude of factors affect health care delivery. Primary preventive dental services address the factors of high cost and labor maldistribution, as most are not costly and many do not require dental personnel for their implementation. However, for the delivery of health care services, regardless of whether they are primary, secondary, or tertiary services, considerations must be given to services that are affordable, available, and accessible. Health care services provided by or for the individual and the community also require complete acceptance and utilization. These factors are not always easily

attained because of variations in the interest, motivation, economic status, and, at times, political inclination of health care consumers, providers, and administrators. Also, the individual and the community may not be knowledgeable about the necessary procedures. An ideal public health measure should address all these concerns of health care delivery.

Experience with the delivery and utilization of health services has advanced a philosophy that the characteristics of an "ideal public health measure" should be: (1) of proven efficacy in the reduction of the targeted disease; (2) medically and dentally safe; (3) easily and efficiently implemented, utilizing a relatively small amount of materials, supplies, and equipment; (4) readily administered by nondental personnel; (5) attainable by the beneficiaries regardless of their socioeconomic, educational, income, and occupational status; (6) readily available and accessible to large numbers of individuals; (7) inexpensive, therefore affordable by the majority; (8) uncomplicated and easily learned by the utilizers; (9) administered with maximum acceptance on the part of the patient(s); and (10) administered with minimum compliance on the part of the patient(s).*

PRIMARY PREVENTIVE DENTISTRY SERVICES

As mentioned earlier, the main emphasis of preventive dentistry is on selecting priorities for the expenditure of efforts and resources for primary preventive services. Accordingly, the subsequent emphasis of this chapter is in this area. For purposes of brevity, this section will address only services targeted toward two of the diseases: dental caries and periodontal disease. Each service is defined and its history, disease prevention effectiveness, implementation and necessary effort, and the required patient acceptance and compliance are described. The services are presented in the following outline.

---

*See references 2, 16, 36, 52, 73, 78, 91.

I. Preventive services provided in the community
   a. Community water fluoridation
   b. School water fluoridation
   c. Fluoride supplement programs
   d. Fluoride mouthrinse programs
   e. School sealant programs
II. Preventive services provided by the dental professional
   a. Pit and fissure sealants
   b. Topical fluoride applications
   c. Plaque control programs
   d. Diet counseling
   e. Dental caries activity tests
III. Preventive services provided by the individual
   a. Fluoride dentifrices
   b. Oral hygiene practices

The "specific protection" services for dental caries (Table 8-2) and the above outline highlight the critical role of fluoride in preventive services. Fluoride effectiveness in caries reduction and its versatility of application cannot be surpassed by any other agent currently available. It can be used systemically, as in community and school water fluoridation and fluoride tablets, and topically, as in solutions, gels, mouthrinses, and dentifrices. Fluoride is most effective when incorporated into the enamel structure during tooth maturation, as in systemic utilization. Topically, it is also incorporated, but to a lesser degree, into the outermost surface of the enamel. Its presence in and on the enamel surface and in the saliva reduces the susceptibility of the tooth surface to dental caries initiation. It has its greatest impact on the smooth surfaces of the teeth and can be administered under the auspices of the community, the individual, or the dental professional.

Caries protection of the pit and fissure surfaces can be achieved through the application of dental sealants. In 1983 a National Institutes of Health (NIH) Consensus Development Conference on Dental Sealants, unanimously endorsed the placement of sealants as a highly effective and safe means of preventing pit and fissure caries.[75] Furthermore, the combined use of sealants and fluorides will provide optimum caries protection.[62] Widespread use of sealants will substantially reduce dental caries below the levels that have already been achieved by fluorides and other preventive measures enabling many adolescents to enter adulthood with caries-free dentitions.

When reading the following sections, the student should keep in mind the properties of an ideal public health measure and refer to Tables 8-2 through 8-5 to attain a relative perspective for each service. Only a few preventive dental services meet this ideal.

Preventive services provided in the community

The community-administered services discussed in this chapter involve participation of key community decision makers and the organization of large numbers of people, resources, and commitments for the purpose of preventing dental caries. Other primary preventive community-administered services exist but have not been shown to be as effective and efficient in disease reduction as the following five caries-preventive services.

Community water fluoridation. Fluoridation is the adjustment of the fluoride content of a community's water supply to an optimum concentration for the prevention of tooth decay. Caries prevalence is reduced by 50% to 65% in the permanent dentition of children who consume fluoridated water from birth.[59] Slightly lower caries reductions are seen in the primary dentition. Fluoridation also benefits adults, as seen in lower decayed, missing, filled (DMF) values, greater tooth retention, and fewer root caries.[92]

The caries-reducing benefits of fluoride in community water were discovered in the process of investigating the cause of "Colorado brown stain," a mottling and staining of the tooth enamel.[68] Studies conducted by Dr. H. Trendley Dean in areas with naturally occurring fluoride demonstrated a direct relationship between community water fluoride levels and enamel mottling (fluorosis) and an inverse relationship between dental caries and community water fluoride levels.[19,20] These studies revealed that in communities with fluoride levels at 1 part per million (ppm), reduction in dental caries experience was substantial, and only 10% of the population had dental fluorosis in the very mildest form (no cosmetic significance). In 1945 a pair of cities, Newburgh and Kingston, New York, began one of the first water fluoridation clinical trials to investigate the hypothesis that central water supplies adjusted for fluoride content were as effective in reducing caries as naturally occurring fluoride in the water. Newburgh adjusted its water supply to 1 ppm of fluoride, and Kingston maintained a natural low level of fluoride. After 10 years of fluoridation, Newburgh children who were 6 to 9 years of age showed reductions of 56.7% in dental caries experience as compared with Kingston children of the same age.[49] This, together with numerous other studies, confirmed the fact that fluoridation had the same properties whether the water supply had natural or adjusted fluoride levels of 1 ppm. This study also showed that there were no medical or dental complications associated with the ingestion of fluoridated water over a period of 10 years.

The U.S. Public Health Service recommends a concentration of 1 ppm of fluoride for optimum safety and caries reduction in a northern temperate climate.[90] In warmer climates where water ingestion is generally greater, the recommended fluoride level is lower (Table 8-6). One part per million equals one milligram (mg) of fluoride per liter, the quantity of water the average person consumes daily in a temperate climate. For maximum effectiveness, ingestion of fluoridated water should begin from birth.

Flouride is easily added to central water supplies by existing dry and solution feeders. This

Table 8-6. Fluoride levels recommended for cool and warm climates

Annual average of maximum daily air temperatures	Recommended control limits (fluoride in parts per million)		
	Lower	Optimum	Upper
50.0-53.7	.9	1.2	1.7
53.8-58.3	.8	1.1	1.5
58.4-63.8	.8	1.0	1.3
63.9-70.6	.7	.9	1.2
70.7-79.2	.7	.8	1.0
79.3-90.5	.6	.7	.8

From the U.S. Public Health Service: Drinking water standards, Washington, DC, 1962, U.S. Government Printing Office. Based on temperature data obtained for a minimum of 5 years.

equipment is maintained and the procedure is supervised by water supply personnel as part of their daily routine. There is no noticeable effect of fluoride on the odor, color, taste, hardness, or pH value of the water. The reduction in dental caries results in decreased costs of dental care for children by 50% to 60%.[92] The cost of water fluoridation varies from $0.06 to $0.80 per person per year depending on the size of the community being served.[83]

Community water fluoridation has emerged as one of the most important public health measures of the twentieth century because of: (1) its high degree of effectiveness in the reduction of dental caries in children who have consumed the water from birth, (2) its safety,[76,87] (3) its ease of implementation, and (4) its low cost.[13,85] The benefits of fluoride are conferred on the entire population serviced by the central water supply regardless of their socioeconomic or educational backgrounds and extend into the adult years. Also, no cooperative effort is required on the part of the individual other than consuming the water regularly.

Despite the abundance of data supporting the benefits of water fluoridation, considerable social and political resistance to the adoption of this method of caries prevention continues.[29,44,50,67] A few of the arguments of antifluoridationists revolve around issues such as the toxicity of fluorides, the expense involved, the alleged interference with commercial activities using water, human rights, and the lack of evidence supporting the value of fluorides. These arguments are all refuted by the evidence presented in innumerable studies.[31,32,63] However, in the United States, community water fluoridation is an issue that requires some type of governmental action for its authorization. This situation places the provision of this unparalleled public health measure into the political arena. Most states require some type of executive decision by appointed or elected officials in order to implement fluoridation. A few states have laws that require fluoridation for communities of varying sizes, and several other states require a referendum.

Approximately 130 million persons, or 55% of the nations' population, receive the benefits of either optimally adjusted or naturally fluoridated water. However, about 77 million other persons do not benefit from fluoridation because their communities do not have fluoridated water systems. Approximately 30 million persons live in areas that lack central water systems and thus cannot benefit from fluoridation.[43]

The dental profession plays a crucial role in the recommendation of community water fluoridation as a public health measure.[28] Numerous pamphlets and books have been written that address a wide variety of issues regarding the fluoridation controversy. These are included in the reference and readings lists at the end of this chapter. The dental professional should be aware of these issues, be prepared to use the vast amount of data available, and be cognizant of the political process that is often needed to implement fluoridation at the community level. In addition, it is vital to the support of fluoridation that dental professionals educate their patients on these issues.

School water fluoridation. In areas without central water supplies, the benefits of systemic fluoride may be attained with the fluoridation of school water supplies. This method is particularly suitable in rural schools where kindergarten through grade 12 may attend class in the same or adjacent buildings. In addition to the systemic effects on developing teeth, school water fluoridation, like community water fluoridation, imparts topical effects on erupted teeth.

In 1954 a school water fluoridation pilot study was initiated in St. Thomas, U.S. Virgin Islands, by the U.S. Public Health Service, Division of Dental Health. The school water was fluoridated slightly over three times the optimum indicated for the community water fluoride, since children are exposed to fluoride on school days only. After 8 years, students showed 22% less caries experience than children at schools that were not fluoridating their water supplies.[57]

Subsequent studies were done with increasing and varying amounts of fluoride. In Pike County, Kentucky, the water supplies of two schools were fluoridated at 3.3 times the optimum, and in Elk Lake, Pennsylvania, the water supply of one school was fluoridated at 4.5 times the optimum recommended level for that area. After 8 years, the children who had attended the study schools had 32.8% (Pike County) and 33.9% (Elk Lake) less caries experience than students who had attended each school prior to fluoridation.[59]

Finally, in Seagrove, North Carolina, after 8 years of school water adjusted at seven times optimum recommended fluoride level for that locale, the students showed approximately 40% difference in caries inhibition when compared to baseline examinations made before the water was adjusted.[46] Participants in the school water fluoridation studies were also examined for dental fluorosis. After 8 years of study in Seagrove, the teeth of 11 of the 134 children examined had "questionable" fluorosis, although none had definite signs of fluorosis.

One limitation of school water fluoridation is

that children are already 5 or 6 years of age when they start consuming the water and some of their teeth have already been calcified. Nevertheless, the entering schoolchild still has a substantial number of teeth that have not yet completely calcified. Study results show that teeth erupting during a school fluoridation program have almost twice the benefit as teeth that have erupted prior to the program's initiation.[46] Another limitation is that children are exposed to fluoride on school days only. To compensate for this intermittent exposure, higher levels of fluoride are recommended.

A school water fluoridation level of 4.5 times the optimum level indicated for community water fluoridation is currently recommended as effective and safe.[21] The results of the Seagrove study showed that dental caries inhibition with a fluoride level of seven times the optimum level recommended for community fluoridation was only marginally greater than a study using 4.5 times the optimum level for the same duration. The authors state that if the results of the Seagrove study are maintained, there would be no reason to use fluoride levels greater than 4.5 times the optimum community level.

The same basic equipment used in community water fluoridation is needed for school water fluoridation. The system must be regularly monitored by a trained school employee to ensure that fluoride is consistently fed into the water to the desired level. Nationally, approximately 168,000 schoolchildren in 500 schools receive fluoride through school fluoridation programs.[83] These programs are primarily in North Carolina, South Carolina, Kentucky, Indiana, and Vermont, although school fluoridation has been reported in 13 states.

Fluoride supplement programs. When it is not possible to adjust water fluoride to optimum levels either in the community or in schools, the use of dietary fluoride supplements should be initiated. Fluoride supplements can be administered at home or in community-sponsored school programs and are available in the form of tablets, lozenges, oral rinse supplements, or for younger children in drops or fluoride-vitamin preparations.

Fluoride supplements function both topically and systemically. The processes of chewing and swishing the tablet or lozenge, and swishing the liquid, topically bathe the tooth surfaces. The subsequent swallowing of the supplement leads to the systemic incorporation of fluoride into the developing tooth structure. For younger children who cannot chew, drops or fluoride-vitamin preparations can be added to beverages such as juice or water. The supplements should not be added to milk because it tends to bind fluoride ions and slow absorption.[83]

Current fluoride supplementation recommendations of the American Dental Association (ADA) and the American Academy of Pediatrics are listed in Table 8-7.[1,2] Recommended fluoride dosage schedules are adjusted according to the age of the child and the fluoride level of the water supply. It should be noted that dietary fluoride is not prescribed when the concentration of fluoride

Table 8-7. Dosage schedule for fluoride supplements recommended by the American Dental Association and the American Academy of Pediatrics

Age (years)	Concentration of fluoride in water (ppm)		
	<0.3	0.3-0.7	>0.7
0-2	0.25 mgF/day	0.0 mgF/day	0.0 mgF/day
2-3	0.50	0.25	0.0
3-13*	1.00	0.50	0.0

Data from American Academy of Pediatrics, Committee on Nutrition: Fluoride supplementation, Pediatrics **77**(5):758, 1986; and American Dental Association, Council on Dental Therapeutics: Accepted dental therapeutics, ed. 39, Chicago, The Association, 1982. (Reproduced by permission of Pediatrics.)
*The American Academy of Pediatrics recommends 16, rather than 13, as the termination age.

in drinking water is greater than 0.7 ppm, nor is it prescribed for infants up to 2 years of age when the fluoride level is 0.3 to 0.7 ppm. It is important for pediatricians and dentists to know the concentration of fluoride in the drinking water of their patients. If uncertainty exists, the local water authority or local or state health department can usually provide accurate information on the concentration of fluoride present. A careful health history should be taken prior to prescribing dietary fluoride supplements to ascertain if the child is taking other fluoride supplements such as vitamin-fluoride combinations.

Dietary fluoride supplementation can inhibit caries to a similar degree as community water fluoridation, if supplementation starts shortly after birth and is conscientiously followed.[26] Caries can be reduced by approximately 25% to 40% when dietary fluoride supplementation is begun at school age.[21]

The objective of obtaining maximum benefits for both the primary and permanent dentition suggests that supplementation should begin shortly after birth and continue until approximately 14 years of age. The ADA's Council on Dental Therapeutics has recommended the continuation of fluoride supplementation until the age of 13. The American Academy of Pediatrics recommends the continuation of supplements to age 16. It is reasoned that the maximum benefits from supplements are during the pre-eruptive phase of tooth development and that after the eruption of the second molars at ages 12 to 14, minimum additional systemic benefits can be attained. There is some evidence to indicate that when systemic supplementation is discontinued there is a gradual diminution of protection against caries. Therefore it has been recommended that after age 13 fluoride treatment should continue with various topical programs that are professionally administered or self-applied.[83]

School-based fluoride tablet programs have been successfully and widely practiced. The tablets are dispensed only on school days, about 150 to 200 days per year, and have imparted a reduction in caries of between 25% to 40%. Similar to water fluoridation, greater benefits are accrued to teeth that erupt after tablet initiation. These programs take little time from the academic schedule and are readily integrated into the daily regimen of a school. Generally a school-affiliated dentist has responsibility for prescribing the tablets, yet actual administration of the supplements can be carried out in the classroom by nondental personnel. Tablets are initiated in the earliest grade for maximum effectiveness, generally kindergarten. The average cost, if materials are purchased in bulk, ranges from $0.25 to $3.60 per child per school year.[51] Because of these characteristics, school-based fluoride tablet programs are regarded as appropriate community-effort programs.

School-based fluoride tablet programs require the initial and continued cooperation of school administrators, teachers, students, and volunteers. The reliance and need for sustained motivation, interest, and cooperation on the part of others do not allow school-based fluoride tablet programs to be regarded as an "ideal" public health activity. However, if fluoride tablets are to be considered as an alternative to water fluoridation, studies have demonstrated that their use in school programs is both effective and practical.[6,24]

Dietary fluoride supplements can also be prescribed by a pediatrician or a dentist for use at home. There is an advantage to home administration of dietary fluoride supplements since supplementation can begin shortly after birth and be given 365 days per year. However, maximum success is dependent on the sustained involvement and motivation of the parents to administer the program daily for 13 years. Continued compliance has been found to be generally poor.[60] Such results have created the incentive to implement school-based tablet programs. These programs instill a routine and schedule whereby the tablets are ingested more consistently, thus maximizing the likelihood of their effectiveness.

Prescribing fluoride supplements to expectant mothers is currently not recommended.[2] The U.S. Food and Drug Administration ruled in 1966 that the evidence did not support the advertising claim that prenatal administration of fluorides would increase the caries resistance of the child and thus banned such advertisements.[34] The efficacy of prenatal fluorides was examined at the American Dental Association's 1980 Annual Meeting, and further research is needed to prove clinical effectiveness.[53]

Fluoride mouthrinse programs. One way in which the topical benefits of fluoride may be attained is by daily, weekly, or biweekly mouthrinsing with a fluoride-containing solution. Many clinical trials have shown that rinsing daily, weekly, or biweekly with dilute solutions of fluoride will reduce the incidence of dental caries by approximately 35%.[48,56] Most of these studies have been conducted in nonfluoridated areas using a neutral sodium fluoride solution. A few studies have shown that in fluoridated areas children who rinse also benefit from the procedure.[17,25]

Mouthrinsing involves a 1 minute swishing of 10 ml of either a 0.2% solution weekly or a 0.05% solution daily. The "swishing" action ensures that the solution passes between the teeth and covers all surfaces of the teeth. The volume of the rinse depends on the age of the patient involved. An adult can easily handle up to a 15 ml rinse, whereas 10 ml is recommended for children in grades 1 through 12 and 5 ml is recommended for kindergarten children. Children below the age of 4 years often cannot control their swallowing reflexes, so this procedure is not recommended for the preschool child.[51] A 0.05% neutral sodium fluoride rinse is now available on the market without a prescription.

Daily, weekly, and biweekly schedules have been used in school-based programs.[72,85] The school classroom procedure basically involves the preparation of the appropriate amount of rinse that is put into paper cups. Each child in the class is given a cup and a napkin. At a designated signal the children take the solution into their mouths and "swish," without swallowing, for 1 minute. The children then expectorate into the paper cups, wipe their mouths with the napkin, and place the used napkins in the cups to absorb the solution. These cups are then collected in a disposable trash bag. This group procedure is recommended for up to 30 to 40 children and can be supervised by nondental personnel such as teachers, parents, or school nurses.[52] The cost of supplies to conduct a fluoride mouthrinse program ranges from $0.60 to over $1.00 per child per year.[51] Approximately 12 million U.S. children are participating in either school fluoride mouthrinse programs or fluoride tablet programs.[51] In some nonfluoridated communities, school programs administer a fluoride tablet daily and a fluoride mouthrinse weekly.

The rinsing procedure can also be implemented at home by the individual patient. This procedure is recommended for the patient who has high caries activity, has exposed root surfaces, and/or is subject to caries-promoting factors. As with the home use of fluoride supplements, the motivation of the adult patient, or of the parent if the patient is a child, is of the utmost importance to the success of this program. Compared to a school-based program, home administration is more costly and less easily monitored.

The results of the recent National Preventive Dentistry Demonstration Program (NPDDP) have created some controversy concerning the cost-effectiveness of school fluoride mouthrinsing programs. In the NPDDP, the effectiveness of regular use of fluoride mouthrinse was considerably lower than reported in other studies.[85] There was little difference between the treatment and long-term comparison groups because of the low incidence of caries in both groups. This issue was addressed in the 1984 "State of the Art

Conference on the Uses of Fluorides in Clinical Dentistry." Carlos[17] states that the extent to which fluoride mouthrinsing has contributed to the recent decline in caries prevalence among children cannot be directly established. However, since fluoride mouthrinsing clinical trials have consistently demonstrated approximately 35% protection against caries, it can be assumed that widespread use of this preventive method has contributed to caries decline. Carlos concluded that fluoride mouthrinsing is a simple, well-accepted, safe and relatively inexpensive adjunct to other methods of caries prevention, including adhesive sealants, fluoride dentifrices and perhaps community water fluoridation, and until it has been clearly demonstrated that caries incidence can be further decreased and maintained at low levels by other, simpler methods, fluoride mouthrinsing will continue to play a major role in efforts to prevent dental caries.[17]

School sealant programs. In 1983 the NIH Sealant Consensus Panel urged practitioners, dental health directors, and dental educators to incorporate the appropriate use of sealants into their practices and programs. Although dental sealants are more expensive than other primary dental caries prevention methods, their effectiveness and specificity for the surfaces shown to be the most susceptible to dental caries and least responsive to other preventive measures provides strong justification for their inclusion in community-based programs.[21]

The use of sealants in individual office settings and in community programs will be discussed in Section Two.

Preventive services provided by the dental professional

The dental profession has the responsibility of supporting, initiating, implementing, and reinforcing community efforts; encouraging, directing, and reinforcing individual efforts; and providing, directly or indirectly, services aimed at preventing oral diseases and promoting oral health. This is a major task, and the following services are some of the primary preventive services that can be provided by the dental professional.

Pit and fissure sealants. The application of dental sealants is a highly effective means of preventing pit and fissure caries, the predominant form of caries in U.S. children. Recent national studies indicate that the prevalence of smooth surface caries is declining, caused mainly by the beneficial effect of water fluoridation and other methods of fluoride delivery.[10,74]

Although the use of topical and systemic fluorides does provide some protection to the occlusal surfaces, the smooth surfaces generally derive greater benefit from fluorides. As a consequence, since the introduction of fluorides, there has been a relative increase in the proportion of occlusal surface caries, with respect to the total caries experience.

In 1971-1974, caries on the smooth proximal surfaces accounted for 24% of caries in 5- to 17-year-old children; this percentage decreased to 16% in 1979-1980 (Table 8-8).[7,84] Conversely, the percentage of occlusal, buccal, and lingual caries increased, so that 84% of all caries in school children now occurs on the occlusal, buccal, and lingual surfaces.[7,84] These surfaces are generally regarded as pit and fissure surfaces. In addition, although caries of all tooth surface types is lower in fluoridated communities compared to nonfluoridated communities, the same high proportion of pit and fissure caries exists in both communities (Table 8-9).[7,84] Therefore caries prevention measures must include the pits and fissures.

A sealant that is firmly bonded to the enamel surface isolates the pits and fissures from the caries-producing conditions of the oral environment. There have been many attempts to reduce the rate of occlusal caries, including the elimination of pits and fissures through the physical removal of sound tooth structure. In 1955 Buonocore developed an acid etching technique

Table 8-8. Relative (percentage) distribution of caries in specific tooth surfaces of U.S. school children

Surface	NCHS* survey 1971-74	NIDR† survey 1979-80
Proximal	24%	16%
Buccolingual	27%	30%
Occlusal	49%	54%
TOTAL	100%	100%

Data from Bohannan, H.M.: Caries distribution and the case for sealants, J. Public Health Dent. **43**(3):200, 1983; Ripa, L.W., and others: Preventing pit and fissure caries; a guide to sealant use, Massachusetts Department of Public Health, Massachusetts Health Research Institute, Inc., Boston, 1986.
*National Center for Health Statistics.
†National Institute of Dental Research.

Table 8-9. Relative (percentage) distribution of caries in specific tooth surfaces of U.S. school children from optimally fluoridated and fluoride-deficient communities

Surface	Fluoridated communities	Fluoride-deficient communities
Proximal	6%	11%
Buccolingual	40%	35%
Occlusal	54%	54%

Data from Bohannan, H.M.: Caries distribution and the case for sealants, J. Public Health Dent. **43**(3):200, 1983; and Ripa, L.W., and others: Preventing pit and fissure caries: a guide to sealant use, Massachusetts Department of Public Health/Massachusetts Health Research Institute, Inc., Boston, 1986.

that enabled plastic resins to adhere to tooth surfaces.[11] By applying a weak solution of phosphoric acid to the tooth surface, enamel mineral is removed both from the surface and within the surface to a depth of approximately 25 microns. This exposes the enamel pores and increases the surface area of the enamel. The result is a bonding surface that is at least 100 times stronger than a nonetched surface.[86]

After the enamel is etched with phosphoric acid, the tooth can retain resins such as those used in anterior proximal restorations. The sealant resin is applied in a viscous, liquid state and enters the micropores, which have been enlarged through acid conditioning. The resin then hardens by using either a self-hardening catalyst, or by applying a light source. The portion of the hardened resins that have penetrated and filled the pores are called *tags*.[41]

Sealants are classified according to the method in which they are cured or hardened. The first generation ultraviolet light-cured sealants helped establish the clinical effectiveness of pit and fissure sealants in preventive dentistry.[84]

Chemically cured sealants have surpassed the retention and thus caries reduction results achieved by ultraviolet light-cured sealants. A rate of 85% complete retention can be expected 1 year after placement of chemically cured sealant, with at least 50% retention after 5 years.[81] One study reported 66% retention of chemically cured sealant after 7 years.[70] Visible light–cured sealants are the most recent type of marketed sealant. Since several brands of visible light–cured sealants have been granted acceptance or provisional acceptance by the ADA, retention comparisons between visible light–cured and chemically cured sealants will be possible in a few years.[84]

The effectiveness of sealants appears equal whether applied by dentists or dental auxiliaries, provided that they have received adequate training (sealant application by dental hygienists and assistants is now permitted by at least 32 state practice acts).[39,80] The operator's technique is the primary determinant of a sealant's retention and, ideally, sealants should be applied with an operator-assistant team.[84] Maintenance of a dry field and avoidance of contamination of the etched surfaces by saliva are paramount. Isolation of the site can be achieved by using a rubber dam or a cottonroll/retraction system.

The selected tooth surface is first cleansed by a flouride-free prophylaxis paste and then conditioned with a phosphoric acid etchant for 60 seconds. This conditioning etches the enamel surface to produce a marked increase in surface area, which renders it more receptive to bonding. The surface is then washed with water and dried with compressed air. Upon drying, a properly etched surface has a frosty appearance in contrast to the glossy appearance of unetched enamel. Using an applicator, the sealant is then flowed over the dried etched surface. The sealant is allowed to polymerize either by itself or by exposure to visible light. The sealant must remain uncontaminated and undisturbed until it is cured to hardness. Setting time will vary according to the sealant used. The teeth are inspected visually and with an explorer after polymerization has occurred. If coverage of the pits and fissures is incomplete, or if there is a surface air bubble, more sealant can be applied if the tooth has remained uncontaminated. Otherwise, the tooth must be re-etched for 10 seconds and washed and dried before additional sealant is added.[38,71]

Questions regarding the possibility of caries progression beneath properly applied sealants have been answered by clinical studies. The ability of bacteria to survive under sealants is impaired because ingested carbohydrates cannot reach them. Several investigators have found that the number of bacteria in deliberately sealed carious lesions decreases dramatically with time.[37,69] Negative or reduced bacterial cultures have been found several years after sealing, and no studies have identified caries progression beneath an intact sealant.[38,71]

The placement of sealants should be limited to previously unrestored pits and fissures. First and second permanent molars are at highest risk to caries and thus will benefit the most from the application of sealant.[8] However, the occlusal surfaces of first and second primary molars, first

and second premolars, and third permanent molars are all potential sites for sealants. Sealants should also be considered where other pits and fissures exist, such as the lingual surfaces of permanent maxillary incisors, buccal surfaces of mandibular molars, and lingual surfaces of maxillary molars.[84]

When selecting teeth for sealants in individual patient care programs, the clinical considerations are occlusal morphology and caries pattern.[84] Teeth with steep cuspal inclines and deep fissures, in contrast to those with shallow cusps and highly coalesced pits and fissures, are ideal choices for sealant application. If the occlusal morphology places the tooth at higher risk to caries, the tooth should be sealed as soon as it has erupted sufficiently to allow adequate isolation for the sealant application procedure. If a patient has many proximal lesions, sealants may still be placed on the occlusal surfaces of caries-free teeth; however, fluoride therapy should be initiated in order to protect the proximal surfaces.

A surface is questionable when the explorer tip sticks in the tooth surface but other evidence of caries, such as softness at the tip of the explorer or a white halo of undermining demineralization, is not present.[84] A restoration is not appropriate since the questionable surface has not been diagnosed as carious; however, the area has an increased susceptibility to caries since bacteria and food particles are easily trapped. A questionable surface is an ideal surface for sealing because the sealant will prevent the surface from progressing from a questionable to a carious status.[84] If an occasional carious lesion is sealed, the lesion will arrest.[37,38,69,71]

Patient education materials may be obtained from the American Dental Association, the American Society of Dentistry for Children, and the National Institute of Dental Research to help inform parents about the nature, safety, and effectiveness of sealants. The materials can be used with a chair-side demonstration of pits and fissures along with an explanation of the atraumatic nature of the sealant procedure. Parents and children should be reminded that sealants are one part of a total caries preventive program that also includes fluorides, brushing and flossing, and a proper diet.

Based upon its 1982 survey of general practitioners and selected specialists in the United States, the American Dental Association reported the average fees for sealant application to be $11.14 per tooth and $27.77 per quadrant.[12] Office costs for sealants can be minimized by delegating the sealant application procedure to auxiliary personnel where legally permitted, selecting sealant products that have the greatest retention rates, and performing a meticulous application procedure to maximize the sealant's retention.[84]

Sealants can also be practically incorporated into community-sponsored preventive dentistry programs for school children. Large-scale school-based sealant programs have been conducted in New Mexico, Tennessee, Minnesota, Kentucky, and Massachussetts.[14,15,22,42]

Since resources are limited, the criteria for participant selection in community sealant programs should incorporate a targeted approach. Criteria for participation in community sealant programs have been recommended and include four levels: community, school, individual, and tooth.[84] Communities with the highest caries levels will receive the greatest benefits from school-based preventive dentistry programs, and both fluorides and sealants should be considered. However, the absence of a fluoride program should not preclude the initiation of a sealant program alone (Table 8-9).[84] Lower socioeconomic schools have more children with higher caries incidence and lower treatment levels than higher socioeconomic schools.[8] These schools can be identified by the large number of children on subsidized lunch programs. Grade level must also be considered. Given the objective of providing maximum benefit to newly

erupted permanent first and second molars, it has been suggested that children in second and sixth grades be included in school sealant programs. These children can be recalled in third and seventh grades to have teeth sealed that were insufficiently erupted in the previous year. Tooth morphology must also be considered. Teeth with deep pits and fissures that tend to catch the point of the explorer should be sealed. Well-coalesced pits and fissures with wide, easily cleaned grooves need not be sealed.

The personnel, schedule, and physical resources of each school must be considered when implementing a school sealant program. Children can walk or be transported to a nearby health department or health center dental clinic to receive their sealant applications. Also portable dental equipment that is sturdy yet light enough to be transported between schools can be used. Portable equipment needed for a school sealant program includes a patient dental chair, operator and assistant stools, extra-oral light, portable dental unit with high-volume suction, air compressor, dryer and filter, dry heat sterilizer, a visible curing unit, and protective glasses if visible light–cured sealant is used. Both chemically cured and visible light–cured sealants are being used in school sealant programs.

Often school sealant programs are conducted with a team approach. Initially, a dentist and recorder using a mirror and explorer examine teeth for caries on the children who returned positive consent forms (in some states dental hygienists are legally permitted to conduct the examinations). The status of the proximal surfaces must be considered. However, the diagnosis of proximal decay is unlikely since newly erupted teeth are targeted in this approach and thus have not been in the mouth long enough to develop proximal decay. Radiographs are not recommended in school sealant programs. Sealant applications should begin as soon as possible following the screening sessions.

Ideally the sealant application sessions are

conducted by an operator and an assistant. Application of sealants by a dental auxiliary is the least costly method of providing this service (if permitted by the state's practice act). The assistant assists chairside during the sealant applications, facilitates the flow of children between the classroom and the treatment room, and maintains records. During the next school year, children who were treated the previous year should be recalled and examined. Sealant should be reapplied to surfaces that have lost their sealant and to eligible teeth that were insufficiently erupted in the previous year.

The cost of sealants in New Mexico's dental disease prevention program was found to be $1.59 per tooth and $7.41 per child.[14] These figures are comparable to the reported costs of $1.20 per tooth and $8.00 per child in a community sealant program in Tennessee.[42] Other programs have reported higher costs ranging from $12.39 to $36.41 per child.[15,23] Factors such as program size, location, available resources, and salary differentials contribute to this variation. Starting a community-based sealant program will require the acquisition of new funds or the diversion of support from other components of an existing preventive dentistry program. However, given the fact that dental caries is now primarily a disease of the pits and fissures is strong justification for the inclusion of sealants in public health programs.

Topical fluoride applications. The previously discussed modes of fluoride administration are conducted by either the community or the individual. The involvement of the dental professional, if at all, is as a supervisor or as a prescriber of the service. Three agents are available for use in professionally applied topical fluoride treatments: sodium fluoride, stannous fluoride, and acidulated phosphate fluoride. These compounds exhibit a similar range of clinical effectiveness when applied to the permanent teeth of children residing in fluoride-deficient areas. Clinical studies in fluoride deficient areas have demonstrated caries reductions of 30% to 40% by the application of solutions of 2% sodium fluoride and 8% stannous fluoride and solutions or gels of acidulated phosphate fluoride containing 1.23% fluoride ion.[35,55,61,79] Topical fluoride applications are effective in the primary dentition; however, caries reductions are not as great as those reported for permanent teeth.[79]

The routine use of professionally applied topical fluoride is not recommended for patients who are lifelong residents of optimally fluoridated communities.[79] The need for professionally applied topical fluoride should be individualized. Patients with higher caries activity are candidates for professional topical fluoride therapy. Because of their low cost-benefit ratio, professionally applied topical fluorides are not recommended for use in school-based preventive dentistry programs. In an attempt to reduce the cost of providing these fluoride preparations and improve their availability, these preparations have been tested through self-application procedures. Fluoride solutions and gels can be self-applied in the home. They are prescribed by the dentist for home use for patients with severe or rampant caries, in areas with or without fluoridated water. Studies with self-applied solutions and gels have shown this procedure to be effective when the treatment is frequently repeated and its use is supervised.[30]

The choice of a topically applied fluoride compound will depend on factors of clinical convenience and cost, patient acceptance, and lack of undesirable side effects, since these compounds are similar in their degrees of clinical effectiveness.[79] Table 8-10 compares and contrasts the three professionally applied topical fluoride solutions. Sodium fluoride requires the least number of total visits; however, the requirement of four visits a few days apart makes it difficult to fit into a private practice schedule. The stannous fluoride application procedure better adapts to the private practice 6-month recall schedule, but the bitter taste, staining proper-

Table 8-10. A comparison of three topical fluorides

	Sodium fluoride (NaF)	Stannous fluoride (SnF₂)	Acidulated phosphate-fluoride (APF)
Concentration	0.2% NaF	0.8% SnF$_2$	1.23% APF
Recommended patients	Children at ages 3, 7, 11, and 13; adults with active caries; adults with exposed root surfaces	Children ages 2 through 12; adults with active caries; adults with exposed root surfaces	Children ages 2 through 15; adults with active caries; adults with exposed root surfaces
Recommended practice	Series of four applications at ages specified above; total of 16 applications	Single application at 6 to 12 month intervals; total of 28 applications	Single application at 6 to 12 month intervals; total of 28 applications
Advantages	Acceptable taste; stable if stored in plastic container and refrigerated	Procedure frequency complies with 6-month recall appointment schedule	Acceptable taste; stable if stored in plastic container; procedure frequency complies with 6-months recall appointment schedule
Disadvantages	Procedures requires four visits to the dentist in a relatively short period of time	Bitter metallic taste; needs to be freshly prepared for each application; not stable in solution; may cause reversible tissue irritations and staining at margins of restorations	None

ties, and instability of SnF$_2$ in solution make it less desirable than the other two solutions. Acidulated phosphate fluoride has none of the disadvantages of either sodium fluoride or stannous fluoride, and its recommended frequency of application makes it the most widely used professionally applied topical solution.

Traditionally, a dental prophylaxis has always preceded the application of topical fluoride. Prophylaxis pastes with and without fluoride have been used for this purpose. Neither type of paste has been found to influence fluoride uptake by the enamel or the degree of caries inhibition. Thus the routine use of a prophylaxis prior to topical fluoride application is no longer recommended.[82] In addition, data from clinical studies do not support the use of fluoride

containing prophylaxis paste alone as an effective caries preventive regimen.[82] However, a thorough prophylaxis may abrade a thin layer of enamel, resulting in the loss of fluoride from the tooth surface. Thus a fluoride prophylaxis paste is indicated in an attempt to replenish the fluoride removed by abrasion during the prophylaxis.

Plaque control. Regular and thorough removal of plaque by dentists and dental hygienists can successfully control periodontal disease. However, success depends on a high level of personal oral hygiene practiced by the patient. Although it is known that the bacterial agents that cause dental caries are harbored in dental plaque, mechanical plaque removal and oral hygiene procedures alone have not proven effective in caries prevention.[4]

Educational programs aimed at refining the plaque removing oral hygiene practices of individual patients can be conducted. A large number of plaque control programs have been described for use in a dental office setting. Chapter 9 describes several plaque control programs that have been conducted for large groups. The outcomes of these studies show that plaque indices are significantly improved at the end of a program; however, long-range evaluations of these programs have shown a relapse in individual plaque scores to almost baseline levels.

Diet counseling. Diet counseling for the dental patient has been recommended as a procedure to be used in the prevention of dental caries. It entails an assessment of the foods a patient selects and eats. Particular emphasis is placed on the ingestion of refined carbohydrates. Studies have demonstrated that the oral environment can be altered by modification in the frequency and consistency of these carbohydrates.[40] The philosophical base of diet counseling has been to assist the patient in recognizing these foods and to make adjustments in accordance with factors that affect the individual's food selection. The suggested modifications are decided on by the patient with guidance from the dental professional. Investigations undertaken by Bowen and colleagues to assess the cariogenicity potential of foodstuffs will greatly enhance the diet counseling procedure.[9]

There are several approaches used in dietary counseling in the dental setting. The most widely used method is that of Nizel. This method adheres to the concept of normal dietary prescriptions with modifications made that focus on the patient's problems and are agreeable to the patient. Nizel suggests three rules to adopt when recommending dietary modifications: (1) the prescribed diet should vary from the normal diet as little as possible; (2) the diet should meet the body's requirements for the essential nutrients as generously as the diseased condition can tolerate it (for example, rampant dental caries might require a reduction in carbohydrates); and (3) the prescribed diet should take into consideration and accommodate the patient's likes and dislikes, food habits, and other environmental factors as long as it does not interfere with the therapeutic or prophylactic objectives.[77]

Dietary modifications and counseling have their greatest success with patients who are motivated and cooperative. Also important are the rapport established with the patients, the degree of individualization given to the patients and their problems, and the opportunity for follow-up assessment. Dietary counseling is highly recommended for patients experiencing a high caries rate or for adolescents, who as a group appear to experience a high caries attack rate. The decision to offer this service to all patients rests with the dental professional and the philosophy of the practice; however, dietary counseling may be more efficient if it is directed to caries-prone patients rather than directed to all patients.

Diet counseling is best undertaken in private practices or clinics. It has been taught in elementary schools, but very little impact in terms of disease reduction has been noted. The information presented in a classroom or large group situation cannot focus on an individual's personal dental problems or provide individualized follow-up assessment. Consequently, diet counseling is not recommended for public health programs.

Dental caries activity tests. Dental caries activity tests, often referred to as susceptibility tests, are primarily used as motivational tools in the dental practice setting to educate the patient to develop habits conducive to the prevention of dental caries. These tests do not predict future caries susceptibility but provide data about the current status of microorganisms in the oral environment. Generally the tests measure the acid-forming ability of microorganisms present in saliva on oral tissue. Tests are available that examine the pH of dental plaque, the acid-buffering capacity of saliva, and the metabolic activity of acidogenic bacteria. Numerous caries activity tests exist and the selection of the appropriate test is based on clinical judgement.

Detailed information pertaining to numerous caries activity tests can be found in most preventive dentistry or clinical practice textbooks. The use of caries activity tests is feasible in the private practice setting. However, these would not be as effective in public health programs because they require individualized patient follow-up and are time-consuming and costly.

Preventive services provided by the individual

The individual plays a pivotal role in the prevention of his/her oral disease and promotion of his/her oral health. A look at the preventive dental services show that the individual acts as both a health care consumer and as a provider. As a consumer, the individual consents to, uses, and demands services. As a provider, the individual self-applies services. To be effective in this dual capacity, the individual needs first to be informed as to when, where, why, and how to obtain or apply the necessary services. Second, the individual needs to actively pursue, use, and demand those services. Individually administered services include diet planning and control, self-examination, proper use of fluoride prescriptions, oral hygiene practices, and use of fluoride dentifrices. The latter two services are described in this section. However, emphasis must be placed on the individual's key role in the appropriate use of fluoride supplements and mouthrinses in a home-based program where these caries preventive modalities are not available elsewhere. These services are described in Section One.

Fluoride dentifrices. Of major interest in preventive dental services is the use of fluoride dentifrices. These products represent a vehicle for topically applying fluoride to the tooth surfaces that is inexpensive, requires no special instructions for use, and can be obtained without a prescription. Caries reductions of 15% to 30% have been reported following the regular home use of fluoride dentifrices containing stannous, sodium, or sodium monofluorophosphate in non-fluoridated communities, regardless of brushing technique and daily frequency of brushing.[45,47] Dentists should recommend that their patients use a fluoride dentifrice that has been accepted by the ADA Council on Dental Therapeutics. Approximately 80% of toothpastes sold in the United States are now ADA accepted fluoride-containing toothpastes.

A 1-gram ribbon of dentifrice contains approximately 1 mg fluoride for most fluoride dentifrices marketed in the United States. Young children should use only small amounts of fluoride-containing dentifrices and should be supervised to ensure that they expectorate and do not swallow the dentifrice. Children under age 5 who habitually swallow dentifrice could develop fluorosis on the permanent incisors.[83] Older children should also be reminded not to swallow the dentifrice.

It has been suggested that school-based brushing programs using fluoride dentifrices would not confer additional protection beyond home usage.[58] The cost-benefit ratio of these school-based programs would render them less beneficial than other alternatives. Therefore home use of these products should be promoted; efforts directed at continued usage for current users, and recommended use for nonusers would be a feasible expenditure of labor and funds.

Oral hygiene practices. Oral hygiene practices involve the thorough daily removal of dental plaque and other debris by toothbrushing and flossing, although mouthrinsing and use of auxiliary aids are also included. The relationship between oral hygiene and periodontal disease has been both statistically and experimentally established. It has been demonstrated that the withholding of hygiene procedures results in the onset of initial gingivitis in mouths that may not have registered periodontal problems in the past. However, once adequate hygiene procedures are reinstated, the gingivitis score decreases.[85] The studies conducted in the area of dental caries and oral hygiene have demonstrated inconclusive results. Presently, definitive statements about such an association cannot be made. However, data do exist that tend to substantiate the association of dental plaque in both dental caries and periodontal disease. A cause and effect relationship has not been established, but plaque can be identified as one of the factors involved in these dental diseases.

Toothbrushing. The present concept of toothbrushing evolved around the beginning of the nineteenth century. Prior to that time, wooden "chewsticks" or a form of toothpicks were used after meals. Apparently the idea of brushing after meals has not changed from earlier times. A once-a-day, albeit thorough, brushing and flossing are minimally sufficient to disorganize and remove plaque; although brushing after every meal is recommended. Flossing is recommended on a once-a-day basis.

The purpose of toothbrushing is to remove the bacterial plaque from the tooth surfaces without injuring the soft tissues. The recommended method of toothbrushing is determined by the individual patient's manual dexterity, motivation, and oral hygiene. Table 8-11 summarizes the commonly recommended toothbrushing methods.* There are two basic directions in which a brush is used: horizontal and vertical. Horizontal brushing utilizes the ends of the bristles, and vertical brushing uses the sides of the bristles. Any other directions in which a brush is used represents a modification of the basic approach. Historically, the most frequently used and recommended method was the roll method. With modifications in technique as an attempt to cleanse the sulcular areas, the Bass method was developed and has become one of the more frequently suggested techniques (see Table 8-11).

*See references 5, 18, 33, 88, and 89.

There are a variety of toothbrushes on the market. These brushes vary in the size of the head of the brush and the length and angulation of the handle. There is no definitive empirical research that statistically or clinically indicates the superiority of one toothbrush over another; however, recent studies have explored this area further. There also has been no evidence to indicate that the powered toothbrush is superior to the hand brush. The type of toothbrush to recommend primarily depends on the individual patient's manual dexterity. The patient's preference and level of oral hygiene are also to be considered. Currently, a soft, multitufted, round-bristled brush is recommended.

Flossing. Toothbrushing can effectively remove plaque from the smooth tooth surfaces, sulcus, and a portion of the interproximal areas. The procedure of flossing is concerned with the removal of plaque in the remainder of the interproximal areas. There are basically two kinds of floss: waxed and unwaxed. The kind to use is a matter of preference. Again, no evidence is available concerning the superiority of waxed as compared with unwaxed floss. Also dental tape is available, which is a ribbonlike aid. The tape is used like the floss but is much larger and bulkier. Generally floss is recommended over tape because of the ease in usage.

Floss is used by wrapping portions around the index fingers of each hand and by using the thumbs. It is then gently guided interproximally between the contact areas to just beneath the gingival margin where it is lightly wrapped around the contact surface and the buccal and lingual surfaces. With a back and forth motion, it is guided coronally along one interproximal surface to the contact point and then repeated on the adjacent interproximal tooth surface in the same interproximal space. This procedure is carried out throughout the mouth. For those areas that do not allow the floss to pass through the contact points, a variety of floss threaders are available for use on the needle and thread principle. The threader is slipped lingually beneath the contact

Table 8-11. Summary of methods for brushing

Method	Bristle placement	Motion	Advantages and disadvantages
Bass[5]	Topically, toward gingiva into the gingival sulcus at a 45-degree angle to the tooth surface	Very short back and forth vibratory; bristle ends remain in the sulcus	Removes plaque from cervical areas and sulcus; small area covered at one time; good gingival stimulation; easily learned
Charters[18]	Coronally, with sides of bristles half on teeth and half on gingiva at a 45-degree angle to tooth surface	Small circular with bristle ends remaining stationary	Cleans interproximal but bristly ends do not go into sulcus; hard to learn; hard to position brush in some areas of mouth; excellent gingival stimulation
Fones[33]	Perpendicular to tooth surface	On buccal a wide circular movement to include gingiva and tooth surfaces; on lingual a back and forth horizontal motion.	Interproximal areas not cleaned; easy to learn; possible trauma to gingiva
Intrasulcular[18]	Apically, toward gingiva into gingival sulcus at 45-degree angle to the tooth surface or toward gingiva, almost parallel to long axis of the teeth	On buccal and lingual—a very short back and forth vibratory or very small circular motion, with bristle tips remaining in the sulcus, then the brush head is rolled toward the occlusal surface; occlusal surfaces cleaned with horizontal stroke	Good interproximal and gingival cleaning; good gingival stimulation; requires moderate dexterity
Physiological[88]	Coronally and then along and over the tooth surfaces and gingiva	Gentle sweeping that starts on teeth progressing over gingiva	Is "physiological"; mimics the passage of food over the gingiva; does not emphasize the interproximal or sulcus areas
Roll	Apically, nearly parallel to the tooth surface then in and over tooth surfaces	On buccal and lingual slight inward pressure at first, then a rolling of the head to sweep bristles over the gingiva and tooth surfaces; occlusal cleaned with horizontal stroke	Does not clean sulcus area; easy to learn; requires moderate dexterity; good gingival stimulation
Stillman[89]	On buccal and lingual—apically at an oblique angle to the long axis of the tooth; ends rest on gingiva and cervical portion of tooth; on occlusal—perpendicular to occlusal surface	On buccal and lingual—slight rotary with bristle ends stationary; on occlusal—horizontal	Excellent gingival stimulation; bristles do not enter sulcus; interproximal area is cleaned when occlusal surfaces are brushed; moderate dexterity required

point and the floss is then employed as usual. Such aids are helpful when the areas beneath a bridge require cleansing.

Mouthrinsing. The purpose of mouthrinsing can be either therapeutic or cosmetic. Therapeutically a mouthwash can be defined as a medicated liquid used for cleansing the oral cavity or treating diseased states of the oral tissues, such as the previously discussed fluoride-containing mouthrinse. General usage of mouthwashes, however, has been for cosmetic purposes. In this endeavor they have been used to remove gross amounts of food debris or to improve mouth odors.

Implications alluding to the germicidal effects of mouthwashes should, however, be regarded skeptically. Mouthwashes that claim to prevent or inhibit the growth of specific bacteria have not been tested in terms of long-range effects. Studies need to be developed that examine the effect on other microflora of the oral cavity. Several agents (for example, chlorhexidine) have been examined that appear to function as de-plaquing mouthwashes; in essence they prevent the formation of dental plaque. To date these mouthwashes are not on the U.S. market because of side effects such as staining of the teeth and tongue.

Auxiliary home care aids. There are a multitude of aids that serve as adjuncts to the basic oral hygiene practices of toothbrushing, flossing, and mouthrinsing. The use of adjunctive aids such as an oral irrigating device frequently addresses a particular problem, which may stem from the difficulty on the part of the patient to reach certain areas or which is specific to the oral condition of the patient. However, these aids only serve as auxiliary services to the basic home care services.

PREVENTIVE DENTISTRY TREATMENT PLANNING

The preceding discussions briefly described some of the currently available primary preventive dental services. The probability of attaining a disease-free oral status is enhanced when any of the previously described efforts are combined. Because a solo method of eliminating dental caries or periodontal diseases is not yet known, the discriminatory selection of multiple preventive services may result in greater disease reductions. The success of each service alone, or of several services together, is dependent on appropriate selection and implementation. This is true of all primary, secondary, and tertiary services. The dental profession must be able to recognize the individual patient's or the community's needs and problems and strategically select the most effective and efficient measures and solutions. This is one of the critical skills in dentistry and involves the process of preventive dentistry treatment planning.

The preventive dentistry treatment planning process is shown in Fig. 8-1. The first step, problem recognition, has two parts. It entails recognition both by the dental professional and the patient or community. Dual recognition enhances future compliance and acceptance on the part of the patient or community to the professional's recommendations. Problem definition, the next step, helps to delineate the scope of the problem and, eventually, the type of measures to be implemented. This is followed by the collection of information relevant to the problem. The nature of this data is dependent on what is already known about the disease, its etiology, and prevention. After sufficient data have been gathered, it is necessary to organize the data for analysis and finally for interpretation or diagnosis. Based on the "scientific" process, a preventive treatment plan is developed with credence given to: (1) the goals to be achieved necessitating a consideration of what level of effectiveness is desired, (2) the ranking of the goals given, (3) the constraints of labor, cost, time, patient acceptance, and patient compliance, and (4) an evaluation of the treatment plan, the achievement of the goals, and the planning process itself.

Problem recognition
by patient/community/dental professional

Problem definition
nature/extent/severity/significance

Problem data collection
host/agent/environmental factors

Problem data analysis

Problem interpretation and presentation

Treatment plan(s) development
goals/priorities/minimum tasks/labor requirements/
cost requirements/constraints identified

Fig. 8-1. Preventive dentistry treatment planning process.

In an attempt to apply the preventive dentistry treatment planning process in conjunction with an understanding of the disease process and how to prevent it, the following model cases are presented. These two case studies describe situations that may be encountered in professional life.

Case study 1. A 24-year-old male who has just completed radiation therapy for head and neck cancer comes to you with a case of rampant caries on the cervical portion of most of his teeth. He is distressed and has not been eating regular meals, and complains of a "dry mouth." Aesthetics and the retention of his own teeth are very important to this young man, who perceives this problem as monumental at the time you see him.

Case study 2. A recent dental screening of all second-grade children in your community by the U.S. Public Health Service revealed a decayed, missing, filled teeth (DMFT) index value twice that for the same age group on a national basis. No one in your community seems to be

aware of the severity of the problem. The fluoride water level in your community is 0.3 ppm. There are three dentists and two dental hygienists in this community of 13,000 individuals.

In both cases, initially the problem must be recognized. Whether it is dental caries or oral cancer, the problem's existence must be acknowledged in a similar fashion by both the dentist and the patient(s). This may seem simple; however, the recognition of dental caries as a problem varies from individual to individual and from community to community. The dentist should ask, "Who perceives the problem as I do, and who perceives it differently?" The 24-year-old man in Case 1 is definitely concerned. However, the community in Case 2 may be unaware and/or unable to afford to remedy the problem. Information, grievances, and preferences should be elicited from those experiencing the problem. If this first step is not accomplished, then the success of any treatment is in question.

Once recognized, the problem should be defined. Problem definition involves the preliminary investigation of all aspects of the problem. What is the nature of the patient's or the community's dental caries? Is this a new or an existing problem? What is the extent of the caries? Are the caries on the smooth surfaces only, on the occlusal surfaces only, or everywhere? Are all of the children in the community affected or only those in certain residential areas? If so, why? How severe are the caries? Does the patient have rampant or arrested caries? Are the anterior teeth as affected as the posterior teeth? Is there an aesthetic problem? Will root canal treatment be indicated? What are the individual components of the community's DMFT? Finally, what is the significance of the problem on the community's list of problems and on the patient's priority list of problems? This process may alert the dentist to certain areas that warrant further examination.

The third step is problem data collection. This involves the careful scrutiny of the host, agent, and environmental factors. What are the host factors? Who are the affected persons? What is their age, sex, race, and socioeconomic, educational, and political background? How long have they lived in the area? Have they had any recent major changes, for example, medical, nutritional, social? What are the agent factors? Are the plaque indices high? Are the individuals maintaining their oral hygiene practices? What are the environmental factors? What is the fluoride level of the water supply? Are there any dental programs offered in the schools? How many dentists and dental hygienists are there in the area? This process further delineates the investigative process and identifies the areas of concern.

The data collected are then analyzed and interpreted, and the most appropriate treatment plan is developed. All the information gathered in the preceding steps is appropriately filtered and analyzed. The interpretation of the situation is dependent on this analysis and should be supplemented by both an evaluation of the literature and of the dentist's and the patient's (or the community's) previous experience with similar problems. The evaluation of the literature should investigate what has been done in similar cases, how effective it has been, who has performed the treatment, and the reasons for the successes or failures.

A thorough evaluation of these factors, together with an assessment of the goals of the patient and the community for dealing with this problem, will help the dentist develop a strategy—a preventive dentistry treatment plan. Priorities are established and questions such as the following are addressed. What are the minimum tasks required for success? What are the labor requirements, both the dentist's and the patient's, to carry out the treatment under consideration? What are the costs? What are the constraints and limitations? How will the treatment plan(s) cope with these barriers? Finally,

can the tasks be executed, the labor be mobilized, the costs be met, and the limitations and constraints be managed? In light of the preferred goals and priorities, two or three feasible treatment plans may need to be developed and considered.

The treatment plan for the 24-year-old man would involve professional efforts, including patient education regarding the dental effects of his radiation therapy, dental sealants, a rigid plaque control program, and restorative treatment for the carious lesions. His individual efforts would include stringent oral hygiene practices and daily self-application of either a fluoride rinse or topical fluoride gel. A dentist, a dental auxiliary, and the patient would comprise the essential labor. There are no present constraints in this case study. However, the lack of money for treatment, lack of manual dexterity, and lack of motivation may be some of the limitations in similar cases. With the latter constraints, alternate treatment plans beyond the minimum essentials need to be developed. The issue of motivation is a difficult one. In this case it is not a problem; in order to prevent it from becoming a problem, constant reinforcement is needed. Finally, as a crucial part of this preventive treatment plan, the physicians should be consulted and informed of the dentist's interest in helping with the appropriate dental treatment of future patients prior to their beginning radiation therapy.

The treatment plan for the second-grade children in the community would involve the implementation of some type of systemic fluoride program, such as community water fluoridation or school water fluoridation, or a school fluoride supplement and/or mouthrinse program. Sealants should also be considered. The fulfillment of this treatment plan would require the utilization of community organization principles, close participation with local government personnel, and actions necessary to institute these programs. A fluoride program is indicated because of the cost-benefit ratio, dental caries prevention effectiveness of fluoride, and the lack of dental personnel in the community. Sealants are indicated because of their effectiveness and specificity for the surfaces shown to be the most vulnerable to caries. In the community described there are limited numbers of dental professionals, and the application of sealants by dental auxiliaries would be highly desirable. Needed restorative services must be provided by dentists.

The development of any preventive dentistry treatment plan entails the careful selection of the measures or services to be provided. Multiple factors must be considered in this selection. These might include the effectiveness of the service in the prevention of disease initiation, progression, or recurrence; the cost of providing the service; the dental and nondental labor needed to administer the service; the ease of implementation of the service; the compliance required on the part of the patient or the community; and the acceptance of the service by the patient or the community. These considerations apply whether the plan is directed toward the individual patient or toward the community.

SUMMARY

This chapter attempts to highlight several preventive dentistry services and concepts. Preventive dentistry is defined as all of dentistry and all of the practices of individuals and communities that affect the oral health status. The importance of cooperative efforts between the individual, the community, and the dental profession in order to attain and maintain optimum oral health is stressed. These efforts are presented in Tables 8-2 through 8-5, which display all preventive dentistry services that can be applied to all levels of prevention for several categories of oral diseases and disorders. Selected primary preventive dental services are briefly described. Finally, the preventive dentistry treatment planning process is discussed and illustrated.

REFERENCES

1. American Academy of Pediatrics, Committee on Nutrition: Fluoride supplementation, Pediatrics 77(5): 758, 1986.
2. American Dental Association, Council on Dental Therapeutics: Accepted dental therapeutics, ed. 39, Chicago, 1982, The Association.
3. American Public Health Association: Review of the national preventive dentistry demonstration program, Am. J. Public Health 76(4):434, 1986.
4. Andlow, R.J.: Oral hygiene and dental caries: a review, Int. Dent. J. 28:1, March 1978.
5. Bass, C.C.: An effective method of personal hygiene, J. La. State Med. Soc. 106:100, 1954.
6. Binder, K., Driscoll, W., and Schutzmannsky, G.: Caries-preventive fluoride tablet programs, Caries Res. 12(suppl. 1):22, 1978.
7. Bohannan, H.M.: Caries distribution and the case for sealants, J. Public Health Dent. 43(3):200, 1983.
8. Bohannan, H.M., and others: Indications for sealant use in a community-based preventive dentistry program, J. Dent. Educ. 48:(suppl. 2):45, 1984.
9. Bowen, W.H., and others: A method to assess cariogenic potential of foodstuffs, J. Am. Dent. Assoc. 100(5):677, 1980.
10. Brunelle, J.A., and Carlos, J.P.: Changes in the prevalence of dental caries in U.S. school children, J. Dent. Res. 61(special issue):1346, 1982.
11. Buonocore, M.G.: A simple method of increasing the adhesion of acrylic filling materials to enamel surfaces, J. Dent. Res. 43:849, 1955.
12. Bureau of Economic and Behavioral Research: Dental fees charged by general practitioners and selected specialists in the United States, 1982, J. Am. Dent. Assoc. 108:83, 1984.
13. Burt, B.A., editor: The relative efficiency of methods of caries prevention in dental public health, Proceedings of a conference at The University of Michigan, June 6-8, 1978.
14. Calderone, J.J., and Mueller, L.A.: The cost of sealant application in a state dental disease prevention program, J. Public Health Dent. 43:249, 1983.
15. Callanen, V.A., and others: Developing a sealant program: the Massachusetts approach, J. Public Health Dent. 46:141, 1986.
16. Carlos, J.P., editor: Prevention and oral health, DHEW Pub. No. (NIH) 74-707, Washington, D.C., 1973, U.S. Government Printing Office.
17. Carlos, J.P.: Fluoride mouthrinses. In Wei, S., editor: Clinical uses of fluorides: a state of the art conference on the uses of fluorides in clinical dentistry, Philadelphia, 1985, Lea & Febiger.

18. Charters, W.J.: Proper home care of the mouth, J. Periodontal. **19**:136, 1948.
19. Dean, H.T., and Elvove, E.: Studies on the minimal threshold of the dental signs of chronic endemic fluorosis (mottled enamel), Public Health Rep. **50**:1719, 1935.
20. Dean, H.T., Arnold, F.A., and Elvove, E.: Domestic water and dental caries. V. Additional studies on the relation of fluoride domestic waters to dental caries experience in 4,425 white children, aged 12 to 14 years, of 13 cities in 4 states, Public Health Rep. **57**:1155, 1942.
21. Dental caries prevention in primary care projects, U.S. Department of Health and Human Services, Public Health Service, Jan. 1985.
22. Disney, J.A.: Personnel and equipment considerations for a community-based sealant program, J. Dent. Educ. **48**(suppl. 2):75, 1984.
23. Doherty, N.J., and Powell, A.E.: Clinical field trial to assess the cost-effectiveness of various caries preventive agents. Final report of contract No. I DE 52449. NIDR, NIH, Bethesda, MD, 1980.
24. Driscoll, W.S., Heifetz, S.B., and Brunelle, J.A.: Treatment and post treatment effects of chewable fluoride tablets on dental caries: findings after 7½ years, J. Am. Dent. Assoc. **99**:817, Nov 1979.
25. Driscoll, W.S., and others: Caries-preventive effects of daily and weekly fluoride mouthrinsing in a fluoridated community: final results after 30 months, J. Am. Dent. Assoc. **105**:1010, 1982.
26. Driscoll, W.S.: What we know and don't know about dietary fluoride supplements—the research basis, ASDC J. Dent. Child. **52**(4):259, 1985.
27. Dunning, J.M.: Principles of dental public health, ed. 4, Cambridge, MA, 1986, Harvard University Press.
28. Easley, M.W., and others, editors: Fluoridation: litigation and changing public policy, Proceedings of a workshop at the University of Michigan, Aug. 9-10, 1983.
29. Easley, M.W.: The new antifluoridationists: who are they and how do they operate? J. Public Health Dent. **45**(3): 133, 1985.
30. Englander, H.R., and others: Clinical anticaries effects of repeated topical sodium fluoride applications by mouthpieces, J. Am. Dent. Assoc. **75**:638, 1967.
31. Erickson, J.D.: Water fluoridation and congenital malformations: no association, J. Am. Dent. Assoc. **93**:981, 1976.
32. Erickson, J.D.: Mortality in selected cities with fluoridated and nonfluoridated water supplies, N. Engl. J. Med. **298**:1112, 1978.
33. Fones, A.C.: Mouth hygiene: a textbook for dental hygienists, Philadelphia, 1934, Lea & Febiger.
34. Food and Drug Administration: Statements of general policy or interpretation, oral prenatal drugs containing fluorides for human use, Federal Register 31(204):13537, 1966.
35. Galagan, D.J., and Knutson, J.W.: The effect of topically applied fluorides on dental caries experience. V. Report of findings with two, four, and six applications of sodium fluoride and of lead fluoride, Public Health Rep. **62**: 1477, 1947.
36. Glossary of evaluative terms in public health, Am. J. Public Health **60**:1546, 1970.
37. Going, R.E., and others: The viability of microorganisms in carious lesions five years after covering with a fissure sealant, J. Am. Dent. Assoc. **97**(9): 455, 1978.
38. Going, R.E.: Sealant effect on incipient caries, enamel maturation, and future caries susceptibility, J. Dent. Educ. **48**(suppl. 2):35, 1984.
39. Groll, L.S.: Training and educational needs in pit and fissure sealant application for graduate dental personnel: continuing education and certification courses, J. Dent. Educ. **48**(suppl. 2):66, 1984.
40. Gustafsson, B.E., and others: The Vipeholm dental caries study: effect of different levels of carbohydrate intake on caries activity in 436 individuals observed for five years, Acta Odontol. Scand. **11**:232, 1954.
41. Gwinnett, A.J.: The search for an ideal sealant. In Viewpoints of preventive dentistry: the role of pit and fissure sealants, Johnson and Johnson Co., Woodbridge, N.J., 1978, Medical Education Dynamics.
42. Hardison, J.R.: The use of pit-and-fissure sealants in community public health programs in Tennessee, J. Public Health Dent. 43:233-1983.
43. Harvey, G.: Centers for Disease Control, Center for Prevention Services, Dental Disease Prevention Activity, Personal communication, Oct. 1986.
44. Hastreiter, R.J.: Fluoridation conflict: a history and conceptual basis, J. Am. Dent. Assoc. **106**:468, April 1983.
45. Heifetz, S.B, and Horowitz, H.S.: Fluoride dentifrices. In Newbrun, E., editor: Fluorides and dental caries, ed. 2, Springfield, IL, 1975, Charles C Thomas, Publisher.
46. Heifetz, S.B., Horowitz, H.S., and Driscoll, W.S.: Effect of school water fluoridation on dental caries: results in Seagrove, North Carolina, after eight years, J. Am. Dent. Assoc. **97**:193, 1978.
47. Heifetz, S.B.: Cost effectiveness of topically applied fluorides. In Burt, B.A., editor: The relative efficiency of methods of caries prevention in dental public health, Ann Arbor, MI, 1978, The University of Michigan.
48. Heifetz, S.B., and others: A comparison of the anticaries effectiveness of daily and weekly rinsing with sodium fluoride: final results after three years, Pediatr. Dent. **4**:300, 1982.
49. Hilleboe, H.E., and others: Newburgh-Kingston caries-fluoride study: final report, J. Am. Dent. Assoc. **52**:290, 1956.
50. Holloway, P.J.: Public attitudes to fluoridation, Royal Soc. Health J. **97**:58, 1977.
51. Horowitz, A.M.: Preventing tooth decay: a guide for im-

plementing self-applied fluorides in school settings, U.S. Department of Health and Human Services, NIH Pub. No. 82-1196, Dec. 1981.

52. Horowitz, H.S.: The prevention of dental caries by mouthrinsing with solutions of neutral sodium fluoride, Int. Dent. J. **135**:353, 1973.

53. Horowitz, H.S., moderator: Perspectives on the use of prenatal fluorides: a symposium, Presented at the annual session of the American Dental Association, New Orleans, LA, Oct. 1980, ASDC J. Dent. Child. **48**:102, March-April, 1981.

54. Horowitz, H.S.: The potential of fluorides and sealants to deal with problems of dental decay, Pediatr. Dent. **4**(4):286, 1982.

55. Horowitz, H.S., and Doyle, J.: The effect of dental caries on topically applied acidulated phosphate-fluoride: results after three years, J. Am. Dent. Assoc. **82**:359, 1971.

56. Horowitz, H.S., Creighton, W.E., and McClendon, B.J.: The effect on human dental caries of weekly rinsing with a sodium fluoride mouthwash, Arch. Oral Biol. **16**:609, 1971.

57. Horowitz, H.S., Law, F.E., and Pritzker, T.: Effect of school water fluoridation on dental caries, St. Thomas, Virgin Islands, Public Health Rep. **80**:381, 1965.

58. Horowitz, H.S., and others: Evaluation of a stannous fluoride dentifrice for use in dental public health programs, basic findings, J. Am. Dent. Assoc. **72**:408, 1966.

59. Horowitz, H.S., and others: School fluoridation studies in Elk Lake, Pennsylvania, and Pike County, Kentucky: results after eight years, Am. J. Public Health **58**:2240, 1968.

60. Katz, S., McDonald, J.L., and Stookey, G.K.: Preventive dentistry in action, Upper Montclair, NJ, 1976, Dental Control Products Publishing.

61. Knutson, J.W., Armstrong, W.D., and Feldman, F.M.: The effect of topically applied sodium fluoride on dental caries experience: IV. Report of findings with two, four, and six applications, Public Health Rep. **62**:425, 1947.

62. Koop, C.E.: Dental sealants, J. Public Health Dent. **44**:126, 1984.

63. Lang, P.: Analyzing selected criticisms of water fluoridation, J. Cand. Dent. Assoc. **47**:3, 1981.

64. Leavell, H.R., and Clark, E.G.: Preventive medicine for the doctor in his community, ed. 3, New York, 1965, McGraw-Hill Book Co.

65. Lutz, B.L.: Preventive dentistry: proposal for definition of terms, J. Dent. Educ. **37**:24, 1973.

66. Mandel, I.D.: What is preventive dentistry? J. Prev. Dent. **1**:25, 1974.

67. Margolis, F.J., and Cohen, S.N.: Successful and unsuccessful experiences in combating the antifluoridationists, Pediatrics **76**(1):113, 1985.

68. McKay, F.S.: Mottled enamel: fundamental problem in dentistry, Dent. Cosmos **67**:847, 1925.

69. Mertz-Fairhurst, E.J., and others: Clinical progress of sealed and unsealed caries. I. Depth changes in bacterial counts, J. Prosthet. Dent. **42**(5):521, 1979.

70. Mertz-Fairhurst, E.J., and others: A comparative clinical study of two pit and fissure sealants: 7-year results in Augusta, GA, J. Am. Dent. Assoc. **109**:252, 1984.

71. Mertz-Fairhurst, E.J., Schuster, G.S., and Fairhurst, C.W.: Arresting caries by sealants: results of a clinical study, J. Am. Dent. Assoc. **112**(2):194, 1986.

72. Miller, A.J., and Brunelle, J.A.: A summary of the NIDR community caries prevention demonstration program, J. Am. Dent. Assoc. **107**:265, 1983.

73. Myers, B.A., editor: A guide to medical care administration, Vol. 1, Concepts and principles, Washington, D.C., 1975, American Public Health Association.

74. National Caries Program, National Institute of Dental Research: The prevalence of dental caries in United States children, 1979-1980, The National Dental Caries Prevalence Survey, U.S. Department of Health and Human Services, NIH Pub. No. 82-2245, Dec. 1981.

75. National Institutes of Health: Dental sealants in the prevention of tooth decay, Consensus Development Conference Statement, Vol. 4, No. 11, U.S. Department of Health and Human Services, Public Health Service.

76. Newbrun, R.: The safety of water fluoridation, J. Am. Dent. Assoc. **94**:301, 1977.

77. Nizel, A.E.: Nutrition in preventive dentistry: science and practice, Philadelphia, 1981, W.B. Saunders Co.

78. Richards, N.D.: Utilization of dental services. In Richards, N.D., and Cohen, L.K., editors: Social sciences and dentistry: a critical bibliography, London, 1971, Federation Dentaire Internationale.

79. Ripa, L.W.: Professionally (operator) applied topical fluoride therapy: a critique, Clin. Prevent. Dent. **4**(3):3, 1982.

80. Ripa, L.W.: Sealants: training and educational needs for dental students and dental auxiliary students, J. Dent. Educ. **48**(suppl. 2):60, 1984.

81. Ripa, L.W.: The current status of pit and fissure sealants: a review, Can. Dent. Assoc. J. **5**:367, 1985.

82. Ripa, L.W.: The roles of prophylaxes and dental prophylaxis pastes in caries prevention. In Wei, S., editor: Clinical uses of fluorides, Philadelphia, 1985, Lea & Febiger.

83. Ripa, L.: A guide to the use of fluorides for the prevention of dental caries, J. Am. Dent. Assoc. **113**(3):502, 1986.

84. Ripa, L.W., and others: Preventing pit and fissure caries: a guide to sealant use, Boston, MA, 1986, Department of Public Health/Massachusetts Health Research Institute, Inc.

85. Robert Wood Johnson Foundation: Preventing tooth decay: results from a four-year national study, Special report no. 2, Princeton, NJ, 1983, The Foundation.

86. Silverstone, L.M.: Fissure sealants: the enamel resin interface, J. Public Health Dent. **43**(3):205, 1983.
87. Smith, F.A.: Safety of water fluoridation, J. Am. Dent. Assoc. **65**:598, 1962.
88. Smith, T.S.: Anatomic and physiologic conditions governing the use of the toothbrush, J. Am. Dent. Assoc. **27**:874, 1940.
89. Stillman, P.R.: A philosophy of the treatment of periodontal disease, Dent. Dig. **38**:315, 1932.
90. U.S. Public Health Service, Public Health Service drinking water standards 1962, P.H.S. Pub. No. 956, Washington, D.C., 1962, Government Printing Office.
91. World Health Organization: Statistical indicators for the planning and evaluation of public health programs, Technical report series, No. 472, Geneva, 1971, The Organization.
92. Young, W.O., Striffler, D.F., and Burt, B.A.: The prevention and control of dental caries: fluoridation. In Striffler, D.F., Young, W.O., and Burt, B.A., editors: Dentistry, dental practice and the community, Philadelphia, 1983, W.B. Saunders Co.

ADDITIONAL READINGS

Aasenden, R., and Peebles, T.C.: Effects of fluoride supplementation from birth on deciduous and permanent teeth, Arch. Oral Biol. **19**:321, April 1974.

American Society of Dentistry for Children and the American Academy of Pedodontics: Rationale and guidelines for pit and fissure sealants, Pediatr. Dent. **5**:89, 1983.

Axelsson, P., Lindhe, J., and Waseby, J.: The effect of various plaque control measures on gingivitis and caries in school-children, Community Dent. Oral Epidemiol. **4**:232, Nov. 1976.

Bell, R.M., and others: Treatment effects in the national preventive dentistry demonstration program, Rand Corporation, No. R-3072-RWJ, Santa Monica, CA, 1984.

Berry, E.A., III, and others: An evaluation of lenses designed to block light emitted by light-curing units, J. Am. Dent. Assoc. **112**:70, 1986.

Binder, K., Driscoll, W.S., and Schutzmannsky, G.: Caries-preventive fluoride tablet programs, Caries Res. **12**(suppl. 1):22, 1978.

Birkeland, J.M., and Torell, P.: Caries preventive fluoride mouthrinses, Caries Res. **12**(suppl. 1): 38, 1978.

Bowen, R.L.: Composite and sealant resins—past, present and future, Pediatr. Dent. **4**:10, 1982.

Burt, B.A.: The future of the caries decline, J. Public Health Dent. **45**(4):261, 1986.

Burt, B.A., Berman, D.S., and Silverstone, L.M.: Sealant retention and effects on occlusal caries after 2 years in a public program, Community Dent. Oral Epidemiol. **5**:15, 1977.

Council on Dental Research: Cost-effectiveness of sealants in private practice and standards for use in prepaid dental care, J. Am. Dent. Assoc. **110**:103, 1985.

Council on Dental Therapeutics: Accepted dental therapeutics, Chicago, 1982, American Dental Association.

Dean, H.T., and others: Studies on mass control of dental caries through fluoridation of the public water supply, Public Health Rep. **65**:1403, Oct. 27, 1950.

Driscoll, W.S.: Review of clinical research on prenatal fluorides, J. Dent. Child. **48**:109, March-April 1981.

Edlund, S.A.: Factors affecting the cost of fissure sealants: a dental insurer's perspective, J. Public Health Dent. **46**(3):113, 1986.

Erickson, J.D.: Mortality in selected cities with fluoridated and nonfluoridated water supplies, N. Engl. J. Med. **298**:112, May 18, 1978.

Forrester, D.J., and Schulz, E.M., editors: International workshop on fluorides and dental caries reductions, Baltimore, 1974, University of Maryland Press.

Frazier, P. Jean: Fluoridation: a review of social research, J. Public Health Dent. **40**:214, Summer 1980.

Frazier, P.J., and Horowitz, A.M.: Priorities in planning and evaluating community oral health programs: family and community health, J. Health Promotion and Maintenance **3**:103, Nov. 1980.

Gish, C.W., and others: Self-application of fluoride as a community preventive measure: rationale, procedures, and three-year results, J. Am. Dent. Assoc. **90**:388, Feb. 1975.

Handelman, S.L., and others: Clinical radiographic evaluation of sealed carious and sound tooth surfaces, J. Am. Dent. Assoc. **113**:751, Nov. 1986.

Heifetz, S.B., and others: Combined anticariogenic effect of fluoride gel-trays and fluoride mouthrinsing in an optimally fluoridated community, Clin. Prevent. Dent. **6**:21, Jan.-Feb. 1979.

Heifetz, S.B., Meyers, R., and Kingman, A.: A comparison of the anticaries effectiveness of daily and weekly rinsing with sodium fluoride solutions: findings after two years, Pediatr. Dent. **3**:17, 1980.

Hormati, A.A., Fuller, J.L., and Denehy, G.E.: Effects of contamination and mechanical disturbances on the quality of acid-etched enamel, J. Am. Dent. Assoc. **100**:34, 1980.

Horowitz, H.S., and Heifetz, S.B.: Clinical tests of dentifrices, Pharmacol. Ther. Dent. **2**:235, 1975.

Horowitz, H.S., Heifetz, S.B., and Law, F.E.: Effect of school water fluoridation on dental caries: final results in Elk Lake, Pennsylvania, after 12 years, J. Am. Dent. Assoc. **84**:832, 1972.

Horowitz, A.M., and Horowitz, H.S.: School-based fluoride programs: a critique, J. Prevent. Dent. **6**:89, April 1980.

Isman, R.: Fluoridation: strategies for success, Am. J. Public Health **71**:717, July 1981.

Jensen, O.E., Handelman, S.L., and Perez-Diez, F.: Occlusal wear of four pit and fissure sealants over two years, Pediatr. Dent. **7**:23, 1985.

Knutson, J.W.: Water fluoridation after 25 years, J. Am. Dent. Assoc. **80**:765, April 1970.

Kunzel, W.: The cost and economic consequences of water fluoridation, Caries Res. **8**(suppl. 1):28, 1974.

Leske, G.S., Pollard, S., and Cons, N.: The effectiveness of dental hygienist teams in applying a pit and fissure sealant, J. Prevent. Dent. **3**(2):33, 1976.

Mellberg, J.R., Peterson, J.K., and Nicholson, C.R.: Fluoride uptake and caries inhibition from self-application of an acidulated phosphate-fluoride prophylaxis paste, Caries Res. **8**:52, 1974.

Miers, J.C., and Jensen, M.E.: Management of the questionable carious fissure: invasive vs noninvasive techniques, J. Am. Dent. Assoc. **108**:64, 1984.

National Institutes of Health: dental sealants in the prevention of tooth decay, Consensus Development Conference Proceedings, Bethesda, M.D., Dec. 5-7, 1983, J. Dent. Educ. **48**:1(supple. 2), 1984.

Newbrun, E.: Cariology, San Francisco, 1977, University of California Press.

Randolf, P.M., and Dennison, C.I.: Diet, nutrition, and dentistry, St. Louis, 1981, The C.V. Mosby Co.

Reeves, T.G.: Water fluoridation: a manual for engineers and technicians, U.S. Department of Health and Human Services, Centers for Disease Control, 1985.

Richardson, A.S.: Parental participation in the administration of fluoride supplements, Can. J. Public Health **50**:508, 1967.

Richardson, J.L.: Mechanical plaque control: a review of the literature, J. Am. Soc. Prevent. Dent. **5**:24, 1975.

Ripa, L.W., Leske, G.S., and Sposato, A.: The surface specific caries pattern of participants in a school-based fluoride mouthrinsing program with implications for the use of sealants, J. Public Health Dent. **45**:90, 1985.

Rock, W.P., and Bradnock, G.: Effect of operator variability and patient age on the retention of fissure sealant resin: 3 year results, Community Dent. Oral Epidemiol. **9**:207, 1981.

Schlesinger, E.R., and others: Newburgh-Kingston caries-fluorine study. XIII. Pediatric findings after ten years, J. Am. Dent. Assoc. **52**:296, March 1956.

Simonsen, R.J.: Preventive resin restorations: three-year results, J. Am. Dent. Assoc. **100**:535, 1980.

Stamm, J.S., and Banting, D.W.: Comparison of root caries prevalence in adults with lifelong residence in fluoridated and non-fluoridated communities (abstract), J. Dent. Res. **59**(Spec. issue A): 405, March 1980.

Szwejda, L.F.: Fluorides in community programs: a study for four years of the cariostatic effects of prophylactic pastes, rinses, and applications of various fluorides, J. Public Health Dent. **32**:110, 1972.

Szwejda, L.F.: Fluorides in community programs: a study of four years of various fluorides applied topically to the teeth of children in fluoridated communities, J. Public Health Dent. **35**:25, 1972.

Wei, S.H.Y., editor: National Symposium on Dental Nutrition: An update on nutrition, diet, cariogenicity of foods and preventive dentistry, Sept. 6-8, 1978, University of Iowa.

Wei, S.H.Y., editor: Clinical uses of fluorides: a state of the art conference on the uses of fluorides in clinical dentistry, Philadelphia, 1985, Lea & Febiger.

SECTION FOUR

COMMUNITY DENTAL PROGRAMS

In 1965, departments of community dentistry responded to President Johnson's "War on Poverty" with new dental programs. Although community-based programs existed long before this time, new impetus was given to these programs with the advent of increased federal funding. This section deals with organized community programs: how they are developed, how effective they are, and the role of the consumer.

Chapter 9 describes programs designed to provide health information or change behavior—dental health education programs. It documents the degree of success of various programs and suggests types of programs that are cost effective.

Chapter 10, on planning community programs, introduces the planning process and involves the student in the case study of a community project. The multitude of pitfalls in the path of the prospective health planner are clearly documented. Methods to effect meaningful change are examined and a step-by-step formula for a successful project is provided.

CHAPTER 9

Dental Health Education

Dental health education for the community is a process that informs, motivates, and helps persons to adopt and maintain health practices and life-styles, advocates environmental changes as needed to facilitate this goal, and conducts professional training and research to the same end.* Health education programs are not isolated events but are educational aspects of any curative, preventive, or promotional health activity. Comprehension of the multifactorial variables in dental disease and their interaction has increased the emphasis now placed on the educational process to assist in achieving desired health outcomes.

It has been well documented in dentistry and other health areas that correct health information or knowledge alone do not necessarily lead to desirable health behaviors.† Both internal and external variables influence whether or not an individual or community will comply with recommended disease prevention, health maintenance, and/or health promotion procedures. The dental health educator must weigh these variables in relation to clinical and behavioral research findings when designing a community program that will be effective in achieving long-term results.

Knowledge of program planning and community organization is thus essential, and skill

development in these areas must be incorporated into the professional preparation of the dentist and dental hygienist. To date, however, development of these skills has received little attention. Recently the American Dental Hygienists Association (ADHA) responded to the growing role of the dental hygienist by developing several self study courses and monographs to foster professional development. The Block Drug Company provided partial funding to the ADHA to support this endeavor. Two of the self-study courses may be particularly helpful for dental professionals with a keen interest in community-based programs catering to the general population, as well as special subgroups within the population. They are: (1) The Dental Health Consultant in Community Based Programs,[5] and (2) Dental Hygiene Care of the Special Needs Patient.[6]

Most professional training is spent on learning specific technical procedures and working with patients on a one-to-one basis. In this situation individual patient motivation is the primary objective of dental health education and unfortunately comprises only a small component of the overall treatment plan. Ideally, this relationship allows the dental practitioner to tailor the preventive prescription to each individual patient's needs, and the patient can identify his/her own short- and long-term dental health goals. Through this process, the dental professional is able to help those patients susceptible to prevention to begin to, if they do not already, internalize the value of good oral health and practice preventive measures. Chambers, however, has

---

*Modified from the definition of consumer health education adopted by the 1975 NIH Fogarty International Center and American College of Preventive Medicine Task Force on Consumer Health Education.
†See references 10, 13, 52, 71, and 72.

concluded that there is strong evidence suggesting that only a limited number of Americans are susceptible to a program of controlling plaque in the home and that a principal factor suppressing this number is that health is not a general habit of living supported by deep-seated values.[10] The role of health educator becomes an essential component in the management of dental disease and in having patients assume responsibility for their own oral health maintenance.

In most cases the same skills that were developed in working with patients on a one-to-one basis are carried over to the community setting. As a result, community dental health programs are usually conducted in much the same manner as individual patient education. Specific educational efforts focus on presenting dental health information and on trying to change an individual's attitudes and behaviors with regard to oral hygiene habits and diet rather than on emphasizing an organized community approach to prevention and control of disease. Emphasis is placed on the correct brushing and flossing techniques to help prevent, or at least control, periodontal disease and on nutritional counseling, sealants, and fluoride therapy for caries control.

Success of these primary health promotion endeavors relies on the individual's development of specific skills and their incorporation into the person's life-style to reduce the prevalence of caries and periodontal disease. This popular approach to disease prevention *alone*, however, has experienced limited success in reducing oral disease and is questioned as being an appropriate focus for public health education.* Utilizing Winslow's definition of dental public health—the science and art of preventing and controlling dental disease and promoting dental health through organized community efforts†—an alternative approach focusing on

*See references 23, 29, 40, 42, 49, 61, and 62.
†Winslow, C.E.A.: The untilled field of public health, Mod. Med. 2:183, 1920.

individual behavior change would be to target health education efforts to community leaders, as suggested by Frazier.[20] This approach would redirect the educational processes to the selection of prevention and control programs that operate at the community level and do not require daily compliance on the part of the individual.

The purpose of this chapter is to present an overview of the current concepts in dental health education and to discuss the transition in educational activities from the traditional approach to current and suggested approaches. By examining three ongoing community programs and examples of other organized community efforts, the student should be able to determine which program goals are appropriate for public health education and possible ways to best accomplish those goals. In addition, areas of recent and recommended educational research will be high-lighted. We hope that previously held beliefs will be challenged and that the extent, complexity, and importance of community dental health education will be better understood.

BASIC CONCEPTS OF DENTAL HEALTH EDUCATION

The content and methodology of health education are derived from the fields of medicine and public health and from the physical, biological, social, and behavioral sciences. Certain concepts and theories developed in these fields have influenced the efforts and practices of health educators. In the area of dental health education, many of the proved theories of behavioral scientists have been either neglected, forgotten, or unaccepted. Given that the goal of dental health education is the prevention and control of dental disease, it would seem apparent that organized efforts aimed at achieving this goal should adhere to the proved theories and concepts relevant to health education activities.

A theory central to all others, since it influences all subsequent activities, is the belief that behavior is learned by individuals, not merely transmitted by one person to another.[71] How individuals learn certain behavior is a complex process that varies with each person. One person may learn a certain dental behavior from a dentist in a one-to-one educational encounter while another person may not. Research has shown that a fundamental error in many dental health education activities is the assumption that increasing a patient's dental health knowledge will help change dental care behavior. This approach, based on a *cognitive learning model*, assumes the following sequence:

Knowledge → Attitude → Behavior change

If this relationship were true, every dental health education program that increased the participants' level of dental knowledge would have resulted in a behavioral change that improved their oral health status over a long period of time. To date, no evaluation of a dental health education program has produced such results.*

An error commonly made with this cognitive approach occurs when the educator fails to assess the learner's level of knowledge before the educational encounter and treats the individual as if he/she were void of any knowlege or past experiences at all. As Yacovone notes, it is important to realize "that the person is already 'behaving' when we encounter him—maybe not as we would like him to, but 'behaving'."[71] In order to successfully influence a person's behavior through health education activities, an understanding of the dynamics of behavior is paramount.

A person's behavior is the result of both internal and external forces. One's beliefs, attitudes, interests, values, needs, motives, expectations, perceptions, and biological factors plus the influence of family, peer groups, and the mass media shape and affect one's actions.[38] Socioeconomic factors such as occupation, education, and income have also been shown to strongly influence dental health practices and should be considered in designing and implementing health education strategies. The interaction of these forces has been illustrated in a dynamic model developed by Young[72] (Fig. 9-1). Considering this model, it becomes evident that a straight-line relationship between the educator's efforts and the learner's behavior does not usually exist as is often assumed. In order to develop an effective dental health education program, the educator must be aware of the interaction of all the forces on the learner. The educator must first assess the learner or learners in order to develop and implement a rational educational program that will result in a sustained behavior change.

A second approach to the educational process is based on a *behavioral learning model*. Realizing that the cognitive approach does not result in developing and sustaining desired behavior practices, this methodology relies on changing the learner's behavior through prescribed activities that present the appropriate skills, behavior, and knowledge with the hope that the desired attitudes will follow. Programs now focus on having students participate in learning brushing and flossing skills as opposed to just having the teacher demonstrate or lecture on the technique. To be truly effective, the educator must assess each learner in order to prescribe activities that are compatible with that learner's life-style. Students will differ in psychomotor development and their oral hygiene practices. In some cases it may not be necessary or desirable to try to change a student's behavior. Once this assessment is completed and the appropriate preventive regimen prescribed when necessary, the learner must be motivated to practice these activities on a daily basis.

Four factors that influence whether or not an individual practices these preventive dental procedures have been identified in research conducted by Rosenstock and later by Kegeles[34,35,54] (1) the individual must feel he/

*See references 10, 13, 49, 52, 57, 71, and 72.

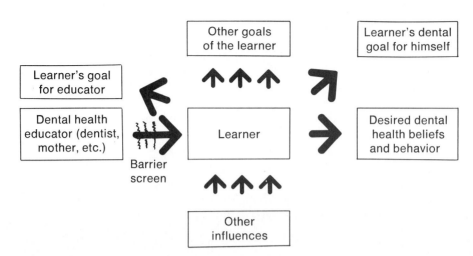

Fig. 9-1. A model of the dental health education process. (Courtesy Young, M.A.C.: Dental health education: an overview of selected concepts and principles relevant to programme planning, Int. J. Health Educ. **13**[1]:2, 1970.)

she is susceptible to dental disease, (2) he/she must perceive dental disease as a serious consequence, (3) he/she must believe that dental disease is preventable, and (4) he/she must attach a certain salience or importance to dental health. If any of these factors are absent, the likelihood of an individual being motivated to adopt and practice the preventive procedure is significantly reduced.

To accelerate improvements in oral health requires an increase in public acceptance of preventive methods. Regardless of the information presented, the public often fails to take the advice of dental professionals and makes decisions based on their own experiences and values.[60]

In dentistry the major obstacle to prevention of dental disease appears to be the perception that the consequences of dental disease are not serious. In most cases dental disease is not life threatening, and a large portion of the population functions without their natural teeth. In a 1973 survey conducted by Opinion Research Corporation for the American Dental Association, the public's chief barrier to prevention of dental disease was identified as the low value many Americans place on regular preventive dental care.[4]

Another factor that affects the ultimate outcome of the educational process is how an individual learns. Learning is not an isolated event occurring in formal educational settings but is a continuous process that can be influenced by many uncontrollable variables. An individual is constantly learning about dental health from many informal sources, such as family, peers, and the mass media. Many times the information gained from these sources is misleading, inaccurate, and directly contradictory to the dental health educator's message.[19] Therefore the educator must be able to assess the impact of these informal messages on the learner in order to develop an appropriate educational program, which should increase the learner's awareness of these informal messages and, hopefully, teach how to critically evaluate their contents.

A third approach to the educational process has been offered by Horowitz; in this approach

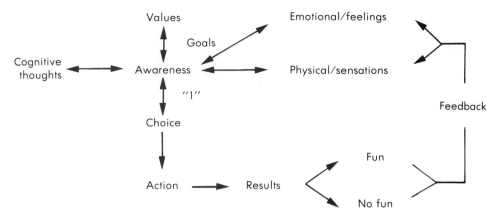

Fig. 9-2. The Self-Care Motivation Model. Diagram indicates the key areas of personal growth and awareness associated with an ongoing process of self-care. (From Horowitz, L.G.: The self-care motivation model: theory and practice in human development, J. School Health **55**(2):59, February 1985. Copyright, 1985, American School Health Association, Kent, OH 44240.)

people are able to make more intelligent choices based on satisfying feelings and outcomes through holistic awareness. This is a whole-person approach to motivating self-care based on values, awareness, choice, and action. The Self-Care Motivation Model addresses elements and functions common to all individuals and underlying all health behaviors. Fig. 9-2 illustrates the dynamics of this approach. It is widely adaptable, comprehensible, and holds promise for integration by a broad range of age and sociocultural groups. The emphasis of this model is on developing comprehensive self-awareness and involves as many human functions in the educational process as possible.[31] In addition to developing The Self-Care Motivation Model, Horowitz has developed related educational curricula to support the dispersal of innovative health education methods and self-care practices in schools and workplaces. The curricula includes units on stress, relaxation, coping skills, health values clarification, health awareness, self-assessment and self-care, as well as positive life-style choice, positive self-image/

esteem; and reinforcement. The curricula emphasizes oral self-care as a starting point within the health education curricula. Through exercises in guided imagery, the learner participates in covert behavior rehearsal, sensitization, and reinforcement (see Fig. 9-2).

Choice making is based on personal awareness of physical, mental, and emotional feedback, which leads to cognitive self-regulation.[28]

Silversin and Kornacki have stated that the media has a role in promoting behavioral change. "Media-based campaigns to promote dental health have been shown to be more effective if they continue over long periods of time, appeal to multiple motives, are coupled with social support, and provide training in requisite skills."[60] In addition, product advertising may influence public opinion and behavior. Budgets for preventive dental health interventions cannot compete with budgets to promote products that are pushed and pulled into the marketplace with huge sums of money. The success of product advertising is based on linking personal satisfaction or enhanced self-esteem with the use of a product. Thus far dental health promotion has not succeeded in linking preventive dental behaviors with motives other than health.[60]

Rubinson has identified parents as the most pervasive intervening variable in school dental health programs. Frequently program developers and evaluators do not consider enlisting the cooperation of parents. Rubinson further states that "the parents will certainly have a direct influence on dental health habits and should be involved with programmatic efforts."[56] The evaluation of dental health programs should be redirected to focus on efforts stressing skill acquisition and reduction of behavioral risk factors through an evaluation plan that is both plausible and realistic in the school setting.[56]

The School Health Education Evaluation (SHEE), conducted in collaboration with the U.S. Centers for Disease Control (CDC), from 1982 through 1984, suggests that exposure to health education curricula in schools can result in substantial changes in students' knowledge, attitude, and self-reported practices.

The SHEE has provided evidence that school health education curricula can effect changes in health-related knowledge, practices, and attitudes, and that such changes increase with amount of instruction. The potential impact of these changes is significant.[68]

In response to this study, many school systems are reevaluating their health curriculum and considering increased integration of health messages throughout the curriculum. Teachers will require additional training to develop greater competency on health issues. In view of budgeting limitations, teachers will continue to be the primary source for the dissemination of health education in our schools with the assistance of health professionals in the community. Students are encouraged to review the ten basic elements that constitute comprehensive school health education as defined in the SHEE study.[14]

The complexity of the variables that must be taken into account in designing a dental health education program to motivate behavioral change for an individual has been briefly discussed. Greater detail and step-by-step procedures can be found in books devoted solely to the techniques of behavior modification and to the social sciences in dentistry.[16,48,69]

HEALTH EDUCATION IN TRANSITION

Dental health education programs for the community have gone through, and will continue to undergo, periods of transition as further study reveals educational methods that will produce desired preventive practices. As was previously discussed, research has shown that behavior is not transmitted; behavior is learned, and in health care, learning requires active participation on the part of the learner. For this reason, the primary objective of most dental health education programs is to motivate individual students to seek the goal of disease prevention and tooth conservation.

Historically dental health education for children has been a high priority for the dental profession because of the high prevalence of dental caries in this age group. As a result, the school system has emerged as the most logical and practical setting to implement large-scale dental health education programs. The school-based dental health program provides an opportunity to reach the largest number of children during early stages of development when habit patterns can more easily be modified or changed. The school setting also provides an environment conducive to learning and reinforcement for a considerable period of time and allows the teachers to use various strategies for inducing children to participate in appropriate preventive dental health actions.[24]

Early school-based dental health programs based on the cognitive learning model primarily consisted of dental professionals and students participating in short-term projects such as National Children's Dental Health Week, high school career days, and one-time visits to elementary and secondary school classrooms. These projects did not seek to incorporate dental health into the school curriculum; they were (and are, in cases where they still exist) seen as an "add-on" activity. Administratively one-time visits present little difficulty and are often welcomed by the teacher and administration; however, reinforcement or evaluation of the dental health lesson is not usually part of the activity. Most reports on dental health education in the classroom agree that the most effective situation is when the classroom teacher works closely with the dental professional. So, regardless of who actually makes the presentation, the teacher can augment and reinforce the oral health concepts and practices. The most significant behavior for the teacher is to be an effective role model of good oral health practices.[39]

Although public interest may be aroused and dentistry's image enhanced, the early school programs, passive and cognitive in nature, were not found to motivate changes in oral health attitudes and behavior.* According to Raynor and Cohen, research in the dental health area suggests that

. . . . there must be something more than motivation per se to establish oral hygiene behavior as a habit. Learning oral hygiene must involve the acquisition of a value, or a change in a value. . . . For adults, this involves change in cognitive structure, but for children, cognitive learning is secondary to motivational learning.[51]

As a consequence, the "show and tell" approach has now evolved into programs of "show and do."

A recent survey of state school health programs by the American School Health Association revealed that only seven states mandate the teaching of dental health and oral hygiene.[9] Un-

*See references 10, 26, 49, 50, 58, and 70.

fortunately, in those seven states requiring instruction on specific health content areas, dental health is given a low priority on the list of required subjects.[64] If dental health education is more than rhetoric and teachers are expected to include it in the curriculum, then adequate teacher training programs are prerequisite.[64] Dental health professionals in the community can serve as valuable resources to the school. Dental health education should be an integral component of all school health education curricula. Regrettably, the majority of dental health education programs were supported through grant funds and many were terminated when funding expired.[41] Unless a strong constituency exists to support dental health programs, continued efforts may be stunted as a result of budgeting constraints.

An interesting by-product of school-based dental health education programs may be the "spread of effect"[12] or the "ripple effect."[33] These terms have been used to describe the impact of school-based health education programs upon parents. Croucher and colleagues conducted an investigation to assess the possible indirect influence of "Natural Noshers"[12] (a school-based dental health education program that emphasizes home activities for skill development) on the dental behavior and knowledge of other family members. "Natural Noshers" contains two distinct dental health messages, one relating to the prevention of gum disease and the other to dental decay. Take-home literature and supplies emphasize these messages. The results of this study indicate that the parents of children who had been taught "Natural Noshers" had reported new dental information more often than the parents in the control group.[12]

In another project, a group of health educators at the University of Maine at Farmington developed a series of health-related games called the "Healthway Arcade."[33] The games were used primarily for a K-3 audience and were structured to address several health issues. "Floss Is the Boss" was a popular follow-along story that utilized repetition, funny sounds, and a variety of motions to cleverly state the importance of flossing one's teeth. Parental feedback indicated that this live arts format was well received and that many youngsters insisted on reciting parts of the story at home for the family. This "ripple effect" is another way of getting a message into the home and community.[33]

Some factors may enhance the success of dental health programs in schools. These include (1) determining who will be responsible for dental health education; (2) involving parents who can provide reinforcement of dental health practices at home; (3) identifying and using community health resources who can contribute their expertise and/or materials to support dental health education efforts; and (4) evaluating the results of the program.[64]

Three programs, based on both the behavioral and the cognitive learning models, will now be described in terms of program development, philosophy and goals, implementation, and evaluation. Findings of formal research investigations as reported in the literature will also be presented for review. The student is asked to keep in mind the desired properties of a good oral public health measure, as defined in Chapter 7, and the planning and implementation strategy and criteria for the prevention of dental caries, as outlined in Chapter 8, when critiquing each program in terms of public health planning.

The students should also be aware that all of the details for each program have not been presented; however, all of the major concepts have been included. Personal contact with individuals in charge of specific programs often results in obtaining information that has not been published. The student is encouraged to contact such individuals if interested in obtaining data not found in the literature.

PRESENT APPROACHES
Learning About Your Oral Health—
a prevention-oriented school program

Development. "Learning About Your Oral Health" was developed by the American Dental Association's Bureau of Dental Health Education and its consultants in response to a request from the 1971 ADA House of Delegates. The program is available to school systems throughout the United States.[11]

Program philosophy and goals. "Learning About Your Oral Health" is a comprehensive program covering current dental concepts. Materials for preschool, primary, and secondary schools have been developed for educators to facilitate the inclusion of preventive dentistry into school health curricula. The primary goal of the program is to develop the knowledge, skills, and attitudes needed for prevention of dental disease.[3] The first priority of the program is to develop effective plaque control knowledge and skills. The next consideration is given to increasing knowledge regarding diet and dental health, with an emphasis on understanding the role of sugar. Other areas that are included at all levels in increasing degree of detail are: the significance of fluoride, oral safety, consumer health concepts, the role of dental professionals, oral health in relationship to total health, and community dental programs.

Program implementation. The program format is divided into five levels with specific content defined for each level. The levels are divided by grades: Preschool (designed for children too young to read); Level I includes kindergarten through grade 3; Level II includes grades 4 through 6; Level III includes grades 7 through 9; and Level IV includes grades 10 through 12.

The core material for each of the five levels is self-contained in a teaching packet that allows the classroom teacher to adapt the presentation to the needs of the students. Each packet includes: (1) a teacher's self-contained guide on "dental health facts" with a new section on handicapped children; (2) a glossary of dental health terms; (3) a curriculum guide featuring content, goals, behavioral objectives, and suggested activities for other classes; (4) five lesson plans for the preschool level and seven or more lesson plans for each of the other levels; (5) four overhead transparencies; (6) 12 spirit masters; and (7) methods and activities for parental involvement.

Supplementary printed material and seven films that specifically coordinate with each level have also been developed. A plaque control kit is also available and contains toothbrushes, disclosing tablets, dental floss, "Eat-Brush-Floss" stickers, and parent and teacher educational pamphlets. In addition, the ADA, in cooperation with the American Cancer Society, has developed and produced a rock video on the dangers of using smokeless tobacco, which is geared for junior and senior high level students, as well as for adult audiences.[4]

Cost of materials. The teaching packet for each level currently costs $8.00 per level. The cost of the plaque control kit for a class of 35 students is $12.95.

Program evaluation. The behavioral objectives provide the basis for evaluating the effectiveness of the lessons at all levels with the exception of Level I and II, which contain a pre- and postknowledge test. It is important to remember that this program was developed for general use and may be adapted in full or in part to complement another ongoing program, such as a fluoride tablet or mouthrinse program.

Formal evaluation. A formal evaluation study of the effectiveness of the ADA's "Learning About Your Oral Health" program was conducted by Oliver L. Ezell, Ed.D., in 1974 and reported during the First National Symposium on Dental Health Education in Schools.[17] The objectives of this study were to determine whether or not there was an improvement in the oral health behavior and attitudes of junior high school students and whether or not the ADA's

Level III program was superior to traditional oral health instruction. The results of the investigation found the ADA's program to (1) more favorably influence oral health behavior than did the traditional approach to oral health education, and (2) effect favorable changes in attitudes toward oral health practices (but not necessarily more so than traditional approaches).[17] The data did not suggest that the ADA's program was effective in improving attitudes toward organized oral health education programs. Dr. Ezell noted several factors that could have influenced these results, such as levels of instructor motivation, possible instructor bias, and levels of instructor capability.

In a second investigation by Donald B. Stone, Ed.D., and colleagues, the cognitive aspects of the ADA's program Level II were evaluated. The target audience was fifth graders, and the primary focus was on determining the value or impact of an intensive in-service training for teachers versus a teacher orientation with minimal exposure to curriculum materials.[63] A test was administered to students within 1 week of the program's completion. The results of this study concluded that there was no significant difference between the mean knowledge scores of students taught by teachers who had received intensive training and students taught by teachers who had received minimal orientation. There was a significant difference between mean knowledge scores of students taught by either of the first two teacher groups and students who had been taught by teachers with no orientation to the program, which may indicate that some teacher orientation to the program is desirable. The Bureau of Health Education and Audiovisual Services revised its program in response to this study to yield the current format.

A third investigation was conducted in 1980 by Rubinson and Peterson, and it was reported in the literature in 1982.[47] The objectives of this study were to determine the effects of the ADA Level IV School Program on the knowledge, attitudes, practices, and dental health status of high school students. The primary instrument employed in this study was an 83-item Dental Knowledge and Attitude Survey that consisted of three major sections: dental knowledge, dental attitudes, and general health attitudes. The generalizability of the results of this study is limited because this study was confined to a specific geographic area, used a specific educational program, and involved schools that offered a one-semester course in health education to sophomores. The following conclusions are based on the results of this study:

1. The ADA level IV program was effective in improving the oral health knowledge of the secondary school students randomly assigned to the experimental groups of this study.

2. The ADA Level IV program produced minor positive changes in dental attitudes, dental locus of control, and health locus of control, none of which were statistically significant.

3. Based on the findings of this study and a review of the literature, high school females generally have higher levels of dental knowledge and more positive attitudes toward dental health than males.

4. The ADA Level IV program had a greater impact on the dental knowledge, dental attitudes, dental locus of control, and health locus of control of females than that of males.

5. There was a low-to-moderate association between secondary students' dental knowledge, dental attitudes, dental locus of control, and health locus of control.

6. The American Dental Association's 1980 Oral Health Teaching and Learning Program for secondary students is an innovative approach to curriculum design and has the potential for contributing to improved dental health teaching and learning.[47]

A fourth investigation was conducted during 1986 to evaluate the effectiveness of the ADA's preschool program. Specifics on this study are currently unavailable.[4]

Texas statewide preventive dentistry program—"Tattletooth Program"

Development. The Tattletooth Program was developed as a cooperative effort between Texas dental health professional organizations, the Texas Department of Health, and the Texas Education Agency through a DHEW (now Health and Human Services) grant to the Bureau of Dental Health, Texas Department of Health. The program was pilot tested in 1975, field tested in spring 1976, and made available in fall 1976 to schools within the state of Texas.[67]

The Headstart and Preschool Program was developed the same way, utilizing a systems approach to curriculum development. The program development was funded in 1978 and it was in use in early 1980.[66]

Program philosophy and goals. Tattletooth relates dental health to the physical, mental, social, and emotional aspects of the individual. Tattletooth focuses on the total person. The Tattletooth Program is based on an educational model that uses the philosophy of Maslow's heirarchy of needs, Lasswell's eight basic human values, and Havighurst's list of development tasks for each age level throughout childhood and adolescence.[65]

The basic goal of the program is to reduce dental disease and develop positive dental habits to last a lifetime. The major thrust of Tattletooth is to convince students that preventing dental disease is important and that they can do it.[65]

Program implementation. In 1985 the Texas legislature required that the essential elements for comprehensive health education curricula identified in the School Health Education Evaluation Project[14] be incorporated into the curriculum statewide and be taught to the state's 3 million children. Oral health is one of the required elements. This legislative action has stimulated a need for the Tattletooth Program statewide.

Texas is divided into 20 Regional Education Service Centers. In September 1985, for the first time, these Regional Education Service Centers employed 13 health coordinators to implement programs in all health areas. It is anticipated that they will assist and possibly handle implementation of the Tattletooth Program.

Teachers are trained to present dental health information and utilize materials developed by curriculum specialists, dentists, hygienists, and teachers. Over the years, teacher training time has been decreased by state law. One of the results is that the teacher training program has been continuously updated and training materials consolidated and refined. Videotapes have been developed for use in training teachers where school staffs have a high rate of turnover.

Dental hygienists generally do the initial in-service training in the school districts and serve as technical experts to provide assistance to teachers. In some remote school districts with only three or four teachers, training can be done by videotape. Although this is less than ideal, the program is implemented with limited resources. It is doubtful that the number of dental hygienists employed will increase in the near future. In fact, the health coordinators may emerge as the individuals responsible for all areas of the health curriculum.

Ten separate lesson plans are available for Prekindergarten through sixth, and junior and senior high school grade levels. Lesson plans contain all the materials and instructions the teacher needs to present a particular lesson. Topics covered in the curriculum include correct brushing and flossing techniques, awareness of the importance of safety, and factual information relating to dental disease, its causes, and preventive techniques. In addition to the curriculum package, supportive materials have been prepared and include:

1. A program overview/administrator's brochure
2. A school nurse brochure
3. A professional awareness kit
4. A public awareness kit

In the spring of 1987 the Bureau of Dental Health held a dental health conference for college and university instructors. It is anticipated that these instructors will begin to prepare college students in teacher preparation classes to implement the Oral Health Program. By training students in the 23 college preparatory programs, it is anticipated that there will be less of a demand for teacher training time and that college students will be motivated and prepared to teach oral health when they get to the classroom.

Cost of materials. In 1976 the Bureau of Dental Health was spending about $1.00 per child for supplies. Since that time state financial resources have steadily declined. Beginning in 1985, the state provided curriculum to new teachers only and schools were asked to purchase their own brushes and floss or get them donated by the parent-teacher organization or some other group. It is anticipated that in the future the Bureau of Dental Health may only be able to provide a single copy for each grade level and the schools will have to make copies for each teacher. The more work a teacher has to do in implementing a program, the greater the chances are that the program will not be implemented. At the same time, nonprofit organizations make available health education materials in attractive kits that are easy to use and accessible. Public health educators are challenged to compete under rigid financial constraints.

Program evaluation. A major field test conducted in 1975 and 1976 studied 15,000 children in 18 educational service regions. Results of a single exposure to the program revealed that:

1. Dental health knowledge levels were significantly increased at all grade levels.
2. Plaque levels were decreased by approximately 15% in a randomly selected sample of 2,142 children.
3. Over 80% of the teachers judged the program to be helpful and effective, but evaluation questions suggested that they felt a need for additional technical help with brushing and flossing.

As the program is implemented, statewide continuous monitoring will take place to ensure that materials are used as intended and that the program takes place in an appropriate classroom situation with a trained school staff and an informed community. In addition, 10% of the children will be examined annually to establish baseline and longitudinal data regarding disease prevalence. The DMFS, PHP, and PMA (which expresses the prevalence of gingivitis) indices will be used to determine any changes in oral health status. It is believed that these dental examinations will, over a period of years, assess and establish the accomplishment of the program's main goal—a substantial reduction of dental disease.

The ongoing evaluation of the Tattletooth Program in 1977 and 1978 had three major goals: (1) to conduct a gross dental screening to obtain an estimate of the prevalence of dental problems and to provide other base-rate data, (2) to conduct an experimental study of dental effectiveness involving a pre- and post-examination design, and (3) to conduct an evaluation of the services provided by trained dental hygienists to determine whether or not the technical help previously requested by participating teachers was provided.

Results of the dental screening, which included 5,071 children in 12 school districts in 5 counties, suggested that dental problems were highly prevalent in this sample and that a preventive program concentrating on proper cleaning is needed. Although most (99%) of the parents were notified about their children's dental problems, only a few (11%) subsequently made appointments with dentists and 8% indicated that they lacked a source of dental care. The experimental dental evaluation indicated that the Tattletooth dental education program is effective in improving cleaning effectiveness, and the teacher questionnaire responses supported the involvement of dental hygienists as a valuable component of the program. The pattern of significant results in the PHP might suggest that more effort be made in the future to teach effective cleaning of molars.[22]

During the spring of 1984, the Texas Department of Health conducted a process evaluation of the Tattletooth school dental health education program. The evaluation was conducted to determine how and if the teachers were implementing the program in the classroom setting.

A questionnaire was mailed to approximately 850 teachers who have implemented the Tattletooth Program in Public Health Regions 5 and 6 of the Texas Department of Health. A total of 515 teachers—representing 106 public schools, 41 school districts, and 41 counties—returned the evaluation questionnaire. The results of the evaluation were very favorable. The teachers were implementing the program at a level that is acceptable to the standards of the Texas Department of Health. The students are brushing their teeth in the classroom approximately 5 times, and the teachers are teaching at least 8 of the 10 Tattletooth lesson plans. In addition, the teacher attitudes toward the teacher training they have received are extremely positive. As program coordinators, the dental hygienists have been effective, and the dental health education in general has been highly successful. Dental flossing and use of disclosing tablets in the classroom are the only facets of the program that the teachers appear to implement on only a minimum basis. The results of this evaluation indicated that the Tattletooth Program benefited the Texas school children.

Parent program

"Dental Health Is a Family Affair" is an education program for parents. It is presented in the following formats: flip chart, slide/tape presentation, and video cassette. The program is coordinated by Texas Department of Health dental hygienists for use with groups such as Headstart parents, school parent groups, local health departments, and clinics.

The content covers dental disease problems

and their prevention as well as diet and a section describing characteristics of children's dental development ranging from prenatal to late adolescence. "Dental Health Is a Family Affair" won the ADA Meritorious Award in Community Preventive Dentistry.

Senior citizen program

Four presentations make up the Senior Citizen's Oral Health program. The presentations are all geared toward noninstitutionalized senior citizens. The first session provides general oral health information. The second presentation consists of a demonstration of brushing and flossing of natural teeth. The purpose of the third session is to demonstrate the proper method for cleaning partials and dentures. In some regions the dental hygienists clean the dentures in the ultrasonic cleaner and label them. During the fourth session, the dental hygienist demonstrates how a person can examine themselves for oral cancer. When possible, a volunteer dentist examines the participants for oral cancer and answers any questions they might have.

In 1985 a pilot project was developed to provide dental care for indigent senior citizens. The Central Area Agency on Aging and the Texas Department of Health, Bureau of Dental Health, were joined by the Central Texas Dental Society to provide treatment for senior citizens. The center identified members needing care and arranged transportation. The Area Agency on Aging Information and Referral Center determined financial eligibility and referred the senior citizens to dentists participating in the program. Dentists donated their services and received limited reimbursement for materials. This program received an Administration on Aging Project Health Award. The Department of Community Affairs and the Department of Health will be expanding the program to three other area agencies on aging. Plans are to extend the program statewide but this is dependent on state financing.[66]

Pre/Post Natal Program

The Pre/Post Natal Program is divided into three parts. The first slide tape or video presentation, "Mom, It's Up to You! Your Health Depends on You!" focuses on dental diseases and their causes, effective oral hygiene aids, drugs during pregnancy, and proper nutrition. It is followed by a demonstration of brushing. The second presentation, "Mom, It's Up to You! Your Baby Depends on You!" discusses fluoride, aids in relieving teething discomfort, nursing bottle mouth syndrome, and brushing and flossing the baby's teeth. This presentation is followed by a demonstration of flossing. In the presentation "Mom, It's Up to You! Your Toddler Depends on You!" the participant learns about primary and permanent teeth, dental accidents, and thumbsucking. Each presentation takes about 15 minutes plus demonstration time.[66]

North Carolina statewide preventive dental health program

Development. North Carolina has a long history of involvement in dental public health and school dental health education. The need for a school dental health education program was realized as early as 1908, when the first scientific paper addressing this subject was presented to the North Carolina Dental Society. Over the past 70 years, many supportive actions have been initiated including fluoridation of community water supplies and comprehensive state surveys of the dental disease problems. In 1970 the North Carolina Dental Society passed resolutions advocating a strong preventive dental disease program embracing school and community fluoridation, fluoride treatments for schoolchildren, continuing education on prevention for dental professionals, and plaque control education in schools and communities.

In 1973 Frank E. Law, D.D.S., M.P.H., prepared a report for the North Carolina Dental Society, which defined the extent of the dental disease problem and resulted in the initiation of a

10-year program to reduce dental disease. The Ten Year Preventive Dentistry Plan had the approval and support of the North Carolina General Assembly. In that same year a coalition of several agencies set up a Steering Committee that was responsible for developing a practical plan for a program in the schools.[7] This was the first statewide program of its magnitude and remains the largest and most comprehensive of all state public health dental programs. Continuation and expansion of the North Carolina Preventive Dentistry Program for Children (NCPDPC) according to the original plan has been made possible through incremental funding from the state legislature. Initial appropriations in 1974 funded 10% of the program. Under the original plan, the program would expand annually by about 10% so that in 10 years the program would include the entire state. A few lean budgetary years hindered progress. Currently the program covers 85% of the state, and there are good indications that the plan will be fully implemented by fiscal year (FY) 1987-88.

In addition to funding appropriations from the state legislature, the Dental Health Section of the Division of Health Service has been awarded grants by the Kate B. Reynolds Health Care Trust. These projects include (1) producing 20 videotapes by July 1987 for use by classroom teachers in teaching dental health; and (2) conducting a statewide oral health survey of a representative sample of North Carolina school children, K-12, during the 1986-87 school year. The results will be analyzed and reported in 1988.[46]

In 1986 the Dental Health Section established specific long-range statewide goals for the next 10 years for the State of North Carolina that reinforce and expand upon those originally started by Dr. Law in 1973.

Program philosophy and goals. North Carolina has established a Framework for Dental Health Education, which is a component of the Statewide Preventive Dental Health Program. Dental health is considered an important part of general health and a condition that can be achieved through the coordinated efforts of the individual, professionals, and the community.[44] The application of organizational skills is critical in gaining both the moral and the financial support of the commuity.

The North Carolina program recognizes primary prevention and education as the most effective means of decreasing dental disease and promoting dental health; fluoride is recognized as the most effective public health measure for preventing dental caries. Priority is given to community water fluoridation, rural school water fluoridation, and weekly fluoride mouthrinse by schoolchildren.

Education for children and adults is also considered a major preventive activity and must be coordinated with fluoride use and regular dental care, diet control, accident prevention, and oral cancer screening to be effective. Young children are the primary focus for education because the earlier a child is reached, the greater the potential for impacting positively on the child's attitudes, values, and behaviors.

The Framework for Dental Health Education was developed to provide health practitioners and others involved in education with a working document to assist them in the development of a comprehensive community dental health education program. The philosophy behind the framework's development relates to a building process, as far as behaviors are concerned, and an internalization of values that relate to dental health in responsibility to self, family, and community. Its purpose is to increase the effectiveness of dental health education as one means of achieving the goals of the Statewide Preventive Dental Health Program. The goal of the Dental Health Section is to provide preventive and educational services for the citizens of North Carolina. Specific long-range goals for the next 10 years are:

A. Goals
* 1. A 25% reduction in dental caries in the population 20 years of age and under;
* 2. A 40% reduction in dental caries in the population 10 years of age and under; and
* 3. A 15% reduction in periodontal disease in the population 20 years of age and under.
  4. Ninety percent (90%) of North Carolinians living on a community water supply will have the benefits of fluoridated water by 1994.
  5. All 100 counties in North Carolina will be served by a preventive dental program by 1988.
* 6. At least 75% of adults should be aware that thorough daily personal oral hygiene and regular professional care are necessary for the prevention and control of dental decay and periodontal disease.
* 7. At least 75% of adults over 50 years of age who are heavy users of alcohol and tobacco should be aware that they are at high risk for developing oral cancer.
* 8. Training in oral cancer screening will be provided by the Office of Nursing, assisted by the Dental Health Section, for local health department staff who screen adults.
* 9. Methods will be developed to target selected adult groups for oral health screenings.
  10. Local health department staff, providing services to mothers and children, will be provided with information and educational materials on nursing bottle decay in 100 counties.

B. Operational objectives
  1. People of childbearing age and newborns
     a. Develop a comprehensive approach to the prevention and control of bottle decay. Joint effort of the Dental Health Section and the Maternal and Child Care Section.
  2. Child health
     a. Provide preventive dental health services for 410,000 children—preschool to grade 8 (fluoride mouthrinse; plaque control).
     b. Provide 60,000 dental care services for approximately 13,000 indigent children—preschool and K-6 grades.
     c. Inspect 250,000 preschool and school-age children and refer approximately 65,000 who need dental care to private practicing dentists.
     d. Provide preventive dental health educational services for 325,000 children—preschool to grade 6.
     e. Provide pit and fissure sealants for 16,000 teeth in school-age children.
     f. Conduct an Oral Health Survey of approximately 7,000 North Carolina school children (K-12) to assess their oral health status.
     g. Establish an inter-agency task force to develop strategies to educate North Carolina school children and their parents about the health risks of smokeless tobacco use.
  3. Adult health
     a. Provide preventive dental health educational services for 40,000 adults.
     b. Develop scripts, with accompanying teacher guides, for 6 video modules and produce 2 teacher training video modules.
     c. Conduct 15 10-hour workshops in preventive dentistry for approximately 325 classroom teachers.
     d. Update 70 dental public health staff in oral cancer screening and provide consultation and technical assistance to public health nurses in oral cancer screening.

---

*Goals are achievable only if adequate dental public health staff are available in the county or district health departments.

4. Community health
   a. Provide funds to assist in the fluoridation of 3 communities and 5 rural
   schools.
   b. Provide funds to train water plant op-
   erators to qualify to fluoridate their respective water supplies.
   c. Provide training and certification for
   school surveillance personnel in 5 new
   schools.
   d. Provide surveillance for 201 communities and 140 schools that fluoridate
   their water supplies.
5. Administration
   a. Provide a continuing education program for state and local dental public
   health staff.
   b. Continue a computer reporting program for community and school fluoridation activities on a monthly basis and
   the fluoride mouthrinse program on an
   annual basis.
   c. Continue the 8-year fluoride combination study of mouthrinse, mouthrinse/
   school water fluoridation, and mouth-
   rinse/community water fluoridation in
   Cumberland and Sampson counties
   (now in its final year).
   d. Provide two (2) orientation and training programs for newly employed state
   and local dental public health staff.
   e. Continue to update/revise section
   manual of procedures, policies, guidelines, and forms through committees
   and task forces of the Section Management Team.
   f. Continue fifth year of formal management development activities staff-
   wide.

Objectives that will facilitate attainment of the
goals include: (1) fluoridation of community
water and rural school water supplies and the use
of supplemental fluorides such as fluoride tablets
and fluoride mouthrinses, (2) health education in

schools and communities, and (3) provision of
public health dental staff in all counties.

Program implementation. In the dental health
status report presented in 1973, dental disease
was found to affect 95% of the total population
and more schoolchildren than any other health
problem.[44] Rozier in 1982 stated that the teenage
population is at greater risk of developing dental
caries than any other age group and that 45% of
children and adolescents show evidence of periodontal disease, almost all of which is reversible.[55] In
1985 the recommendations of Dr. Frank Law
had been implemented in 20 communities with
fluoridated water supplies, 144 rural schools with
fluoridated water supplies, and 1,053 schools
that were implementing a fluoride mouthrinse
program, and in a new and expanding service,
dental sealants were applied to 11,000 teeth.[46]
The comprehensive nature of the problem's
definition is reflected in the uniqueness of the
program, which is designed to reach several
segments of the population—young children,
parents, teachers, dental professionals, and
community leaders.

To reach the children, public health dental
staff provide the training of and consultation to
those who work with preschool children and
Maternal and Infant Programs; for example,
elementary school teachers and parents. Teachers are believed to be the key in the educational
program, and to improve their capability for
teaching and reinforcement of sound dental
principles they receive preservice, in-service,
and follow-up training to cover dental health
concepts, practice oral hygiene skills, and integrate dental health into the curriculum.

The coordinated effort of the consultant team
of dentists, hygienists, and health educators is
extremely important in program implementation. The activities of the consultant staff (made
available to all public health dentists and hygienists) provide for continuity in program planning
and implementation. With 48 public health dental hygienists and 17 public health dentists work-

ing in county programs, it is important that consultative services necessary for program growth be available to them. Also, the consultants serve in a capacity that helps to tie together the individual county programs and needs of staff through statewide conferences and so on, in this way retaining and promoting the philosophy of the statewide preventive dental health program.

Several teaching aids are available for North Carolinians, such as the Teacher's Guide to a Preventive Dental Health Program, Guidelines for Planning a Teacher Workshop in Preventive Dental Health, and leaflets and handouts on nutrition, sugar, fluoride, toothbrush storage in the classroom, and reading food labels. In addition, the Division of Health Services has a film library containing some 30 films on dental health, which are free on loan to any school in the state; the videotapes currently under development will also be available. (*Note:* Because of budget limitations and the Dental Section policy, materials are only made available to educators in North Carolina.)

Table 9-1 provides an overview of the total program integrating the three components. It also illustrates the focus of education for parents, dental professionals, and community leaders.

North Carolinians believe that one reason their community dental health program has been so successful is the total support of the North Carolina Dental Society. It was the Dental Society, in 1973, that went before the legislature to seek the funding for the statewide program. It is believed that through screening, identification of third party funding, and referral, as well as other public health activity, children can be referred to the private sector for the dental care that is needed.

Program evaluation. Evaluation has been and will continue to be a necessary ongoing process to measure the effectiveness of specific areas and the total dental health program. Because of the program's comprehensive nature, various ad-

ministrative levels participate in the evaluation process. Some of the evaluations that have been conducted since the first Ten Year Preventive Dentistry Plan are as follows[44]:

1. The replication of the 1963 Fulton-Hughes survey (in 1976). Data collected are being used to evaluate long-range goals and objectives.
2. A survey of schoolchildren in Ashville, North Carolina, where the community's water supply had been fluoridated for 10 years. The survey revealed a 53% reduction in decayed, missing, and filled permanent teeth for children who had 10 years experience drinking fluoridated water.
3. A survey of schoolchildren at the Happy Valley School in Caldwell County, North Carolina, where the school water supply had been fluoridated for 8 years. The results of this survey indicated a 34% reduction in decayed, missing, and filled permanent teeth for children who had 8 years experience drinking school fluoridated water.
4. A survey on the use of sealants in a Public Health Dental Program, where a very high retention rate of 84% after 4 years was found.
5. A statewide oral health survey of school-age population is currently underway. The specific objectives of the project are (1) to describe the oral health status and factors associated with this status by recording survey participant's (a) DMFT's, DMFS's for primary (deft, dfs) and permanent dentition, (b) number of teeth sealed with dental sealants (c) extent of gingivitis, (d) restorative and exodontic treatment needs; (2) to determine the extent, type, and frequency of use of smokeless tobacco products, patterns of use, and knowledge of harmful effects; (3) to develop a mechanism for continuous monitoring of disease levels as part of ongoing program regardless of

Table 9-1. Schematic presentation of preventive dental health program in North Carolina

Agencies involved	Target audiences, by priority	Approaches
Department of Public Education Department of Human Resources, Dental Health Section	1. Teachers and staff of preschool programs and elementary schools, grades K-6	In-service training for teachers on the job Preservice training in teacher training institutions Public health dental consultation Coordination with public health Maternal and Child Health programs Provision of educational materials
North Carolina Dental Society University of North Carolina School of Dentistry	2. Students in preschool and elementary grades K-6	Fluoridation of community water supplies Fluoridation of rural school water supplies Fluoride by topical application, mouthwash, and so on Educational programs in school and materials Remedial dental service to selected children
North Carolina Dental Hygienists' Association North Carolina Dental Assistant's Association North Carolina Association of Local Health Directors	3. Parents of students K-6	Educational work with parent groups such as P.T.A. Head Start Educational work with agricultural extension clubs, 4-H, and other farm and civic groups Use of mass media for education Work through public health personnel such as health educators, nurses, and public health programs such as Maternal and Child Health
	4. Dentists and auxiliaries including students	Continuing education in preventive dentistry and public health via seminars, workshops, conferences, and so on Basic training to include school and community dental health education Representation on Steering Committee
	5. Community leaders, official and lay	Public health dental consultation Use of mass media for education Work with clubs and groups

From North Carolina Department of the Preventive Dental Health program, Human Resources, Division of Health Services

additional funding appropriateness; (4) to establish a Policy Advisory Committee to the Dental Health Section to study survey results and to make recommendations on program effectiveness and planning for North Carolina Dental Health Section to the year 2000. Once analyzed, the results of this survey may affect program planning for dental health nationwide.

In addition to these surveys, the effectiveness of an education program in changing knowledge, attitudes, values, and practices of students will be evaluated over a long period of time. Effects of the educational program may not become evident for 15 to 20 years; however, the results are expected to be positive (see Table 9-2).[44]

SUGGESTED APPROACHES

Each of the community dental health education programs that has been described was chosen for three reasons. First, these programs are some of the most widely known and reported

Items in dental health program, by priority	Sources of funds
1. Fluoridation of community water supplies	Regular budget from state funds to cover salaries, supplies, office supplies, and so on
2. Fluoridation of rural school water supplies	State funds appropriated beginning 1986 for the preventive dental health program to provide:
3. Use of fluoride via special programs such as mouthrinse, topical applications	One Public Health Dental Hygienist in each of North Carolina's 100 counties
4. Dental health education in preschools and elementary schools, including preservice and in-service training for teachers/staff	Supplies and equipment for the above Public Health Dental Hygienists
5. Dental education for consumers to include parents and community leaders via agencies such as agricultural extension, industry, civic clubs, and mass media	Fluoridation of community and rural school water supplies via matching funds for equipment and assistance with installation and maintenance
6. Support services such as:	Other staff: three public health educators and two dental hygiene consultants to work with Public Health Dental Hygienists and Public Health Dentists as a team for educational and clinical services
Provision of public health dental staff, health educators, maintenance staff	Other services such as statistical assistance for research, artwork, photography, film rental/purchase
Provision of supplies/equipment for dental staff	
Production/distribution of educational training aids	
Kate B. Reynolds Health Care Trust, a North Carolina Foundation, provides funding for grant proposal to develop and produce 8 teacher training video modules and guides, 12 video modules and guides for classroom instruction, and copy 200 sets of video modules (K-3, 4-6) and 15 sets of teacher modules by June 30, 1987.	
7. Coordinated planning among agencies such as the North Carolina Dental Society, Steering Committee for a Preventive Dental Health Program for North Carolina Children, and Dental Health Section of the Department of Human Resources	

in North Carolina Schools, Raleigh, NC.

in the literature; second, they represent a variety of approaches to dental health education; and third, they illustrate the range of success that can be expected to be achieved given their programmatic structure and goals. Utilizing the criteria that are presented in Chapters 7 and 8, several issues for discussion should become apparent. For instance, if we assume that the goal for a dental health education program for the community is to reduce the prevalence of dental caries, which of the programs, if any, are using the most cost-effective and clinically proven preventive measures? Which of the programs are using evaluation criteria that will measure caries experience? Which of the programs have determined their priorities based on the collection of data gathered through a formal needs assessment? And which programs are easily implemented and administered?

Answers to these questions begin to identify the inherent weaknesses in the majority of the programs, which to a large extent have lost sight

Table 9-2. Summary of dental health education programs in terms of development, program

Name of program	Characteristics of program	
	Development	Philosophy and goals
Learning About Your Oral Health—ADA, Bureau of Dental Health	Request from ADA's House of Delegates in 1971 Bureau of Dental Health and consultants	Comprehensive program covering Preschool, K-12 Goal—develop knowledge, skills, and attitudes to prevent disease Priority—plaque control knowledge and skills
Texas Department of Health, Tattletooth Program, Parent Program, Senior Citizen Program, Pre/Postnatal Program	Cooperative effort of professional organizations, Texas Department of Health Resources, Texas Educational Agency Funded by DHEW grant to Texas Department of Health Resources, Central Area Agency on Aging	Goal—reduce dental caries and develop positive dental habits to last a lifetime Program tries to convince students that preventing dental disease is important and they can do it Program focuses on dental health as a part of total health
North Carolina Statewide Preventive Dental Health Program	North Carolina Dental Health Section, Dental Organizations, Department of Public Education, University of North Carolina School of Dentistry plus support of General Assembly Based on the documented needs assessment of North Carolina citizens	Prevention and education are major activities Priority—young children Goals: 1. 25% reduction in dental disease in population 20 years of age and younger 2. 40% reduction in dental disease in population 10 years of age and under 3. 15% reduction in periodontal disease in population 20 years of age and under Long-range plan for development and use of dental health materials in competency-based curriculum entitled "Framework for Dental Health Education"—emphasizes role of classroom elementary teacher for integrating dental health education into curriculum

philosophy and goals, implementation, costs, and evaluation

Characteristics of program		
Implementation	**Costs**	**Evaluation**
Five levels with core material for teachers to adapt to needs of students Overheads and spirit masters are included Films, videotapes and plaque control kits are available Dental hygienists serve as technical consultants for school districts and promote dental education for expectant women, parents, and senior citizens Supportive materials are available for teachers and program hygienists	$8 for teaching packet $12.95 for plaque control kits for 35 students Film and videotape rental costs vary	Levels I and II—pre- and postknowledge tests Behavioral objectives provide basis for teachers to develop evaluation mechanisms
Statewide implementation plan Teachers are trained to present dental health information for school-age population Health coordinators role emerging to include oral health	Estimated at less than $1.00 per child; State legislated budget	Field testing Statewide continuous monitoring of material use
Ten Year Preventive Dental Health Program 1973 (revised 1986) Priorities are community and rural school water fluoridation and fluoride mouthrinse Public health dental staff provides training and consultative services to teachers, parents, professionals, and community Several teaching adjuncts are available; curriculum videotapes and guides currently under development	State budget includes salaries	Comprehensive survey of dental disease in 1976 and 1986-87 Statewide oral health survey funded by Kate B. Reynolds Health Care Trust Survey of school children after 10 years of community water fluoridation and 8 years of rural school water fluoridation Clinical evaluation of school health program educational aspects will be evaluated over a long period of time

of the disease prevention/tooth conservation goal. In these cases the primary objectives emphasize motivating a group of students to practice positive health behaviors as if they were individual patients. Success is based on long-term behavior change, which is very difficult to obtain and may not be practical for dental public health.* As concluded at a 1973 Conference on Prevention and Oral Health sponsored by the Fogarty International Center for Advanced Study in Health Sciences and the National Institute of Dental Research, "mechanical procedures for plaque prevention do not offer a promising solution to the problem of control of dental diseases for the population at large."[8] In addition, a clear-cut cause-and-effect relationship between dental plaque and caries has not been clinically proven in human populations. The Research Committee of the American Association of Public Health Dentists in their report, "Programs for the Mass Control of Plaque: An Appraisal," states[32]:

> On theoretical grounds, it may appear evident that the daily, thorough removal of plaque should have a marked effect on reducing the increment of new carious lesions. As this report attempts to point out, however, this supposition cannot be supported with clinical evidence.

Yacovone has also noted that "Some authorities in community health feel that prevention will only be successful when individual behavior is eliminated."[71] If this is the case, then community educational efforts must focus on those disease prevention strategies that require the least compliance on the part of the individual. This would require a reorientation to health education and its goal, as well as redirecting the educational efforts to community leaders in an attempt to improve the oral health status through organized community efforts.[20]

This is not to say that school-based educational programs should be eliminated or are not val-

uable; it does, however, indicate the need for further behavioral research and the need for communities to decide which of the preventive programs and which of the strategies or measures now employed in each program should take priority. If community leaders are expected to make these decisions, then they must be given the tools to do so. This would necessitate a new role or new responsibilities for the community dental health educator. Frazier states that the appropriate educational methods for this target group are those designed to (1) provide accurate information about the relative merits of various disease prevention and control measures, and (2) stimulate group decision making and action regarding the adoption of effective organized programs.[20]

A question that must be examined if these new responsibilities are to be assumed is, Are community dental health educators presently prepared and willing to adopt this new role? Hunter's study indicates that dental hygienists feel "capable of providing services for DMF surveys, plaque control programs for community groups and fluoride self-application programs."[32] The dental hygienists surveyed, however, reported lower feelings of competence in areas of health legislation and in serving as an officer or committee member of the national dental hygiene association, both of which require organizational skills and leadership ability.[32] Frazier speaks of the possibility of an alternative educational role in which "the community-based hygienist could become skillful in organizing meetings, conducting seminars and workshops for decision-makers, opinion leaders and community groups. . . ."[21] The development of these organizational skills would require appropriate educational experiences, which dental and dental hygiene students presently do not receive as part of their professional training. These skills might best be learned through required field experiences in the community dentistry or public health courses.

---

*See references 1, 8, 10, 20, 25, 26.

Although students generally participate in school-based community programs, other types of organized community efforts should serve as viable field experience alternatives. The following are several issues that require professional support and involvement and are currently receiving national attention:

1. Water fluoridation
2. Frequency of use, types of product used, patterns of utilization, and knowledge about the harmful effects of smokeless tobacco
3. Efforts by the consumer-interest group, Action for Children's Television, to restrict advertising of cariogenic foods directed at children
4. Prohibition of confectionary food sales in schools
5. Participation in the development and implementation of the Health Systems Agency's health system plan where applicable

The need for active participation in these areas cannot be overemphasized. Visible support and action in the community, for instance, can make the difference in whether or not a referendum for water fluoridation is passed.[15,18,27,39] Two examples illustrating this point are the defeat of the referendum to continue water fluoridation in Flagstaff, Arizona, in March 1978 and the passage of the referendum in Seattle, Washington, in 1973.

Fluoridation, in each of these cases and in most cases, has proved to be a highly emotionally charged issue. In Flagstaff, organized opponents to water fluoridation, namely the National Health Federation (NHF), held public forums and disseminated large amounts of propaganda. The usual tactic was to link fluoridation to cancer. Other arguments, that fluoridation is unconstitutional, fluoridation is a form of medication, and fluoridation is contrary to the right of "free choice of health care," were also cited.[43] To combat these unscientific charges and the

emotional fervor with which they are made, it is incumbent on all dental professionals in the community, and students during their training, to familiarize themselves with the NHF and other antifluoridation groups strategies and the documented evidence refuting their claims. It is also a professional responsibility to educate the voters, community leaders, and agencies regarding the benefits of fluoridation and regarding the movements opposed to fluoridation, which pose a danger to the oral health of the community. In the Flagstaff, Arizona, case, an initial survey indicated that the referendum would pass 2 to 1; however, the NHF was able to reverse this prediction by creating an illusion of scientific controversy. Fortunately in Seattle, Washington, the opposition was not as active or successful. Here the dental profession focused on building a broad base of community support; it educated people to understand the working of the ballot and on how to vote. Fifteen days before voters went to the poll, dental and dental hygiene students along with community volunteers actively campaigned door-to-door for fluoridation. This successful strategy should be examined by communities where fluoridation is an issue. Success at one point in time does not mean that at some future date the decision could not be reversed, as it was in Flagstaff. Dental professionals must continue to be visible in the community to reinforce the benefits of fluoridation and the decision made by the voters. Dental health education must be provided on a continuous basis if it is to serve as a means for health promotion.

Student activities and degree of involvement in each of the other three listed areas may vary from state to state. An examination of existing legislation and accreditation standards for primary and secondary schools can provide students with "ammunition" to assist communities in improving their oral health. Action taken by the Alabama Dental Association to eliminate the sale of sweets in local schools led to their discovery of the Southern Association of Schools' accreditation standard, which prohibits the sale of sweets in schools, and resulted in its enforcement. The standard was not being enforced by the Accrediting Division of the Department of Education because it did not have a working definition of the word *confection*. The Alabama Dental Association and Alabama Nutrition Council were able to provide the needed definition as well as a list of acceptable snack foods. This effort should serve as an example of what can be accomplished and it identifies activities in which students can certainly become involved.[59]

Educational experiences in these areas will afford students the opportunity to begin developing necessary organizational and planning skills. Only through working with dental and other professional societies, state and local agencies, and community leaders and decision makers can an organized community effort be effective in preventing and controlling dental disease.

RESEARCH

The most promising avenue to improving oral health lies in the prevention of dental disease.

The National Institute of Dental Research (NIDR) National Caries Program conducted an 11-year study beginning in 1972 to determine the long-term effects of the combination of student-applied fluoride agents (fluoride mouth-rinsing, fluoride tablets, and fluoride toothpaste) among schoolchildren living in a rural area with low concentrations of fluoride in the drinking water. In school participating students ingested a 1 mg fluoride tablet and rinsed weekly with a 0.2% sodium fluoride solution. The children also received fluoride dentifrice and toothbrushes for home use throughout the calendar year. In 1983, dental examinations of study participants aged 6 to 17 years, who had continuously participated in the program for 1 to 11 years, depending on school grade, showed a mean prevalence of 3.12 DMFS, which was 65% lower than the corresponding score of 9.02 DMFS for children of the same ages at the baseline examinations. The preventive program inhibited decay in all types of surfaces: 54% in occlusal surfaces, 59% in buccolingual surfaces, and 90% in mesiodistal surfaces.[30]

In a second study conducted by NIDR National Caries Program, the effects of supervised daily dental plaque removal by children were evaluated for a 3-year period. This study was initiated in 1973 in a rural fluoride-deficient community. Approximately 480 children in grades 5-8 were initially included in the study to determine the effect on oral hygiene, gingival inflammation, and dental caries from supervised daily flossing and brushing in school. A fluoride-free dentifrice was used. In June 1976 final examinations were conducted using the same indices and examiners. "In the treatment group, the mean plaque and gingival scores at program completion were 18% and 29% lower, respectively, than at baseline. The differences in plaque and gingival scores were statistically significant. However, differences between groups disappeared during summer vacation. The increment of dental caries was lower in the treatment group but not significant either for teeth or for surfaces."[29]

Another research project was conducted to test the effectiveness of dental health education in the workplace. The American Dental Association's Bureau of Health Education and Audio Visual Service, Councils on Dental Care Programs, and Dental Health and Health Planning, and the ADA Health Foundation Research Institute worked cooperatively with several agencies in the state of Maine on this initial effort to determine the impact of health education in the work setting on dental health status. The program objectives were as follows[2]:

1. To design an educational program for adults that would develop the knowledge, skills, and attitudes needed for the pre-

vention of dental disease for themselves and their families
2. To motivate adults to seek regular dental care for themselves and their families
3. To determine the type of educational interventions that were appropriate for the workplace setting
4. To determine the extent to which dental professionals could be involved in workplace programs
5. To determine the impact on the dental health status of the target population

The Maine Workplace Project was conducted from 1982 to 1985 with data collection and analysis continuing into 1986. Preliminary results are still incomplete; however, a representative from the ADA who is responsible for coordinating study results indicated that the ADA will eventually develop a protocol for dental health education in the workplace based upon this study.[3]

The National Preventive Dentistry Demonstration Program (NPDDP), carried out between 1976 and 1983, was the largest, most comprehensive school-based preventive dentistry program ever conducted anywhere. Its purpose was to determine the costs and effectiveness of several types and combinations of generally accepted school-based preventive dental procedures in order to provide the data base for developing the most effective modern school-based preventive dental program. The preventive procedures selected included five general categories: (1) fluorides (topical and systemic), (2) sealants, (3) diet regulation, (4) plaque control, and (5) classroom health education. The major findings from this program were the following:
1. There was a sharp decline in the prevalence of dental caries from the late 1970s to the early 1980s.
2. The application of dental sealants is the most effective preventive measure of those utilized in the program.

3. Community water fluoridation is effective in reducing dental caries.
4. Classroom-based preventive measures are ineffective.[36,53]

The study was reviewed and critiqued by a Review Committee of the American Public Health Association. Although the committee had reservations as to the specific design of the study as well as the analytical methods applied, there is general consensus that the first three findings of the study appear to be correct. The fourth finding is considered questionable because of possible flaws in study design.

The NPDDP suggests several elements of dental research that need improvement or greater emphasis. The profession should adopt a more conservative attitude when projecting the expected benefits from the practical application of preventive measures whose merit is supported by only a few clinical trials conducted by a limited number of investigators. Many clinical trials conducted by totally independent investigators should be mandated before any preventive measure is regarded as safe, effective, and efficient.

It is imprudent to neglect basic research while pushing ahead with practical application. The lack of basic research on the mechanism of fluoride action in the prevention of dental decay and in the production of enamel fluorosis was evident from this study. Several of the modes of application of the agent may have been duplicating rather than reinforcing, each other.

Greater attention should be given to monitoring the prevalence of dental diseases so that up-to-date indices are available that will further delineate characteristics of populations to be studied. There is a need for maintenance of an established pool of skilled clinical investigators who would be available to take part in large-scale national clinical trials. Also there is a need to foster new research leading to improved clinical trial methodology, reduced cost, and possibly the reduction in the size of groups to be studied.

As a result of this study, two additional areas of research have been identified: (1) There is a definite need to develop and apply better outcome measures for the evaluation of the effectiveness of school dental health education programs; and (2) more research is needed to identify the significant characteristics of groups susceptible to dental diseases.[36]

Given that fluoridation is highly cost-effective and requires no behavior change on the part of the individual to produce its effects, future research should explore strategies for increasing its acceptance.[60]

Further details regarding the American Dental Association's pilot program and each of the other research projects can be obtained from the organizations involved.

SUMMARY

An analysis of the information presented in this chapter leads to several conclusions regarding the status of and future for community dental health education programs. We have seen that the traditional educational activities based on either the cognitive or behavioral models of learning cannot alone be effective in achieving the goal of disease prevention and control. Techniques developed and refined for educating an individual patient differ from those that should be applied to the community. Behavioral research and expert opinions agree that educational methodologies have not yet been developed that can be successfully applied to the community at large. Given the variance in human limitations, questions must be answered regarding the possibility or practicality of concentrating resources on trying to discover an educational strategy that could be applied equally to all and the possibility of changing the perception of dental disease so that persons will seek early detection and treatment for problems.

Dental health education programs for the community should be applicable to all segments of the population and should be developed through appropriate program planning and implementation criteria. A needs assessment should be conducted to define the extent of the problem and serve as baseline data and to determine program objectives and priorities, alternative solutions, and evaluation guidelines. Evaluation must be an ongoing and integral component of the plan; it must focus on measuring the program's effectiveness in terms of disease reduction, not merely increased knowledge or improved performance level. Longitudinal behavioral studies should be conducted to validate the cost-benefit and cost-effectiveness of each program.

Existing curriculum and field experiences for dental and dental hygiene students must be reexamined and revised in light of the new responsibilities these professionals must assume in the community setting. Students should be educated in community organization, group dynamics, program planning and implementation strategies, effectiveness of community preventive measures, and community decision-making processes and the necessary communication, management, and leadership skills.

Research must continue in order to develop, test, and evaluate new combinations of preventive programs and to evaluate the effectiveness of any new strategies for community dental health education. More must be known about the relationship between plaque and dental caries and about the acquisition of oral health as a value. Community programs must use the approaches most likely to succeed against known barriers to receiving dental care and maintaining good oral health.

If the success of dental health education programs in schools is judged by effectiveness based on knowledge, attitudes, and skill acquisition, evaluators of such programs must be held accountable for conducting evaluation studies in a manner appropriate to these predetermined general objectives.

Dental health education in schools can be more of a priority, however, that involves the efforts of many people. Universities and colleges charged with the responsibility of preparing school personnel must include dental health as a component of the curriculum. School districts also need to explore ways of including dental health education on a permanent basis. Parents must be encouraged to support dental health activities through reinforcement at home and can also join other health professionals in demanding that dental health education be a mandatory component of health education in every curriculum.

There are several major changes taking place that will affect the dental profession and the oral health of the public: a reduction in tooth decay, an increased awareness of the prevalence of periodontal disease, changes in population demographics that may affect the prevalence of root caries, periodontal conditions and oral cancer in association with advancing age, and finally an alarming increase in the use of smokeless tobacco among American youth. Future planning in community dental health education will include the targeting of preventive measures for specific subgroups with documented unmet needs within the general population. Innovative programs for persons with developmental disabilities residing in the community and in state institutions, as well as programs for the elderly (ambulatory, homebound, and institutionalized) have been developed. Creativity and resourcefulness in future program planning are essential in view of our finite resources, especially funding, which is so crucial to program development, implementation, and evaluation.

REFERENCES

1. American Association of State and Territorial Dental Directors: Policy statement: resolution on preventive dentistry, March 1974, The Association.
2. American Dental Association: Ask higher dental priorities at AMA-Kennedy meeting, ADA Leadership Bull. 7(16), 1978.
3. American Dental Association: Health education at the worksite, Maine project report, Chicago, 1986, ADA Bureau of Health Education and Audio Visual Service.
4. American Dental Association: Learning about your oral health: a prevention-oriented school program, Chicago, 1986, American Dental Association, Bureau of Health Education.
5. American Dental Hygienists' Association: Self-study course: the dental health consultant in community-based programs, Chicago, 1983, The Association.
6. American Dental Hygienists' Association: Self-study course: dental hygiene care of the special needs patient, Chicago, 1983, The Association.
7. Bivins, E.C.: History and development of dental public health in North Carolina, Report prepared for the North Carolina Department of Human Resources, Division of Health Services, Dental Health Section, March 1974.
8. Carlos, J.P., editor: Prevention and oral health, Fogarty Internationaol Center Series on Preventive Medicine, vol. I, DHEW Pub. No. NIII 74-707. U.S. Department of Health, Education and Welfare, Public Health Service, National Institute of Health, 1973.
9. Castile, A.S., and Jerrick, S.J.: School health in America, ed. 2, Atlanta, GA, 1979, U.S. Department of Health, Education and Welfare, American School Health Association.
10. Chambers, D.W.: Susceptibility to preventive dental treatment, J. Public Health Dent. 33(2):82, 1973.
11. Cozort, P.J., and Sheffrin, S.: Learning about your oral health, Paper presented at the First National Symposium on Dental Health Education in Schools, Chicago, October 1975, American Dental Association, Bureau of Health Education.
12. Croucher, R., and others: The "spread effect" of a school-based dental health education project, Community Dent. Oral Epidemiol. 13:205, 1985.
13. Davis, M.S.: Variations in patients' compliance with doctors' orders: analyses of congruence between survey responses and results of empirical investigations, J. Med. Educ. 41:1037, 1966.
14. Davis, R.L., and others: Comprehensive school health education: a practical definition, J. Sch. Health 55(8): 335, 1985.
15. Domoto, P.K., Faine, R.C., and Rovin, S.: Seattle fluoridation campaign 1973—prescription of a victory, J. Am. Dent. Assoc. 91(3):583, 1975.
16. Dworkin, S.F., Ference, T.P., and Giddon, D.B.: Behavioral science and dental practice, St. Louis, 1978, The C.V. Mosby Co.
17. Ezell, O.L.: Evaluation of the American Dental Association's prevention-oriented program in a school health education setting, Paper presented at the First National

Symposium on Dental Health Education in Schools, Chicago, October 1975, American Dental Association, Bureau of Health Education.

18. Frankel, J.M., and Allukian, M.: Sixteen referenda on fluoridation in Massachusetts: an analysis, J. Public Health Dent. **33**(2):96, 1973.

19. Frazier, P.J., and others: Quality of information in mass media: a barrier to the dental health education of the public, J. Public Health Dent. **34**(4):244, 1974.

20. Frazier, P.J.: The effectiveness and practicality of current dental health education programs from a public health perspective: a conceptual appraisal, Paper presented at the Dental Health Section Symposium, American Public Health Association's Annual Meeting, Miami Beach, FL, October 1976.

21. Frazier, P.J.: A new look at dental health education in community programs, Dent. Hygiene **52**(11):535, 1978.

22. Fructer, D.A.: An evaluation of the Tattletooth dental program covering ongoing evaluation, 1977-1978, Report prepared for the Bureau of Dental Health, Texas Department of Health, 1978.

23. Gravies, R.C., and others: A comparison of effectiveness of the "Toothkeeper" and a traditional dental health education program, J. Public Health Dent. **35**(2):81, 1975.

24. Haefner, D.P.: School dental health programs, Health Educ. Monogr. **2**(3):212, 1974.

25. Heifetz, S.B., and Suomi, J.D.: The control of dental caries and periodontal disease: a fundamental approach, J. Public Health Dent. **33**(1):2, 1973.

26. Heifetz, S.B., and others: Programs for the mass control of plaque: an appraisal, J. Public Health Dent. **33**(2):91, 1973.

27. Hirakio, S.S., and Foote, F.M.: Statewide fluoridation: how it was done in Connecticut, J. Am. Dent. Assoc. **75**:174, 1967.

28. Horowitz, L.G.: The self-care motivation model: theory and practice in human development, J. Sch. Health **55**(2):57, 1985.

29. Horowitz, A.M., and others: Effect of supervised daily plaque removal by children: results after third and final year, J. Dent. Res. (special issue) abstract no. 85, 1977.

30. Horowitz, H.S., and others: Combined fluoride, school-based program in a fluoride-deficient area: results of an 11-year study, J. Am. Dent. Assoc. **112**(5):621, 1986.

31. Horowitz, H.S., and others: Evaluation of a combination of self-administered fluoride procedures for the control of dental caries in a nonfluoride area: findings after four years, J. Am. Dent. Assoc. **98**(2):219, 1979.

32. Hunter, E.L.: Volunteerism of dental hygienists, Dent. Hygiene **52**(11):535, 1978.

33. Kamholtz, J.D., and Wood, B.: Competing with Ronald McDonald, Cap'n Crunch and the Pepsi Generation, J. Sch. Health **52**(1):17, 1982.

34. Kegeles, S.S.: Why people seek dental care: a review of present knowledge, Am. J. Public Health **51**:1306, 1961.

35. Kegeles, S.S.: Why people seek dental care: a test of a conceptual formulation, J. Health Hum. Behavior **4**:166, 1963.

36. Klein, S.P., and others: The cost and effectiveness of school-based preventive dental care, Am. J. Public Health **75**:382, 1985.

37. Levy, G.F.: A survey of preschool oral health education programs, J. Public Health Dent. **44**(1):10, 1984.

38. Lewin, K.: Field theory in social science, New York, 1951, Harper and Brothers.

39. McNeil, D.R.: Political aspects of fluoridation, J. Am. Dent. Assoc. **65**(5):659, 1962.

40. Meskins, H.M., Martens, L.V., and Katz, B.J.: Effectiveness of community preventive programs on improving oral health, J. Public Health Dent. **38**(4):302, 1978.

41. Mulholland, D.N.: A comprehensive dental health education program, J. Sch. Health **48**(4):225, 1978.

42. Nasi, J.: Stakes of measures to prevent periodontal disease: effectiveness and practicality in community programs, Paper presented at the American Public Health Association's Annual Meeting, Miami Beach, FL, October 1976.

43. National Health Federation: This is the National Health Federation, leaflet.

44. North Carolina Department of Human Resources, Division of Health Services, Dental Health Section: A ten-year report, p. 72, 1985.

45. North Carolina Department of Human Resources, Division of Health Services, Dental Health Section: Program report—FY86, Program plan—FY87:5, 1986.

46. North Carolina Department of Human Resources, Division of Health Services, Dental Health Section: 1986 conjoint report.

47. Peterson, F.L., Jr., and Rubinson, L.: An evaluation of the effects of the American Dental Association's dental health education program on the knowledge, attitudes, and health locus control of high school students, J. Sch. Health **52**(1):63, 1982.

48. Pipe, P., and others: Developing a plaque control program, Berkeley, CA 1972, Praxis Publishing Co.

49. Podshadley, A.G., and Shannon, J.H.: Oral hygiene performance of elementary school children following dental health education, J. Dent. Child. **37**(4):293, 1970.

50. Podshadley, A.G., and Schweikle, E.S.: The effectiveness of two educational programs in changing the per-

formance of oral hygiene by elementary school children, J. Public Health Dent. **30**(1):17, 1970.

51. Raynor, J.F., and Cohen, L.K.: School dental health education. In Richards, N.D., and Cohen, L.K., editors: Social sciences and dentistry: a critical bibliography, London, 1971, Federation Dentaire International, p. 275.

52. Raynor, J.F., and Cohen, L.K.: A position of school dental health education: behavioral influences on oral hygiene practices, J. Prev. Dent. **1**(2):11, 1974.

53. Review of the national preventive dentistry demonstration program, Am. J. Public Health **76**(4):434, 1986.

54. Rosenstock, I.M.: Why people use health services, Milbank Memorial Fund Q. **44**:94, 1966.

55. Rozier, G.R., and others: Dental health in North Carolina: a chartbook, Department of Health Policy and Administration School of Public Health, University of North Carolina, Chapel Hill, NC, p. 51, 1982.

56. Rubinson, L.: Evaluating school dental health education programs, J. Sch. Health **52**(1):26, 1982.

57. Sacket, D.L., and Haynes, R.B.: Compliance with therapeutic regimens, Baltimore, 1976, Johns Hopkins University Press.

58. Shiller, W.R., and Dittmer, J.C.: An evaluation of some current oral hygiene motivation methods, J. Periodontal. **39**(2):83, 1968.

59. Shorey, N.L.: Using state policy to affect dental health education: vending, Paper presented at the Second National Symposium on Dental Health Education in Schools, Miami Beach, FL, Chicago, October 1977, American Dental Association, Bureau of Health Education.

60. Silversin, J., and Kornacki, M.J.: Acceptance of preventive measures by individuals, institutions, and communities, Int. Dent. J. **34**:170, 1984.

61. Smith, L.W., and others: Teachers as models in programs for school dental health: an evaluation of "The Toothkeeper," J. Public Health Dent. **35**(2):75, 1975.

62. Stamm, J.W., Kuo, H.C., and Neil, D.R.: An evaluation of the "Toothkeeper" program in Vermont, J. Public Health Dent. **35**(2):81, 1975.

63. Stone, D.B., Mortimer, R.G., and Rubinson, L.: An evaluation of the cognitive aspect of the American Dental Association's learning about your oral health teaching and learning program, level II, Paper presented at the First National Symposium on Dental Health Education in Schools, Chicago, October 1975, American Dental Association, Bureau of Health Education.

64. Taub, A.: Dental health education: rhetoric or reality? J. Sch. Health **52**(1):10, 1982.

65. Texas Department of Health: Tattletooth for the school nurse, Austin, TX, 1976.

66. Texas Department of Health: Preventive dentistry program, Austin, TX, 1986.

67. Texas Department of Health: Tattletooth program: statewide implementation plan, Austin, TX, 1986.

68. U.S. Department of Health and Human Services, Public Health Service Center for Disease Control, Morbidity and Mortality Weekly Report: Current trends—the effectiveness of school health education **35**(38):593, 1986.

69. Weinstein, P., and Getz, T.: Changing human behavior: strategies for preventive dentistry, Chicago, 1978, Science Research Associates, Inc.

70. World Health Organization: Dental health education, technical report series no. 449, Geneva, 1970, The Organization.

71. Yacovone, J.A.: Translating research in the social and behavioral sciences for more effective use in community dentistry, J. Public Health Dent. **36**(3):155, 1971.

72. Young, M.A.C.: Dental health education: an overview of selected concepts and principles relevant to programme planning, Int. J. Health Educ. **13**(1):2, 1970.

CHAPTER 10

Planning for Community Programs

René Dubos has pointed out that most of human history has been a result of accidents and blind choices. When a crisis occurs, our solutions are immediate and involve piecemeal efforts rather than considered and thoughtful planning. The need to develop our ability to predict, plan, and thus *prevent* the same crisis from recurring should have the highest priority.[4]

WHY PLAN?

As part of our role as health professionals, we will be called on to assist health agencies and organizations in developing plans for obtaining dental care. We now need to develop our own abilities to take our dental expertise and channel it into the areas of policy development, decision making, and program planning in a system more complex than the one with which we are familiar in the private dental office. This complex system may take the form of a community, an organization, a corporation, or an institution. The system can be better understood if we look on it as a patient, possessing certain needs and characteristics. Because we are dealing with more than one individual, planning a program for a community or institution requires a deep understanding and analysis of the system as a whole as well as of the individual members that make up the system.

Planning dental care for the patient

The steps the dentist takes when seeing a *patient* for the first time can be compared to the steps a planner takes when viewing a *system* for the first time. When a new patient walks into the dental office, he/she is given a complete medical and dental history. This provides background information on the patient's health, history of diseases, and drug reactions, as well as the patient's history of dental care. In addition, information on the patient's ethnic background, degree of education, and financial status may indicate the patient's attitude about dental care, the type of dental care he/she wants, and how that care will be financed. A clinical examination with the use of radiographs further reveals the type and the quality of dental care received and identifies any existing conditions or disease requiring treatment. For the dentist, these steps *assess the needs* of the patient.

The next step is to identify and diagnose the problems. Perhaps the patient requires full mouth reconstruction to restore the mouth to optimum functioning. The dentist reviews *with* the patient the ideal plan as well as acceptable *alternatives* based on the patient's wants and financial limitations. Once the patient accepts the treatment plan and the method of payment, the plan is ready to be *implemented*.

The dentist selects the appropriate person to perform the necessary services from a staff of specialists and designs a realistic *timetable* to coordinate who will do what first, second, and so on until treatment has been completed.

When treatment has been completed, the patient is placed on a 6-month recall and returns to have an *evaluation* of the care that was rendered. Any modifications or adjustments are done at this time. The patient is then placed on a maintenance plan and returns periodically for a routine examination. This becomes an *ongoing* process for the patient and the dentist. The difference between the planning steps for an individual patient and the planning steps for a community is that when dealing with more than one individual at a time, the steps become more complex. The box on p. 182 compares the provision of dental care for a private patient with that for a community.

Planning dental care for the community

Usually a planner is contacted because a problem has been identified within the community, for example, a high incidence of nursing bottle caries among young children. The planner, like the dentist, begins by conducting a *needs assessment* of these children and their families. Included in the needs assessment will be the population's health problems and beliefs, ethnic makeup, diet, education and socioeconomic status, number of children with nursing bottle caries, and the severity of the disease. Again, this information will help the planner in determining an appropriate plan.

Once the information has been gathered and analyzed, the planner, along with the community, *sets priorities* for dealing with the problem. The planner may decide that the first priority is to treat all existing nursing bottle cases within the community, followed by reeducating the mothers and fathers of these children and those individuals who recommended sweetening the contents of the children's bottles. The planner then sets a reasonable goal to reduce the incidence of nursing bottle caries within that community within a specified time period and proposes methods or objectives to accomplish the goal.

Next, the planner identifies what resources are available to the community. Who will provide the treatment, how will the care be financed, and where will the care be provided? If too many *constraints* exist (for example, no

transportation available to bring the children to the dental office or a lack of funds necessary to provide the treatment), then the planner has to consider alternative strategies to accomplish the intended goal. The planner might identify and recruit volunteer dentists or dental students to treat the children at no cost to the community.

Once the decision is made and approved by the community, it is ready for *implementation*. An implementation timetable is developed to provide a schedule for putting the plan into action.

After the children have been treated, a 6-month follow-up examination is instituted to evaluate the effectiveness of the plan. At that time, the planner addresses questions such as the following: How many children identified as having nursing bottle caries were treated? How many dropped out of treatment, and if so, why did they? How many developed new nursing bottle caries? The answers to these questions will help the planner to modify and adjust the program according to the needs of the community.

The steps taken by a dentist to plan a course of action for the patient are a simplified version of the steps taken by a planner to plan for a community. However, because of time, cost, or labor limitations, the planner may find it necessary to modify the plan by considering various options that will ultimately reach the same end.

Who are the individuals who do the planning? There are many kinds of planners; some have been professionally trained and/or educated, while others have received on-the-job experience within their organization. There are two perspectives to planning: planning by individuals within the system/organization and planning by those brought into the system/organization from outside. A planner hired from within the system is usually an individual whose work responsibility is to plan for the system on a full-time basis. The advantage of hiring from within is that the planner already has a true understanding

---

A COMPARISON OF THE PROVISION OF DENTAL CARE
FOR A PRIVATE PATIENT AND FOR A COMMUNITY

Private patient	Community
1. The dentist conducts a dental and medical *history* and a clinical *examination* of the patient.	1. The planner conducts a *survey* of the community's structure and dental status.
2. The dentist *diagnoses* the oral health of the patient.	2. The planner *analyzes* the survey data of the community.
3. The dentist develops a *treatment plan* based on the diagnosis, the priorities, the patient's attitude, and the method of payment for the services.	3. The planner develops a program plan based on the analysis of the survey data, the priorities and alternatives, the community's attitudes, and the resources available.
4. The dentist obtains patient consent for treatment.	4. The planner obtains community approval of the plan.
5. The dentist selects the appropriate labor to provide the care: dentist, specialist, laboratory technician, dental hygienist, dental assistant.	5. The planner selects the appropriate labor to implement the program: dentist, dental hygienist, dental assistant, dental technician, nutritionist, health educator, school teacher, social worker, health aides, public health nurses.
6. The dentist selects the appropriate *dental service* for the patient: preventive services, restorative services, endodontic services, and so on.	6. The planner selects the appropriate activities for the community: community water fluoridation, school-based fluoride rinse programs, comprehensive dental services, oral cancer screening and referral programs.
7. The dentist evaluates the treatment rendered to the patient: clinical examination, radiographs, patient oral hygiene, patient satisfaction.	7. The planner evaluates the community program: comparison of baseline survey with subsequent survey, attainment of goals and objectives, cost-effectiveness of activities, appropriateness of activities, community satisfaction.

Modified from Young, W., and Striffler, D.: The dentist, his practice, and the community, Philadelphia, 1969, W.B. Saunders Co.

of the issues and operation of the system, including the subtleties of that system. This knowledge enables the planner to more quickly begin making decisions regarding appropriate action. The disadvantage, however, is that the planner may already have acquired certain biases about the system that could influence his/her objectivity.

The planner brought in from outside is usually an individual who contracts to work for the company or agency on a consulting basis for a short period of time. The planner's job is to assist the organization in its planning by formulating a new proposal and/or making recommendations for changing an existing plan. The advantage of this type of planner is that he/she potentially brings to the organization a fresher outlook, less bias, and a greater sense of objectivity than someone from the inside. The drawback is that the planner requires more time to reach a level of understanding of the system sufficient to plan an appropriate course of action.

One of the most important concerns for any planner should be to take into consideration the human element. Statistics alone do not tell the whole story. For example, a planner who reviews the health labor statistics on a multiethnic community and who sees that, overall, sufficient numbers of practitioners work within the community may think that the community does not need any new practitioners. A closer examination of the practitioner/patient populations may reveal that the practitioners are primarily of a certain ethnic background and do not like treating patients of different ethnic backgrounds of which there are a great number in the community. Thus, there may be large subgroups of the population who do not have *access* to dental care, even though statistically there are enough dentists available in the community. While statistics can be most useful in analyzing data, a planner must be aware of their limitations.

PLANNING: A DEFINITION

E.C. Banfield presents a basic definition of the term *planning:* "a plan is a decision about a course of action." In other words, a plan is a systematic approach to defining the problem, setting priorities, developing specific goals and objectives, determining alternative strategies and a method of implementation.

There are many types of health planning. Each varies according to the factors affecting the health system, such as the geography of a region, the sociocultural background of the population, economic considerations, and the political situation.

Some types of health planning, as outlined by Spiegel and associates, include the following[8]:

1. *Problem-solving planning* involves the identification and resolution of a problem.

An example of problem solving was the appearance of dental fluorosis among residents of a community in Colorado. This enamel disorder was identified through a scientific study of possible causative factors.

2. *Program planning* entails designing a course of action for a circumscribed health problem. School-based fluoride rinse programs are an example of designing a course of action for the problem of dental caries within a community setting.

3. *Coordination of efforts and activities planning* aims to increase the availability, efficiency, productivity, effectiveness, and other aspects of activities and programs. This often involves an adjustment process such as a merger or a closing of services and facilities. An example of this is the closing of obstetric and pediatric wards in hospitals located in areas with a declining birth rate.

4. *Planning for the allocation of resources* involves selecting the best alternative to achieve a desired goal when the amount of resources is limited. Planners are called on to allocate the budget, the labor, and the facilities in a system so that it may meet existing needs and demands. An example of this is the decision by a state government with limited financial resources for the provision of dental services to cut services to medically indigent adults based on the cost-effectiveness of providing preventive dental care to a younger population.

5. *Creation of a plan* involves the development of a blueprint or proposal for action containing recommendations and supporting data. It is common for a commission or special task force to be created to prepare the plan. A state health plan that describes the health status and the distribution of health services for the population in that state is a good example of such planning.

6. *Design of standard operating procedures*

requires planners to come forth with a set of standards of practice or criteria for operation and evaluation. This can be a result of legislation or can be created voluntarily by the parties concerned. Guidelines for evaluating the quality of dental care as part of a quality assurance program for an insurance company is one example.

This chapter describes various types of health planning but concentrates specifically on the program-planning process. This process of program planning uses a systematic approach as seen in Fig. 10-1 and should be used as a guide to solving a particular problem. The process can be compared to the ability of a jazz musician to take the notes of a standard musical scale and use them to create a unique melody. In a similar fashion, a planner uses the program-planning steps to create a plan that is unique for the specific situation or system.

The process of planning is dynamic. Within a fluctuating and ever-changing system, the process itself must remain fluid and flexible, responsive to the presentation of new factors and issues.

This chapter will discuss the components of program planning and focus on the various options available to the planner. Let us first discuss the initial step in the planning process—conducting a needs assessment.

CONDUCTING A NEEDS ASSESSMENT

There are several reasons why a planner should conduct a needs assessment. The primary reason is to *define* the problem and to *identify* its extent and severity. Second, it is used to obtain a profile of the community to ascertain the causes of the problem. This information will help in developing the appropriate goals and objectives in the problem solution.

Another important reason to conduct a needs assessment is to evaluate the effectiveness of the program. This is accomplished by obtaining baseline information and, over time, measuring the amount of progress achieved in solving the specific problem.

Suppose the planner designed a program to administer fluoride tablets to all school-aged children in a given community. To determine how effective a fluoride tablet program is in terms of reduction of dental caries, the planner would first take a baseline needs assessment of the caries rate among the schoolchildren prior to implementing the fluoride tablet program. After the initial assessment, the program is implemented. To measure the effectiveness of such a preventive regimen, the planner would then make periodic assessments of the schoolchildren at various time intervals and compare these results with the initial assessment.

Conducting a needs assessment for a community can be a very costly endeavor, with respect to funds, labor, and time. If the funds are not readily available, there are several options for the planner.

One option is to coordinate with the research activities of other agencies interested in obtaining similar health information on the given population. For example, a neighborhood health center may be involved in conducting a health survey of all the residents living in a defined geographic area.

Another method is to investigate surveys that have been done in the past by other organizations. Frequently, dental surveys are conducted through research departments of dental schools, through local and state health departments, or by the local health systems agencies (HSAs). If no surveys have ever been done, the planner may either want to solicit the assistance of these agencies and organizations or inform them that a survey will be conducted. This will avoid overlap or duplication of activities.

Whether the planner conducts his/her own survey, combines efforts with others, or utilizes information from past surveys, it is important to consider what type of information is needed and how it should be obtained.

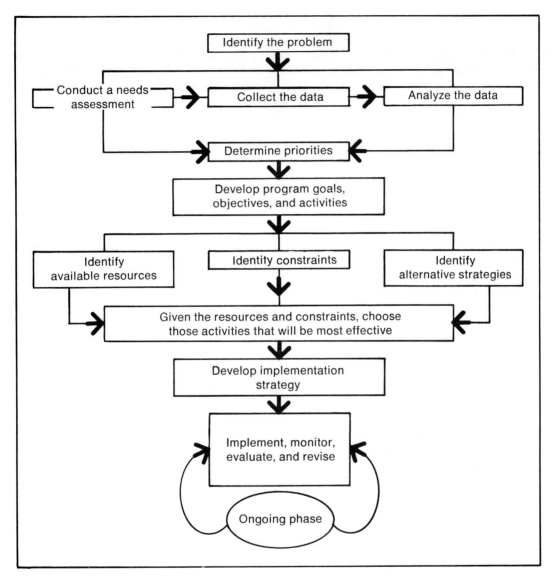

Fig. 10-1. Planning and implementation strategy—flow chart.

Data can be obtained by various techniques such as survey questionnaires or clinical examinations or more informally through personal communications. The technique the planner chooses is based on who is to be examined. Factors the planner should consider are the number of individuals involved, the extent and degree of severity of the problem, and the attitudes of the individuals to be surveyed. The greater the number of individuals to be examined, the more formal the survey. If the problem is clinical, as opposed to attitudinal, a more clinical examination might be recommended. If the planner wants to interview a small group of individuals on their attitudes and feelings about a particular issue, a personal communication might be more appropriate.

To gather general information on a population, a *population profile* should be obtained. Such a profile includes the following:

1. Number of individuals in the population
2. The geographic distribution of the population
3. The rate of growth
4. The population density and degree of urbanization
5. The ethnic backgrounds
6. The diet and nutritional levels
7. The standard of living, including types of housing
8. The amount and type of public services and utilities
9. The public and private school system
10. A general health profile
11. The patterns and distribution of dental disease

To gather epidemiological data on the patterns and distribution of dental disease, the planner can use a clinical examination (Fig. 10-2), review patients' dental records, or consult the National Health Survey for data on a population residing in a similar geographic region with similar characteristics.

In addition to assessing the incidence and the distribution of dental disease, the planner needs to inquire into the history and current status of dental programs in the community. Questions to ask should include those listed below:

1. What types of programs currently exist?
2. Are these programs oriented toward prevention, treatment, education, research, or combination?
3. Who or what organization is responsible for the planning, implementation, and/or administration of the program(s)?

4. How successful have those responsible been?
5. What was the community's acceptance of such a program?

The planner must learn the way in which policies are developed and decisions are made within the community to better understand the community as a whole, especially if he/she is new to the community. He/she needs to explore the following areas:

1. Who are the financial leaders (bankers, business people) and who are the political leaders (mayor, city council, other public officials)?
2. Who sets the policies for the community?
3. What is the organizational structure of the community?
4. What are the community leaders' attitudes toward oral health and community dental programs?

Once the planner learns how the community operates, he/she needs to examine the types of resources that are available to the community to successfully implement a program. These include the *funds*, the *facilities*, and the *labor*. The following questions might be asked:

1. Funds
   a. What is the source of funding at the state and local level for dental care?
   b. Is third party coverage available to the community through the workplace?
   c. Is federal funding available through special eligibility programs?
   d. Are private funds available through foundations or endowments?
2. Facilities
   a. Where is the closest major medical center?
   b. What specialty services does it provide?
   c. What dental facilities exist and where are they located (in public schools, health centers, hospitals)?
   d. How well are the facilities utilized by the population?
   e. Are the facilities easily assessible to the population served?
   f. Are the provided dental services handled

appropriately, adequately, and efficiently?

  g. Is the equipment adequate and running efficiently?

  h. How many operatories are available?

  i. How many dental laboratories are available?

3. Labor

  a. How many active licensed dentists, hygienists, and assistants are available?

  b. How many laboratory technicians are available?

  c. How many expanded function dental auxiliaries are available?

  d. How many dental and dental auxiliary schools are located nearby?

  e. How many active community health aides are available?

  f. How many public health nurses are available?

  g. How many school nurses are available?

  h. How many public health hygienists, voluntary health agencies, and nutritionists are available?

When planning a dental program for a community or institution, it is important for the planner to determine where the population obtains water and the fluoride status of that water. In certain regions of the country, particularly in rural areas, many persons obtain their water from either individual wells or nearby rivers, lakes, or streams. The amount of fluoride in the water sources might indicate to the planner that a fluoride supplement program may not be necessary for that community. If individual wells are being used the planner would need to get a report on the fluoride status of each well, since wells may be receiving their water from different sources.

If a community is obtaining water from a central area, the planner needs the following information:

1. What type of drinking water is available to the community?

2. What is the fluoride content of the water?

3. Does the water contain optimum levels of fluoride?

4. What efforts, if any, have been made in the past to gain fluoridation?

5. What are the attitudes of the community, the dental profession, and decision makers toward fluoridation?

6. What are the laws in regard to fluoridation?

7. Is a referendum possible or required?

8. Are the school's water supplies fluoridated?

In order to avoid duplication of fluoride administration, the planner also should inquire into the type of fluoride being administered to individuals in the private office, the schools, and the health centers.

1. Do the local dentists or physicians prescribe fluoride supplements to their patients?

2. Do the schools (preschool, parochial, public) have a fluoride tablet or rinse program?

3. Do the health centers or hospitals administer fluoride to their patients?

4. Do fluoride brush-in programs exist in the schools? If so:

5. How often do children brush with a fluoride toothpaste?

6. How successful have these programs been and how are they supported?

All the information presented in this section can easily be obtained through the various survey instruments discussed. If, however, a survey cannot be conducted, the necessary information on an institution or a community can also be obtained through other means. This approach will require the planner to investigate all available sources that might have data relevant to the population and/or the community. Such sources include the local, state, and federal agencies and private organizations.

In a small community, one can find a tremendous amount of information on the community's residents by visiting the local health department. The local health department maintains statistics on the population's health status, morbidity and mortality, general health problems, and health service utilization. A trip to the chamber of commerce and town hall will provide useful information on the community profile including population distribution, age breakdown, in-

WHO COMBINED ORAL HEALTH AND TREATMENT ASSESSMENT FORM   Sheet 1

Note: 1. No codes to be changed.   2. Unused sections to be cancelled by diagonal lines

Examination

(1) [J 2] (5)   (6) [ ] (7) Registration (8) [ ] (11) Number
Study Number   Date 19   Number   [ ] (for (12) duplicates)

PERSONAL AND DEMOGRAPHIC INFORMATION

Sex   M = 1   F = 2 . . . . (13) [ ]   Name . . . .
                             family   other

Age in years . . . . (14) [ ] (15)   Geographic location . . . . (18) [ ] (19)

Ethnic group . . . . (16) [ ]   Examiner . . . . (20) [ ]

Occupation . . . . (17) [ ]

SERVICE UTILIZATION

Q. 1 Did you obtain dental care in the last 12 months?

                    NO = 0   (21) [ ]   CODE CATEGORIES FROM RESPONSE (1 to 6, 9)
                    YES = 1   See list in criteria (p. 1)

If YES Q. 1(a) For what reason?   (22) [ ]   CODE CATEGORIES FROM RESPONSE (1 to 5)
                                     See list in criteria (p. 1)
    Q. 1(b) Who treated you?   (23) [ ]
                                       CODE CATEGORIES FROM RESPONSE (1 to 9)
If NO   Q. 1(c) Why not?   (24) [ ]   See list in criteria (p. 2)

Q. 2 Is anything wrong with your teeth, gums or mouth now?

                            (25) [ ]   CODE CATEGORIES FROM RESPONSE (0 to 4, 9)
                                       See list in criteria (p. 2)

Q. 2(a) Do you want any dental advice or treatment?

                    NO = 0   (26) [ ]
                    YES = 1

If you do Q. 2(b) What sort of advice or treatment do you want?

                            (27) [ ]   CODE CATEGORIES FROM RESPONSE (0 to 9)
                                       See list in criteria (p. 2)

DISORDERS OF MUCOSA TEETH AND BONE AND OTHER CONDITIONS

       ABSENT = 0, PRESENT, NO TREATMENT
   RECOMMENDED = 1, PRESENT, TREATMENT
            RECOMMENDED = 2   OTHER CONDITIONS

ORAL MUCOSAL DISEASE   (28) [ ]   Titles to be entered as needed, from results of pilot study
Specify
Disease . . . . (31) [ ]
Treatment . . . .

DEFECT OF TEETH   (29) [ ]
Specify
Defect . . . . (32) [ ]
Treatment . . . .

DISORDERS INVOLVING BONE
Specify   (30) [ ]   . . . . (33) [ ]
Disease . . . .
Treatment . . . .

PROSTHETIC STATUS   DENTURE REQUIREMENTS
   NO   DENTURE = 0, DENTURE WEARING = 1   NIL = 0, NEW DENTURE REQUIRED = 1
         DENTURE NOT WEARING 2   REPAIR, RELINE OR REMODEL 2
    UPPER JAW   LOWER JAW   LOWER JAW   UPPER JAW

(34) [ ] (35) [ ] (36) [ ] (37) [ ]   (38) [ ] (39) [ ] (40) [ ] (41) [ ]
   full   partial   full   partial   full   partial   full   partial

WHO 5-297 ORH (6/76) 40000

Fig. 10-2. An oral data collection instrument. (From World Health Organization/ Division of Dentistry. USPHS: An international collaborative study of dental manpower in relation to oral health status, Document 2. Geneva, 1977.)

WHO COMBINED ORAL HEALTH AND TREATMENT ASSESSMENT FORM   Sheet 2

Note: 1. No codes to be changed.   2. Unused sections to be cancelled by diagonal lines

(1) J 2 ____ (5) Date 19   (6) ☐☐ (7) Registration (8) ☐☐☐ (11) ☐   Examination Number (12) ☐
Study Number   Number   (for duplicates)

PERIODONTAL STATUS   Absent = 0   Present = 1

SOFT DEPOSITS	max. (42) ☐☐	(44)	
	mand. (45) ☐☐	(47)	
CALCULUS	max. (48) ☐☐	(50)	
	mand. (51) ☐☐	(53)	
INTENSE GINGIVITIS	max. (54) ☐☐	(56)	
	mand. (57) ☐☐	(59)	
ADVANCED PERIODONTAL INVOLVEMENT	max. (60) ☐☐	(62)	
	mand. (63) ☐☐	(65)	

NB. Central segments include cuspids and incisors left and right segments include molars and premolars

PERIODONTAL TREATMENT REQUIREMENTS

(66) ☐

NONE	0
Oral Hygiene Instruction	1
Prophylaxis and OHI	2
Periodontal therapy (no extraction)	3
Treatment with 1 or more extraction	4
Full extraction	5

DENTOFACIAL ANOMALIES

WHO Criteria
condition (specify) . . . . (67) ☐

treatment . . . . (68) ☐

Other criteria (to be specified)
condition (specify) . . . . (69) ☐

treatment . . . . (70) ☐

CONDITIONS NEEDING IMMEDIATE ATTENTION   ABSENT = 0   PRESENT = 1

RELIEF OF EXISTING PAIN OR INFECTION   (71) ☐   TREATMENT OF PULPALLY INVOLVED TEETH (73) ☐

TREATMENT FOR LESIONS LIKELY TO CAUSE PAIN OR INFECTION IN THE IMMEDIATE (72) ☐ FUTURE   OTHER (SPECIFY) . . . . (74) ☐
. . . .
CARD NO. (80) 3

DENTAL CARIES STATUS AND TREATMENT OF TEETH

		55 54 53 52 51 61 62 63 64 65		
		18 17 16 15 14 13 12 11 21 22 23 24 25 26 27 28		
CARIES	(13)	☐☐☐☐☐☐☐☐☐☐☐☐☐☐☐☐	(28)	CARIES
TREATMENT	(29) R	☐☐☐☐☐☐☐☐☐☐☐☐☐☐☐☐	(44)	TREATMENT L
		85 84 83 82 81 71 72 73 74 75		
		48 47 46 45 44 43 42 41 31 32 33 34 35 36 37 38		
CARIES	(45)	☐☐☐☐☐☐☐☐☐☐☐☐☐☐☐☐	(60)	CARIES
TREATMENT	(61)	☐☐☐☐☐☐☐☐☐☐☐☐☐☐☐☐	(76)	TREATMENT

DENTAL CARIES

	PRIMARY	PERM.	TREATMENT	
SOUND	A	0	NONE	0
DECAYED	B	1	RESTORATIONS	
FILLED & CARIES FREE	C	2	1 surface	1
FILLED WITH PRIMARY DECAY	D	3	2 surface	2
FILLED WITH SECONDARY DECAY	E	4	3 surface	3
PRIMARY TEETH MISSING DUE CARIES < 9 yrs	M	–	> 3 surface or crown	4
PERMANENT TEETH MISSING DUE CARIES (UNDER 30 YEARS ONLY)	–	5	EXTRACTION FOR	
PERMANENT TEETH MISSING ANY REASON OTHER THAN CARIES (UNDER 30 YEARS ONLY)			caries	5
			periodontal disease	6
	–	6	dentures	7
PERMANENT TEETH MISSING ANY REASON (30 YEARS & OLDER)	–	7	other reason	8
UNERUPTED TOOTH	–	8	OTHER (specify)	9
EXCLUDED TOOTH	X	9	CARD No. (80)	4

Fig. 10-2, cont'd. For legend see opposite page.

come, educational levels, school systems, and transportation.

In a larger community where health information may not be as readily accessible as in a small community, a good source for data is the health systems agency (HSA). HSAs are federally mandated health planning agencies that develop specific plans to address the health problems of a designated region. HSAs have data on health statistics of a population and health resources available in a given district. The state health department can also provide health related information for all communities, cities, and towns within the state.

The federal government has large volumes of health statistics data from many of its agencies. The most familiar and widely used sources of data are the National Health Surveys and the U.S. Census Bureau. These sources provide longitudinal and comparative data regarding large population groups. Because of the magnitude of the data gathering for these surveys, they are usually conducted once every 10 years. Consideration of the publication date of such data and its relevancy and applicability to specific populations is important.

Other sources for obtaining such data are research studies and investigative reports. Many of these studies are funded by government agencies and are conducted by local organizations, research companies, or consulting groups. A considerable volume of data is usually generated from these reports. A computer literature search (MEDLINE) may be helpful. The National Library of Medicine provides these computer searches for a nominal fee. Most medical libraries affiliated with universities also provide this service.

Once the data are obtained, the information must be analyzed before it can be put into a plan of action. Let us examine the data presented below and consider ways of using the information to develop an appropriate program.

Analysis of data: a case study

BACKGROUND. Tide Water is the fifth largest city in Massachusetts and is situated in the southeastern section of the state on the shore of Deep Water Bay. Excellent water resources and deep-water shipping potential brought industrial growth to Tide Water, and it became the "spindle city of the world" as the cotton industry flourished. Native granite was used to construct multi-story factories, some of which are still in use. This prosperity ended quickly when the cotton manufacturers moved to the South in the 1930s and 1940s. The problem of vacant mill space, in addition to the depression, made Tide Water's economic situation one of the worst in the country. Tide Water was able to make a strong recovery with a growing garment industry, which replaced the cotton mills and other manufacturers and provided a more diversified industrial base.

The following information is available about Tide Water:

POPULATION
1980 census: 96,988 persons
Ethnic and racial characteristics
1. Foreign born: 16%
2. Foreign stock: 48%
3. Race: White 99%
         Black .5%
         Other .5%
4. Density (persons per sq. mile): 2,946

AGE DISTRIBUTION

	Total male	Total female
Under 5 years	4,223	4,047
5 to 14 years	8,120	7,893
15 to 19 years	3,782	4,028
20 to 64 years	23,992	27,458
Over 64 years	4,902	8,453

EDUCATION*
Median number of school years completed: 8.8
Persons completing high school or more: 25.6%
Persons completing fewer than 5 grades: 13.3%

PERSONAL INCOME

Salary	Families
Less than $1,000	616
$1,000 to $2,999	2,341
$3,000 to $4,999	2,988
$5,000 to $6,999	3,922
$7,000 to $8,999	4,474

*Figures reflect a large immigrant population, principally Portuguese.

$9,000 to $11,999	5,761	
$12,000 to $14,999	2,838	
$15,000 to $24,999	2,079	
$25,000 to $49,999	407	
$50,000 or more	95	
Total families	25,521	
Median income	$8,000	

TRANSPORTATION

Bus service: intra- and intercity

Taxi service: 3 companies, with a total of 65 radio equipped cabs

Highways and streets:
4 major highways (2 N-S; 2 E-W)
600 miles of streets 99% paved

FLUORIDE STATUS. Tide Water has a community water supply that has been fluoridated since 1976.

HEALTH RESOURCES (LABOR). 140 physicians
43 dentists

FACILITIES

2 hospitals (725 bed capacity)

1 community health center (diagnosis, primary health dental care, education and prevention; sliding fee)

Mental health centers (many facilities, in-/out-patient clinics and residencies; free and sliding scale fee)

Venereal and tuberculosis (free)

Alcohol and drug programs (free)

15 nursing homes (1150 bed capacity, representing all levels of care)

GOVERNMENT

City size: 33 square miles

Mayor/council form (Mayor, 2 yr. term; Councilmen [9], 2 yr. term)

Democrats: 31,311

Republicans: 4,875

Independents: 10,204

EDUCATIONAL FACILITIES

20 day-care centers (50% free and/or sliding fee)

	Number	Enrollment
Public Schools		
Elementary	32	10,007
Middle	1	982
Junior high school	2	1,852
Academic high school	1	1,948
Girls' vocational high school	1	214
Total	37	15,003

	Number	Enrollment
Parochial schools		
Catholic elementary	15	3,379
Catholic high school	2	992
Other		
Regional/technical high school		
County agricultural high school		
Colleges		
Community college: offers wide range of courses, many in health disciplines		
Southeastern University: 4-year programs in most areas		

It is important to first look into the *socioeconomic structure* of the community and determine the type of employment that exists. Tide Water has a large, industrial, garment area. This leads to the following questions: Is there a high percentage of industrial workers, and if so, are they union employees? If this is the case, are they provided with a comprehensive health benefits package, including the provision of dental care? This information is important because it tells whether or not this population might be able to afford dental care through their jobs.

The *population breakdown* shows a large percentage of Portuguese living within the community. This indicates that possible cultural and language issues should be considered. In addition, the age distribution indicates that the highest proportion of people are between 20 and 60 years of age, or in the age bracket for the adult working population. There is a large population of school-aged children between the ages of 5 and 19 years living in the community. The age distribution of a community is important to consider, since it tells where the target groups are and thus sets up certain priorities for planning. For example, if the majority of the population was of middle to older age, it would not be effective to design a program that would only affect a young population, such as the implementation of school-wide fluoride rinse programs.

The *educational status* of a community provides two perspectives for planning. It first tells the educational level, in years of schooling obtained, by the majority of community members; second, it may indicate what the community's values are toward obtaining an education. Planning a health awareness program centered around an educational institution would only be successful if people are attending schools and value the information they receive there.

Knowing the *median income* of a community is very important to a health planner because it indicates the population's ability to purchase health services. If a segment of the population's income falls below poverty level, those individuals would be eligible for federal and state medical assistance programs (provided the individual states participate in such a program) thus making health services financially accessible to these individuals.

Health care must be geographically accessible as well as financially accessible if people are going to utilize it. A look into the community's public *transportation system* will provide the planner with information regarding a population's ability to get to health care services. This is especially true for rural communities where roads are unpaved and public transportation is scarce.

Looking at the *health care facilities* in the communities will tell the planner what type of services are being provided, the amount of services, and the cost of receiving those services.

The *labor data* give information as to the number of dentists providing care. (The federal government has developed certain labor to population ratios that indicate whether or not a population is considered to be residing in a medically underserved area.) However, just looking at the number of dentists in the community will not give the planner a true picture of whether or not there is a sufficient number of dentists within the community to provide services to the population residing there.

Although there may be an adequate number of dentists in the community, the planner must question whether or not the dentists are avail-

able to provide the care. How long does it take to get appointments? What are their hours (for example, do they work after 5 PM and/or on the weekends)? In addition to knowing the number of dentists, it is necessary to consider *what types* of services are being provided *to whom*, as well as *for what cost*.

Another consideration is the type of practice. Do the dentists accept third party payments or Medicaid payments? Do they provide comprehensive services including preventive care? Do they provide dental health education to their patients?

Knowing the *fluoride status* of a community is also essential for dental planning. In the case study community profile it states that water has been fluoridated since 1976. This indicates that those children born from 1976 on will receive maximum benefits from the fluoridated water. However, it is safe to say that those children born prior to 1976 may need additional attention with other fluoride measures.

In most cases, the *politics* of the community will determine the direction the program will take. A conservative town government attempting to cut costs may be opposed to programs that provide prosthetic services to the medically indigent or elderly. Each *local* government's policies may vary in its methods of instituting new programs, allocating funds, hiring personnel, or setting priorities. In addition, the politics of *state* government will also shape the overall direction taken by the communities within the state.

By looking at the educational system of a community, the planner can determine the number of schools, the enrollment for each, and the distribution of children among the schools within the community. This information can assist the planner who is developing a school-based program for the community. The public and the parochial schools are the ideal settings for dental programs. Moreover, as in countries like New Zealand, schools also serve as excellent vehicles for providing routine dental care.

The educational facilities should be designed appropriately to accommodate such programs. Teachers, parents, and school administrators should be in support of the programs and, most importantly, the need must exist among the school-aged population to warrant such programs. In this particular community with the high percentage of Portuguese children, the schools can be a good meeting place to use to open communication channels with the families and offer support services when needed.

If the planner is designing a dental treatment program for a specific population that is not receiving any care, there are methods developed by the Indian Health Service to convert the survey data into specific resource requirements for treating the population. The Indian Health Service (IHS) is a federal agency within the Public Health Service. IHS has been involved with extensive surveys on the oral health status of American Indians. One method it has developed with the use of specific oral health surveys assesses the dental disease prevalence among the population and translates that data into time and cost estimates to treat the population. These surveys for disease prevalence include the decayed, missing, filled (DMF) index, the Periodontal Index, and the Oral Hygiene Index—Simplified (OHI-S). In addition to determining the dental need, IHS also assesses treatment needs, which include prosthetic status, periodontal status, orthodontal status, oral pathology status, and restorative status.

By using a mathematical model, dental resource requirements can be computed and projected over a period of time. The data are then translated into time, labor, and facility requirements.

The basic measurement is time. Clinical dental services requirements and labor capability both can be expressed in time units. Various time requirement studies have been done by the Indian Health Service to determine the amount of chair time that is necessary to complete a clinical service. This unit of time is called a service minute. For example:

Clinical service	Time required in service minutes[10]
A complete oral examination	10
A prophylaxis	17
Single surface amalgam	10

Labor and facility requirements

The number of dentists and dental auxiliaries as well as of facilities and operatories necessary to treat the population is determined by obtaining the total number of service minutes required for a given population. For example, a random sample of a population was examined and calculations showed that 70,000 service minutes would be required per year to treat approximately 60% of that population. Based on that figure, the amount of staff required to provide approximately 70,000 service minutes would be 1 dentist and 2 dental assistants.[10] The number of operatories needed to accommodate the above dental staff for maximum efficiency would be 3.[10] The ratios (1 dentist to 2 dental assistants to 3 operatories) have been derived from efficiency studies by the Indian Health Service.

This evaluation is highly statistical. Statistics can set parameters to the problem, but the values and attitudes of persons are equally important. The planner must take into consideration the sociocultural interests or the psychological readiness of a people to want or use health services. If the community does not agree on which of the array of statistics represents the community's priorities, little will be done to translate the need identified in the data into effective programs.

DETERMINING PRIORITIES

"Priority determination is a method of imposing people's values and judgments of what is important onto the raw data."[8] The method can be used for different purposes such as for setting priorities among problems elicited through a needs assessment. It also can be used for ranking the solutions to the problem.

Few dental public health programs meet all of the dental needs of the population. With limited resources, it becomes necessary to establish priorities so as to allow the most efficient allocation of resources. If priorities are not determined, the program may not serve those individuals or groups who need the care most.

Certain factors should be considered in determining priorities. For example, a problem that affects a large number of people generally takes priority over a problem that affects a small number of people. However, if the problem is common colds affecting a large number of people competing with swine flu affecting few people, then the more serious problem should take priority.

Given the community profile and analysis of dental survey data, how are priorities established? At this point, the community should be involved to assist in the establishment of these priorities. A health advisory committee or task force representing consumers, community leaders, and providers should be established to assist in the development of policies and priorities. Planning with community representation will aid in the program's implementation and acceptance.

When setting priorities for a community, the planner must ask, How serious is the problem and what percent of the population is affected by it? The number of individuals affected most by the problem would be the group to which the program would be targeted.

However, when the problem is dental disease there is generally more than one target group that is affected. The following are target groups commonly associated with high-risk dental needs:

1. Preschool and school-aged children
2. Mentally and/or physically handicapped persons

3. Chronically ill and/or medically compromised
4. Elderly persons
5. Expectant mothers
6. Low-income minority groups (urban and rural)

If the community decides to address the problem of dental caries first, there are specific groups that are more susceptible to dental caries, such as preschool and school-aged children and low-income minority groups. The planner then begins to develop plans geared to an identifiable population group.

When the target group has been identified (based on the dental problem), the type of program should be established. To do this, the planner begins to set program goals and objectives.

DEVELOPMENT OF PROGRAM GOALS AND OBJECTIVES

Program goals are broad statements on the overall purpose of a program to meet a defined problem. An example of a program goal for a community that has an identifiable problem of dental caries among school-aged children would be "To improve the oral health of the school-aged children in community X."

Program objectives are more specific and describe in a measurable way the desired end result of program activities. The objectives should specify the following:

1. What: the nature of the situation or condition to be attained
2. Extent: the scope and magnitude of the situation or condition to be attained
3. Who: the particular group or portion of the environment in which attainment is desired
4. Where: the geographic areas of the program
5. When: the time "at" or "by" which the desired situation or condition is intended to exist

An objective might state "By 1990 more than 90% of the population aged 6 to 17 years in community X will not have lost any teeth as a result of caries, and at least 40% will be caries-free." This is known as an *outcome objective* and provides a means by which to quantitatively measure the outcome of the specific objective. This approach helps the evaluator and the community know both where the program is and where it hopes to be with respect to a given health problem. It also aids in establishing a realistic timetable for reducing or preventing principal health problems.

Second, objectives are the specific avenues by which goals are met. *Process objectives* state a specific process by which a public health problem can be reduced and prevented. For example:

By 1990 community X will have a public fluoride program to guarantee access to fluoride exposure via:
1. Fluoridation of the public water supply to the optimum level
2. Appropriately monitored fluoridation of school water supplies in areas where community fluoridation is impossible or impractical
3. Initiation of the most cost-effective topical and/ or systemic fluoride supplement programs available to all schools if both (1) and (2) are impossible
4. Provision of topical fluoride application for persons with rampant caries and use of pit and fissure sealants where indicated[5]

Once the problem has been identified and program goals and objectives have been established describing a solution to or a reduction of the problem, the next step is to state how to bring about the desired results. This area of program planning is referred to as program activities, and it describes how the objectives will be accomplished.

Activities include three components: (1) *what* is going to be done, (2) *who* will be doing it, and (3) *when* it will be done. For example:

Activity no. 1: Beginning January 1, 1980, two dental hygienists will be hired to administer a self-applied fluoride rinse program within the public school systems.

Activity no. 2: On March 1, 8, 15, 22, and 30, 1980, a series of 2-day training workshops for parent volunteers will be conducted by the two hygienists at selected public schools in community X.

When planning these program activities, careful consideration should be made to the type of resources available as well as to the program constraints.

Resource identification

Selection of resources for an activity, such as personnel, equipment and supplies, facilities, and financial resources, must be determined by consideration of what would be most effective, adequate, efficient, and appropriate for the tasks to be accomplished. Some criteria that are commonly used to determine what resources should be utilized are listed below:
1. Appropriateness: the most suitable resources to get the job done
2. Adequacy: the extent or degree to which the resources would complete the job
3. Effectiveness: how capable the resources are at completing the job
4. Efficiency: the dollar cost and amount of time expended to complete the job

As discussed previously in the chapter, obtaining the community profile will provide the planner with valuable information on available resources. The type of resources one would need when developing a dental program and the sources from which they can be obtained are listed in the box on p. 196.

Identifying constraints

When planning any program, there are usually as many reasons *not* to do something as there are reasons to do something. The former are usually considered to be roadblocks or obstacles to achieving a certain goal or objective. What

---

RESOURCE IDENTIFICATION WORKSHEET

Resource	Source
Personnel	
Sponsors or supporters	American Dental Association, public health organizations, professional organizations, industry, health consumer groups, government, labor, media, business, foundations, public schools
Clinical providers	Dentists, dental hygienists, dental assistants, dental technicians, social workers, health aides, public health nurses, physician's assistants, nutritionists
Nonclinical	
Planning	Health planning agencies
Clerical	Volunteers, students, unemployed persons, parents
Educational	Professional organizations, universities
Analytical	Universities, consulting firms
Equipment	
Dental units and instruments	Dental supply companies, dental and dental hygiene schools, renovated public health clinics, hospitals, federal government depositories
Typewriters, calculators, filing cabinets	Business, industry, civic groups, hospitals
Supplies	
Office supplies	Consumer groups, industry, business, government
Dental supplies	Dental supply companies, dental products companies
Dental health education materials	American Dental Association, other professional organizations, public health agencies, dairy councils, local, state, or federal agencies, i.e., National Institute for Dental Research, Center for Disease Control
Facilities	Hospitals, health centers nursing homes, public schools, union clinics, public health clinics, industry, Health Maintenance Organizations

---

should be determined at this point are the most obvious constraints to meeting program objectives. By identifying these constraints early in the planning, one can modify the design of the program, thereby creating a more practical and realistic plan.

Constraints may result from organizational policies, resource limitations, or characteristics of the community. For example, constraints that commonly occur in community dental programs include limitations of the state's dental practice act, attitudes of professional organizations, lack of funding, restrictive governmental policies, inadequate transportation systems, labor shortages, lack of or inadequate facilities, negative community attitudes toward dentistry, and the population's socioeconomic, cultural, and educational characteristics. The community's source of water (the type and location), the lack of fluoride in the water, or the community's dental health status are also viewed as constraints to program planning. In addition, the amount of time available to complete a project is considered a constraint if that time is too limited to attain the program goals.

One of the best ways to identify constraints is

to bring together a group of concerned citizens who might in some capacity be involved in or affected by the project. As a group that is familiar with the local politics and community structures, they not only can identify the constraints but can also offer alternative solutions to and/or strategies for meeting the goals.

ALTERNATIVE STRATEGIES

Being aware of the existing constraints and given the available resources, the planner should then consider alternative courses of action that might be effective in attaining the objectives. It is important to generate a sufficient number of alternatives so that out of that number at least one may be considered to be acceptable.

The planner must beware of those alternatives that sound good on the surface but may have certain limitations when closely examined. With limited resources, the planner needs to consider the anticipated costs and the effectiveness of each alternative. A classic example is the use of preventive measures in a community setting. If, for example, the community refused to fluoridate the central water supply, or if a community received its water from individual wells, the planner would look at the alternative preventive measures available in relation to dental caries and the cost savings in terms of needed treatment.

If the preventive measure was considered to be cost-effective as well as practical to implement, the planner would choose the measure as the best of the alternatives. Table 10-1 describes the various types of preventive measures, the ages most affected by dental caries, the effectiveness of such a measure, the cost per year to provide it, the practicality of implementation, and the priority for intervention.

IMPLEMENTATION, SUPERVISION, EVALUATION, AND REVISION

This chapter has concentrated on the planning process: identifying the problem, determining priorities, defining the goals and objectives, identifying the resources and constraints, and considering the alternatives for implementation. The process of putting the plan into operation is referred to as the implementation phase. This phase is ongoing in situations where close supervision and evaluation of the program will ensure effective operations.

The implementation process, like the planning process, involves individuals, organizations, and the community. Integrating all the external variables as depicted in Fig. 10-3 to achieve comprehensive planning and implementation requires what the author terms an *ecologic* approach.[3] Only through teamwork between the individual and the environment can the implementation be successful.

Developing implementation strategy

An implementation strategy for each activity is complete when the following questions are answered:

1. Why: the effect of the objective to be achieved
2. What: the activities required to achieve the objective
3. Who: individuals responsible for each activity
4. When: chronological sequence of activities
5. How: materials, media, methods, techniques to be used
6. How much: a cost estimate of materials and time

To develop an implementation strategy, the planner must know what specific activity he/she wants to do. The most effective method is to work backward to identify the events that must occur prior to initiating the activity. The National Heart, Lung and Blood Institute has developed a *Handbook for Health Professionals and Consumers on Strategies for Designing and Implementing a High Blood Pressure Program in the Community*, which provides examples of implementation strategies that can be applied to

Table 10-1. Criteria for prevention of dental caries

Intervention	Age(s) affected	Cost per year	Effectiveness	General practicality as public health measure	Priority for intervention (1 = high; 11 = low)
Community water fluoridation	All	$.10 to $.40 per capita	50% to 70%	Excellent	1
School water fluoridation	4 to 18 yr	$.30 to $1.24 per child	40%	Good	2
School fluoride supplements (tablets, drops)					
At home	0 to 14 yr	$4.00 to $15.00 per person	20% to 35% depending on regularity of use	Poor	6
In school	4 to 18 yr	$6.00 to $8.00 per person (with paid lay supervisors)		Fair	3
School fluoride mouthrinse program	4 to 18 yr	$6.00 to $8.00 per person (with paid lay supervisors)	30% to 40%	Fair	3
Topical fluoride treatment (professionally applied for dental service programs)	4 to 20 yr 20+ yr (on incidence)	$8.00 to $30.00 per person depending on age and amount of treatment	20% to 40%	Poor	9
Brush-in-school program (high-fluoride toothpaste)	4 to 18 yr	$.25 treatment public program	Incomplete evidence	Fair-poor	11
Control of detrimental school foods	4 to 18 yr		Unknown	Fair	7
Adhesive tooth sealants	6 to 12 yr	$3 to $10 per tooth depending on number of applications	Fair to poor depending on number of applications	Poor	10
Labeling of sweets (FTC)	All	Unknown	Unknown	Fair	8
Regular dental visits	All	$8.00 to $12.00 per visit		Always recommended	—
Dental health education and promotion Infant Preschool Schools Working individuals Retirees	All	Low per person	Unknown	Fair to poor depending on access to target population	4
Influence of mass media re: news events	All	Negligible	Unknown	Fair	5

Modified from Allukian, M.: Effective community prevention programs (In De Paola, D.P., and Cheney, H.G., editors: Handbook of preventive dentistry, Littleton, MA, Publishing Sciences Group, Inc., 1979) and Massachusetts Department of Public Health, Preventive dentistry for Massachusetts report, 1979.

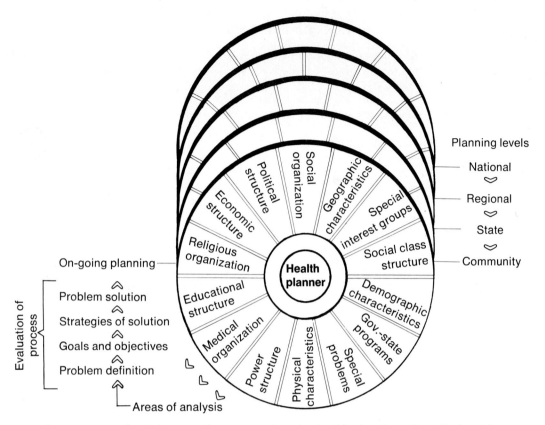

Fig. 10-3. An ecological approach to comprehensive health planning. (From Bruhn, J.G.: Planning for social change: dilemmas for health planning, Am. J. Public Health **63**:604, 1972.)

any type of health program. The box at the top of p. 200 lists rules for implementation strategy development. By reviewing these rules and the example activity worksheets that follow, the details of operating a program will become clear to those responsible for instituting the program.

Monitoring, evaluating, and revising the program

Once it has been implemented, the program requires continuous surveillance of all activities. The program's success is determined by monitoring how well individuals are doing their jobs, how well equipment functions, and how appropriate and adequate facilities are. Before problems arise in any of these areas, adjustments must be made to fine-tune the program.

Evaluation, both informal and formal, is a necessary and important aspect of the program. Evaluation allows us to (1) measure the progress of each activity, (2) measure the effectiveness of each activity, (3) identify problems in carrying out the activities, (4) plan revision and modification, and (5) justify the dollar costs of administering the program and if necessary, justify seeking additional funds.

Each objective should be examined periodically to determine how well it is meeting the

RULES FOR IMPLEMENTATION

1. Specify clearly the activity (who does what for whom).
2. Be sure someone is responsible for the whole activity and coordinates individuals who may carry out the different tasks.
3. Identify all the preparatory steps prior to doing that activity (e.g., prepare training manual, prepare materials, write article, acquire equipment, train volunteers, determine treatment protocol).
4. List steps in the order in which they must occur.
5. Check for missing steps which need to be added.
6. Determine when (date) each step should begin and end.
7. Check your dates to make sure the correct amount of time has been allowed.
8. Consult with organizations affected by the activity; identify potential problems, opportunities, etc.
9. Specify what resources will be needed and their source.
10. Specify what constraints will need to be addressed.
11. Make sure all people involved know what is expected of them and by when.

From National Heart, Lung and Blood Institute: Handbook for improving high blood pressure control in the community, Washington, DC, 1977, U.S. Government Printing Office, p. 36.

ACTIVITY WORKSHEET

(Example A)

Activity: State Heart Association develops and distributes training manual for patient educators.

Resources (to be used): Heart Association funds, staff, and materials with assistance from community-wide Patient Education Committee.

Constraints (to be addressed): Must be completed by 7/30/77. Must be accepted by majority of committee. Is highest priority of Heart Association.

Implementation strategy:

(who does what)	(when)
1. Committee develops methodology	11/10/76
2. Heart Association (HA) educator prepares draft manual	12/10/76
3. Committee reviews draft manual	12/20/76
4. Nine practicing educators review draft manual	1/10/77
5. HA educator prepares final draft	1/31/77
6. Commercial artist prepares graphics	2/15/77
7. Nine practicing educators test manual	4/15/77
8. HA educator evaluates test and makes revisions	5/15/77
9. Committee approves manual	6/1/77
10. HA gets manual printed	6/30/77
11. Manual is distributed to nurses and health educators	7/30/77
12. HA educator evaluates training manual	7/30/77

From National Heart, Lung and Blood Institute: Handbook for improving high blood pressure control in the community, Washington, DC, 1977, U.S. Government Printing Office, p. 33.

ACTIVITY WORKSHEET (Example B)

Activity: County Health Services Center will screen and treat inner city hypertensive residents who normally use that center, beginning 11/15/76.

Resources (to be used): County funds, staff, and facilities.

Constraints (to be addressed): Inner city residents are suspicious of Center staff. Residents discourage any follow-up efforts. Must begin by 1/1/77.

Implementation strategy:

(who does what)	(when)
1. Director of Ambulatory Services develops proposal for detection/treatment center	1/1/76
2. County Board funds proposal	3/1/76
3. County renovates facilities	6/1/76
4. Director hires staff, including administrator and medical director	6/15/76
5. Administrator and medical director develop protocols and procedures, including special efforts to overcome suspicion and follow-up problems	8/15/76
6. Administrator acquires equipment and supplies	8/15/76
7. Data specialist develops patient records forms	9/15/76
8. Nurse educator develops education materials	9/15/76
9. Nurse educator along with medical director trains staff and volunteers	10/1/76
10. Administrator tests methods and materials with inner city residents	10/15/76
11. Staff begins detection and treatment services to inner city residents	11/15/76
12. Administrator evaluates detection and treatment services	11/15/76

From National Heart, Lung and Blood Institute: Handbook for improving high blood pressure control in the community, Washington, DC, 1977, U.S. Government Printing Office, p. 37.

program goals. The objective should be stated in measurable terms so that a comparison can be made of what the objective intended to accomplish and what the objective actually accomplished.

Evaluation should also address the quality of what is being done. For example, if one of the activities were placing pit and fissure sealants on specific teeth of school-aged children, an evaluator would want to assess how well that sealant was placed, the appropriateness of the tooth chosen, and the time involved in placing the sealant on the tooth.

The attitudes of the recipients of the program should be examined to determine whether or not the program was acceptable to them. There are

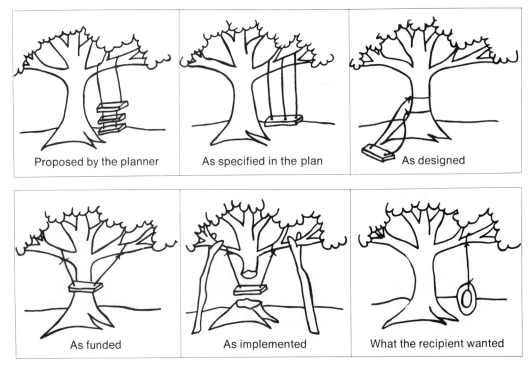

Proposed by the planner

As specified in the plan

As designed

As funded

As implemented

What the recipient wanted

Fig. 10-4. A perspective on planning.

many programs that are considered successful by those who run the program; however, the people who have been the recipients of the service may have wanted something very different. Fig. 10-4 illustrates this point and gives us perspective on planning by showing the concept of the planner, the actual plan, the design, the constraints involved, the alternative strategy, and finally what in fact the recipient wanted in the first place.

SUMMARY

Merely hanging up a shingle is no longer all that is necessary for a health care provider to deliver health services to a given community. Consumers of health care are more involved than ever before in learning about the types of health care they should be receiving, and are actively questioning the choices available to them. We as health professionals need to be responsive to consumers.

We must be prepared to meet the challenges of the 1990s through the development of good planning skills. These skills can then be used to achieve such goals as the following:

1. The construction of well-planned and accessible health facilities
2. The selection of appropriate, well-qualified, and sensitive health personnel
3. The provision of appropriate and effective health services
4. The time and the funds to adequately provide the needed care
5. The active participation of representatives of those communities/organizations/individuals that will be the recipients of the given health care

Only through fully understanding the needs of the community, the organization, and the individual can we begin to coordinate our planning efforts to develop acceptable, appropriate, and effective health care programs today and for the future.

REFERENCES

1. Allukian, M.: Effective community prevention programs. In De Paola, D.P., and Cheney, H.G., editors: Handbook of preventive dentistry, Littleton, MA, Publishing Sciences Group, Inc., 1979.
2. Blum, H.L.: Note on comprehensive planning for health, Berkeley, CA, 1968, Comprehensive Health Planning Unit, School of Public Health, University of California.
3. Bruhn, J.: Planning for social change, Am. J. Public Health 63:7, 1972.
4. Dubos, R.: So human an animal, New York, 1968, Charles Scribner's Sons.
5. Model standards for community preventive health services: a report to the U.S. Congress for the Secretary of Health, Education and Welfare, August 1979.
6. Provision of dental care in the community, University of Michigan, School of Public Health, Ann Arbor, 1973, Proceedings from the third annual course in dental public health, Waldenwoods Conference Center, Hartland, MI, May 22-26, 1966.
7. Schulbert, H., and others: Program evaluation in the health fields, New York, 1969, Human Sciences, Inc.
8. Spiegel, A., and others: Basic health planning methods, Germantown, MD, 1978, Aspen Systems Corporation.
9. Striffler, D.: Surveying a community and developing a working policy: the administration of local dental programs, University of Michigan, School of Public Health, Proceedings from fifth workshop on dental public health, Ann Arbor, 1963.
10. U.S. Department of Health, Education and Welfare, Public Health Service: Dental program efficiency criteria and standards for the Indian Health Service, 1974.
11. U.S. Department of Health, Education and Welfare, Public Health Services, National Institutes of Health, National Heart, Lung and Blood Institute: Handbook for improving high blood pressure control in the community, DHEW Pub. No. 78-1086. Washington, DC, 1977, U.S. Government Printing Office.
12. World Health Organization/Division of Dentistry, USPHS: An international collaborative study of dental manpower systems in relation to oral health status, Document 2. Geneva, 1977.
13. Young, W., and Striffler, D.: The dentist, his practice, and the community, Philadelphia, 1969, W.B. Saunders Co.

RESEARCH AND EVALUATION IN DENTAL CARE

Dentistry is referred to both as an art and as a science. The art of dentistry relates to skill in the less tangible aspects of dental care: judgments and esthetics, the proper contouring of restorations, the gentle touch in the manipulation of a curette, the chairside approach to the patient, and developing patient motivation toward oral hygiene.

The science of dental care involves knowledge acquired through research and evaluation and requires the use of tools such as biostatistics to assist in the development of new information. Biostatistics enables the analysis of data in a systematic fashion and thus the processing of data that can be used to improve the state of dental health of individual patients and the community. Chapter 11 introduces some fundamental concepts in biostatistics in order to permit the student to evaluate programs and the research literature.

Chapter 12 further develops the concept of program evaluation that was introduced previously. Chapter 10 described the process of program development and touched on the evaluation of programs; Chapter 12 analyzes the process of evaluation and gives the student tools with which to improve a program.

Chapter 13 provides a substantive overview of research activities in dentistry, as well as useful guidelines for carrying out a research study. Clinical and social science research is emphasized, and a clear point-by-point method is provided for each type. A brief discussion on how to read the research literature is also included.

CHAPTER 11

Introduction to Biostatistics

Familiarity with biostatistics or the mathematics of collection, organization, and interpretation of numerical data having to do with living organisms is essential for today's health care professional. Many people, however, are statistic shy. It is the goal of this chapter to make clear the basics of biostatistics and to make the reader more comfortable with their usage.*

Dental health professionals have a variety of uses for data: in designing a health care program or facility, in evaluating the effectiveness of an ongoing program, in determining the needs of a specific population, in evaluating the scientific accuracy of a journal article—to name just a few. These data are helpful only to the extent that they may be ordered and interpreted. Therefore, what has been established is a system of managing data using various techniques. Two statistical techniques are generally accepted: *Descriptive statistical* techniques enable an individual to describe and summarize a set of data numerically; *inferential statistical* techniques provide a basis for making a generalization about the probable results of a large group when only a select portion of the group has been observed. Inferential statistics are used to generalize results to a larger population of interest, while descriptive statistics attempt only to generalize the group actually studied.

Before elaborating on terms relating to descriptive and inferential techniques, it is necessary to identify what is meant by the terms *population* and *sample*.

A *population* is any entire group of items (objects, materials, people, and so on) that possess at least one basic defined characteristic in common. Examples of populations might be all dentists, all U.S. citizens, all periodontally involved teeth, all individuals in a given school, or all patients treated at a particular private office. It is often impossible to collect information from an entire population because of the size of the population or because of such limitations as finances, time, or distance between population members. In cases where it is impossible to collect data on the entire population, complete and reliable information can be collected from a representative portion of the population called a *sample*. By observing and measuring a sample, it is possible to obtain information and make statements about the total population.

Statistics is a science that describes data for the purpose of making inferences about a population from which the data are obtained. When we collect a specific piece of information—data—from each member of a population, we obtain a characteristic of the population called a *parameter*. Similarly, when we collect a piece of information from each member of a sample, we obtain a characteristic of the sample called a *statistic*. Since most studies are conducted using samples, statistics are most commonly used. Using statistics (characteristics of a sample), we try to infer what the parameters (characteristics of a population) will be.

---

*A complete treatment of biostatistics is not possible in this text. The interested reader is referred to standard texts listed in the bibliography of this chapter which cover this material in detail.

SAMPLING

Samples, by definition, cannot have exactly the same characteristics of a population. However, a sample truly representative of the population can be obtained by using probability sampling methods and by taking a sufficiently large sample.

A *random sample* is defined as one in which every element in the population has an equal and independent chance of being selected. The following example will illustrate two random sampling procedures: Assume a population of 5,000 seniors is in the predental program at 50 universities. Each senior class has 100 pre-dental students divided into 5 equal sections of 20 students each. The objective is to determine the grade point average (GPA) of each predental student by selecting a representative sample of 1,000 students (that is, a sampling ratio of one fifth, or 20%). A simple random sample to select the 1,000 students would be completed in the following manner. A list of 5,000 students needs to be compiled and numbered 1 through 5,000. A numbered tag is prepared for each student and from the 5,000 well-mixed tags, 1,000 are drawn by a lottery. After each selection the tag is replaced and another tag is drawn. This is the most basic random sample approach.

A similar procedure may be applied for selecting a random sample using a table of random numbers, which can be found in most statistics textbooks. For this example, it would be necessary to use four columns of digits in the tables so that each student, 1 through 5,000, would have an equal probability of being selected. Selection would begin by blindly identifying a number on the table that corresponds to a member of the total population (1 through 5,000). The selection process continues by taking numbers horizontally or vertically until the desired sample size is reached. Repeated numbers are omitted when encountered during sample selection in both procedures.

Random sampling is the procedure of choice whenever possible. It prevents the possibility of selection bias on the part of the researcher. What if GPA is related to school? A simple random sample may not ensure representation of the entire population of predental students. It may be necessary to select individuals according to certain strata or subgroups to diminish the chance of sample fluctuation. This method of selection is called *stratified sampling*. It is accomplished by randomly selecting a proportionate number of subjects from each subgroup for the sample. In the preceding example, the subgroup would be the university attended. Therefore, to produce a *stratified random sample*, one would (1) prepare a list of students at each of the 50 universities and (2) draw at random one fifth of the students at each university. Since the sampling ratio is used in each stratum, there is a proportional allocation by school. This eliminates the possibility of sampling bias that could result by selecting at random giving no consideration to school.

Another type of sampling is the *systematic sample*. A systematic sample is not a true random sample because everyone may not have an independent chance of being selected. This type of sample is usually obtained by drawing a number and then selecting every nth individual, for example, having a list of names and deciding to test every even numbered person on the list. All odd numbered names are systemically excluded.

Two types of samples that may introduce serious bias in estimating population parameters are (1) the judgment sample and (2) the convenience sample. In a *judgment sample*, someone with knowledge of the population may select a sample in arbitrary ways to represent the population. In a *convenience sample*, a group is chosen because it happens to be convenient and may represent the population; for example, one classroom within a school is selected because the teacher gives permission to work with his/her pupils, or the patients at a particular private office are used because the dentist allows access to his/her patient list. Results relating to that particular classroom or that particular dentist's office may be valid, but when generalized to include the larger population of school classrooms or dentists' offices, their reliability is questionable.

Once a sample has been selected, *raw data* are collected and consideration must then be given to data analysis. *Data analysis* requires the application of statistical tests to data for the purpose of organizing, describing, and summarizing findings. Among the steps that may be applied in data analysis are the following:

1. Organizing data from lowest to highest
2. Constructing a frequency distribution
3. Grouping and regrouping data, based on relevant information
4. Tabulating scores
5. Constructing tables and graphs for efficient communication of obtained results

DESCRIPTIVE DATA DISPLAY
Frequency distributions

Often, to better explain data that have been collected, they are grouped according to the variable they measure and are ordered into an array. An *array* is simply a group of scores ar-

ranged from lowest to highest score. It can be organized into a *frequency distribution* by tabulating the frequency with which each score occurs. Three types of frequency distributions may be employed—ungrouped, grouped, and cumulative. The following example will illustrate the use of these statistical methods.

Envision a school brushing program where a dental hygienist is responsible for keeping a record of the students who voluntarily brush each day. After a period of 50 days, he/she wants to present the data to the program director. This is an ideal situation for the use of descriptive statistics. Here are a few of the ways the information could be presented to the program director.

An *ungrouped frequency distribution* of the number of students per day is presented in Table 11-1. Here, the variable of interest is the number of students. Therefore, number of students is listed down the left hand margin of the table from highest to lowest, and the frequency of days is listed along the right hand margin. The ungrouped frequency distribution is used to organize data obtained from small samples (less than 30). A *grouped frequency* distribution is used to arrange data from large samples (more than 30) when the scores are numerous and fairly close together. Table 11-2 illustrates the same data as Table 11-1. However, a specific number of students per day cannot be examined using Table 11-2.

Table 11-1. Ungrouped frequency distribution of students seen during the 50-day brushing program

Students	Frequency of days	Students	Frequency of days
99	1	86	—
98	—	85	—
97	3	84	3
96	—	83	4
95	4	82	2
94	3	81	1
93	2	80	—
92	2	79	1
91	—	78	3
90	6	77	1
89	1	76	4
88	3	75	1
87	2	74	3

Table 11-2. Group frequency distribution of the students seen during the 50-day brushing program

Students	Frequency of days	Cumulative frequency
95-99	8	50
90-94	13	42
85-89	6	29
80-84	10	23
75-79	10	13
70-74	3	3

A *cumulative frequency distribution*, also shown in Table 11-2, is similar to the previously discussed frequency distribution tables but displays the frequency of scores up to and including any given value in the distribution of data. This distribution is used to condense large arrays of data.

It is important to point out that whenever data are grouped or consolidated some information becomes lost. For instance, the use of Table 11-2 alllows the reader to determine the number of days in which 94 to 97 students participated in the tooth brushing program. However, the exact number of days that 94, 95, 96, and 97 students appeared cannot be determined. Table 11-1— ungrouped data—must be used for that purpose.

Graphing techniques

Graphing represents another alternative in displaying descriptive data pictorially and allowing rapid assimilation of findings by the reader. A general rule for constructing graphs along the X and Y axes is that the vertical Y axis usually represents the frequency of scores occurring along the scale of measurement, while the X axis respresents the scale that measures the variable of most interest.

A *bar graph* is a two-dimensional pictorial display of data that are discrete in nature.

A *histogram* is a graphic representation formed directly from a frequency distribution. It is a display where the horizontal (abscissa) and vertical (ordinate) axes of a graph are formed

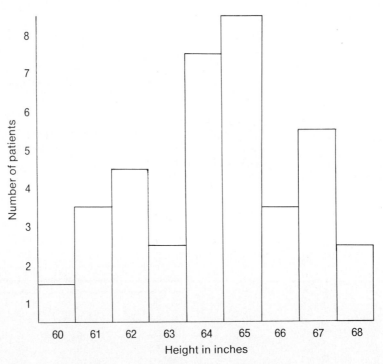

Fig. 11-1. Histogram of patient height.

according to the scale values and the frequencies of the distribution, respectively. A histogram consists of a set of rectangles whose base is on the horizontal axis and that extends in height along the vertical axis proportional to the frequency. If the points are widespread, a double bar (//) or a double curved line (≈) is used to indicate breaks in the graph. Graphically, a histogram is similar to a bar graph except that rectangles touch one another in a histogram (see Fig. 11-1).

When the concern is to depict the continuous nature of the data, a line graph called a *frequency polygon* is used. To construct it, one would place a point at the center of each rectangle found in a histogram and connect each point with a straight line. Polygons are used the most frequently of all graphing techniques, and often polygons are superimposed on a line graph to pictorially display two or more distributions in one figure (Fig. 11-2).

When presenting material in tabular form, the table should be able to stand alone. That is, correctly presented material in tabular form should be understandable even if the written discussion of the data is not read.

The following presentation outlines the display of data in graphic or tabular form*:

1. The contents of a table as a whole and the items in each separate column should be clearly and fully defined. The unit of measurement must be included.

---

*Hill, A.B.: Principles of medical statistics, ed. 7. London, 1961, Lancet Ltd., pp. 56-58.

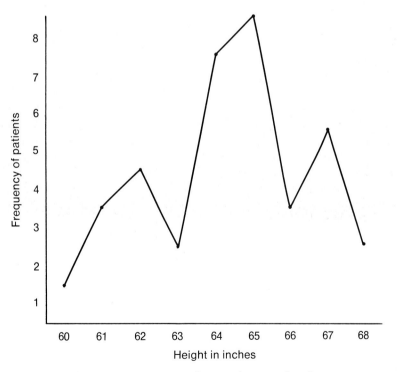

Fig. 11-2. Frequency polygon of patient height.

2. If the table includes rates, the basis upon which they are measured must be clearly stated . . . death rate percent or per thousand or per million as the case may be.
3. Whenever possible, the frequency distributions should be given in full. These are basic data from which conclusions are being drawn, and their presentation allows the reader to check the validity of the author's arguments.
4. Rates or proportions should not be given alone without any information as to the numbers of observations upon which they are based. By giving only rates of observations and omitting the actual number of observations or frequency distributions, we are excluding the basic data.
5. Where percentages are used it must be clearly indicated that these are not absolute numbers. Rather than combine too many types of figures in one table, it is often best to divide the material into two or three small tables.
6. Full particulars of any exclusion of observations from a collected series must be given. The reasons for and the criteria of exclusions must be clearly defined.

Figures (graphs) are used for a different purpose than are tables. Figures are the presentation of material in a simplified manner to clearly illustrate a particular set of data. A major concern in the presentation of both figures and tables is readability. Tables and figures must be clearly understood and clearly labeled so that the reader is aided by the information and not confused. The student is again directed to standard biostatistic tests for a formal discussion on summarizing data in graphic and tabular form. Also, standard writing style manuals generally contain discussions on the formal display of tables and graphs.

Measures of central tendency

The display of data in graphic or tabular form may be found tedious, time-consuming, and unwieldy when it is not necessary to look at every piece of data but rather at a summary that can describe the total collection of data using just one number. Three measures in common use describe the central tendency of a distribution of scores: the mode, the mean, and the median.

The *mode* is that value that occurs with the greatest frequency. It is possible for a distribution to have more than one mode when two or more values have equally large frequencies. From Table 11-1 it can be seen that the highest frequency is 6, and one value has a frequency of 6. Therefore, 90 is the mode for this distribution. The primary value of the mode lies in its ease of computation and in its convenience as a quick indicator of the central value in a distribution. Beyond this, its statistical users are extremely limited.

The measure of central tendency, called the *mean,* is the same as an arithmetic average that one learns to calculate in the elementary grades. It is computed by adding a list of scores and then dividing by the number of scores. The symbol for mean is a capital letter X with a bar above it $(\overline{X})$. The mean is by far the most common measure of central tendency used to describe a set of data, since it fluctuates least from sample to sample and is sensitive to any change in any score in the distribution. The presence of a few extremely high or extremely low scores can change the value of the mean considerably.

The *median* is that point that divides the distribution of scores into two equal parts, that is, the point at which 50% of the scores lie above it and 50% lie below it. For example, given the scores 1, 3, 5, 6, 8, 9, 10, the median is 6, because two equal-sized parts (1, 3, 5 and 8, 9, 10) are above and below 6. The median is not affected by extreme scores in a given direction and is more stable than the mode.

An area in which the median is most often used and clearly illustrates its advantage over the mean or the mode is salary, or dollar, values. For illustrative purposes, suppose seven dental hygienists and two dentists work in a productive private office. Their salaries are as follows:

$75,000	$28,500	$22,300
$72,000	$26,000	$22,300
$29,000	$25,000	$22,300

The owner of the office declares that the average member's salary is $35,822—the mean. The business manager declares in a later report that the average salary is $22,300—the mode. Neither person has intentionally reported false results. Both have used a measure of central tendency. However, the statistical tool reported was the one best suited to the reporter's objective rather than the one that best described the data—in this case, the median. In this illustration the median is $26,000. This value gives a much clearer picture of where the salaries lie for the individual in the middle of the salary range. The mode in this example was extremely low compared with the majority of salaries and the mean was influenced by two extremely high salaries.

Variability. Measures of central tendency indicate the typical performance for a group. However, this is not enough information to describe a distribution of scores. How widely scores are dispensed around that central point must also be known. Suppose Dr. A has a class of dental hygienists whose mean intelligence quotient (IQ) is 110. Some students in this class have IQs of 80 to 90 while others have IQs of 130 to 140. Dr. B's class of hygienists also has a mean IQ of 110, but the lowest is 100 and the highest is 124. The two hygiene classes have the same mean; however, we can see that the abilities of one class are definitely different from those of the other class because we know something about the spread of scores around the average.

Three terms are commonly associated with variability: range, variance, and standard deviation. The *range* is the difference between the high score and the low score in a distribution. In Table 11-1 the range is 25 (99 to 74). Often, ranges are stated as lowest and highest score, that is, the range is 74 to 99. The range has the advantage of being easy to calculate. However, it is unstable and affected by one extremely high or extremely low score. Also, only two scores are considered and these happen to be the extreme scores of the distribution. Standard deviation and variance have much more utility than the range.

The *variance* is a measure of the average deviation or spread of scores around the mean. The variance, as the standard deviation, is based on each score in the distribution. It is possible to have zero variance. However, it is impossible to have negative variance. Zero variance would occur when all scores in a distribution are equal, for instance, when everyone gets 100% as a test score, or when everyone in a group has the same weight or height. The following steps show how the variance is calculated:

1. Obtain the mean of the distribution
2. Subtract the mean from each score (deviation scores)
3. Square each deviation score
4. Add these squared deviation scores
5. Divide the sum by the number of cases added

Standard deviation of a set of scores is simply the positive square root of the variance. Table 11-3 illustrates the calculation of variance and standard deviation for using the IQ scores of 10 students.

The variance and the standard deviation are relatively easy to interpret. The greater the dispersion of scores from the mean of the distribution, the greater will be the standard deviation and the variance. A large standard deviation indicates a wide dispersion around the mean. In interpreting the following statistics one can see

A. $\overline{X} = 60$ $s = 4$
B. $\overline{X} = 60$ $s = 9$
C. $\overline{X} = 60$ $s = 21$

group A to be the most homogeneous group with

Table 11-3. Calculation of variance and standard deviation for sample of 10 students

IQ scores X	Deviation from mean $(X - \bar{X})$	(Deviation)² $(X - \bar{X})^2$
109	− 2	4
99	−12	144
123	12	144
116	5	25
131	20	400
98	−13	169
116	5	25
89	−22	484
128	17	289
101	−10	100
1110 = Sum of IQs	0	1784 = Sum of the deviation squared

111 = Mean IQ

Variance $(s^2) = 1784 \div 10 = 178.4$

Standard deviation $(s) = 13.36$

a small standard deviation and therefore small dispersion around the mean. Group C is the most heterogeneous group, with $s = 21$ indicating a major spread of scores around the mean.

Normal curve. The normal curve is one of the most utilized frequency distributions in biostatistics. It is a bell-shaped curve that is symmetrical around the mean of the distribution. The normal curve may vary from rather narrow distributions that are pointy in the center to wide distributions whose center is flat. The mean of the distribution is the focal point from which all assumptions and statements may be made. The mean is used for two reasons: (1) most distributions do not have a zero point to be used as a starting point (what is zero intelligence?), and (2) the normal curve theoretically does not touch the baseline at any point because of the remote possibility of an extreme score in the distribution. Curves that meet the criteria for normality can be separated into areas under the curve. See Fig. 11-3 for an example of this separation.

The total area bounded by the curve is 1, or 100%. A curve that meets the criteria of normality has the mean equal to the median that is equal to the mode. The total area is broken into segments of single units (one standard deviation). As indicated in Fig. 11-3, the portion of the area under the curve between the mean and one standard deviation is 34.13% of the total area. The same area is found one unit below the mean. Similarly, two units above and below the mean cut off an additional 13.59% of the area under the curve and so on for three standard deviations. Area under the curve can best be understood by imagining a test that is administered to a large group of students. When the tests are scored, the distribution will probably take the form of a normal curve. In that case, 34.13% of the students who took the test would score between the mean and one standard deviation above the mean, another 13.59% would score between the first and second standard deviations, and 2.21% would score between the second and third standard deviations. Thinking of the area under the curve in terms of percent of persons makes it easier to interpret the distribution of the normal curve.

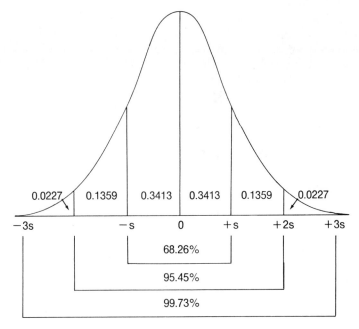

Fig. 11-3. The normal frequency curve.

SIGNIFICANCE RELATED TO INFERENTIAL STATISTICS

With large populations, it is often impossible to study each member in the group because of time, cost, and so on. Instead we select a sample from the population and from that sample attempt to generalize to the population as a whole. In using inferential statistical procedures (trying to infer about a larger group than our sample), we must deal with statistical probability—the mathematical assumption that a certain situation will occur according to chance a specific portion of time. For example, if a coin is flipped an infinite number of times, by chance the coin will come up heads 50% of the time and tails 50% of the time.

The main thing to remember in inferential statistical procedures is that we are trying to generalize about a larger group than the one for which we actually have data. If we have a good sample, our generalization will be accurate; if our sample is poor, we will be hampered in our ability to generalize to the population. For example, suppose we are interested in determining the general status of a patient's oral health. We could examine each tooth of an individual and then make our judgment. However, if we had 1,000 persons to examine in a limited time we might look for an alternative method. Perhaps we would select four teeth, one from each quadrant, and then base our decision regarding the oral cavity on results of examining those four teeth. In this case, we have taken a sample of four teeth from the population of 32 teeth. Our assessment of the oral cavity will be accurate if the teeth we have chosen are the best representatives of teeth in each quadrant. Needless to say, we should be certain to examine the same four teeth of each individual when making our assessment.

Another more detailed example may serve to clarify the use of inferential statistical procedures: A graduate student in public health wishes to implement a community-based education program for a group of urban mothers. He finds through the literature that an education program has been offered to a similar group of mothers using an entirely different approach. He is interested in testing how much the participants in his program learn as compared with the other program. Assume both groups started with the same knowledge level. The student tests the mothers and compares the mean result of his program with that obtained in the other program; he finds that his group tests higher, but he is not sure if it is such a difference that he can clearly say his program is better. There is a procedure available called Student's t-test that allows the graduate student to compare the mean results from his program to the mean results of the other program. The purpose of using Student's t-test is to determine the probability that the difference between the two means is real and not a result produced by a chance difference. What this public health student wishes to find is a statistically significant difference between mean 1 and mean 2, that is, the mean produced by his program and the mean produced by the other program.

The distinction between statistically significant and practically significant results is important. For example, in the case just discussed, two programs are offered in health education and one is found to produce greater test scores among participants than the other, say 5 points greater. Based on test results, the program of choice is the one producing the greater score. Suppose this program, which produces a 5-point gain, also costs $100 more per participant to produce. In all likelihood a group of decision makers might decide that $100 per participant is too high a price to pay for the "moderate" gain; although the greater test scores were statistically significant,

statistically better, the difference between program results was not practically significant. Pragmatic decisions play a much greater role in research than many scientists are willing to admit.

CORRELATION AND INFERENTIAL STATISTICS

The science of statistics has given us a large number of tests that can be applied to public health data. Only a few of these will be discussed in this section. Discussions will center on the chi-square test, the calculation of the coefficient of correlation, and Student's t-test. Each is best adapted to data of a certain type. An understanding of the tests will guide an individual toward the efficient collection of data that will meet the assumptions of the statistical procedures particularly well.

Chi-square test

The chi-square test is based on the comparison of the observed measurement of a given characteristic and the expected measurement if the sample differs in no way from what is expected by chance. The chi-square statistic (X^2) measures the discrepancy between observed and expected frequencies by adding together all values of:

$$\frac{(\text{Observed number} - \text{Expected number})^2}{\text{Expected number}}$$

The X^2 test is set up in such a way that the original number of cases entering into each sample becomes part of the calculation and affects interpretation of the answer. Therefore, all observations play an equally important role, whether negative or positive. A zero observation is as important as a large positive or negative value.

Chi-square will equal zero if all comparisons between observed and expected values are zero. The accurate interpretation of χ^2 depends on the computation of a figure called the *degrees of freedom*. This indicates the number of cells in a two-dimensional grid that can be filled independently without the totals for the problem being incorrect. It is calculated by subtracting 1 from the number of rows and 1 from the number of columns in the grid and then multiplying these figures together:

$$(r - 1) \times (c - 1) = df$$

After calculating the χ^2 value and the degrees of freedom, the next step is to use a master table and find the numbers closest to the value computed for χ^2 in the line of the table that represents the figure for degrees of freedom. Having located the number, one then follows to the head of the column and reads the probability of chance occurrence of such a value of χ^2.

The following problem illustrates the procedure for calculating the chi-square value. Suppose we are interested in whether or not vaccination, apart from whether it has only prophylactic effect, reduces the severity of any actual attack of smallpox. Chi-square could be used to determine whether or not vaccination has an effect.

First we must discuss several areas illustrated in Table 11-4. In order to perform χ^2 analysis it must be possible to place each piece of information into only one cell. For instance, an individual who was never vaccinated could not be placed in both the abundant and the sparse categories. This would cause one person to be counted twice and invalidate our results. Next, expected frequencies must be determined before we are able to make comparisons with the observed frequencies. The formula for calculating expected frequency is: $e_{ij} = (Tr \times Tc)/N$, where e is the expected frequency of cell ij, Tr is the total for row r, Tc is the total for column c, and N is the total frequency. Table 11-5 provides an example showing the expected frequencies used in Table 11-4 and how they were calculated.

The master table value for χ^2 with 2 degrees of freedom is 5.99 at the 5% confidence level. Since our calculated value was 230.17, we have determined that there is a statistically significant difference between what was expected by chance and what actually occurred. Therefore,

Table 11-4. Calculation of chi-square

	Hemorrhagic or confluent	Abundant	Sparse	Row totals
Observed frequencies				
Vaccinated within 10 yr of attack	10	150	240	400
Never vaccinated	60	30	10	100
Column total	70	180	250	500
Expected frequencies				
Vaccinated within 10 yr of attack	56	144	200	400
Never vaccinated	14	36	50	100
Column total	70	180	250	500

$$\chi^2 = \frac{(10 - 56)^2}{56} + \frac{(150 - 144)^2}{144} + \frac{(240 - 200)^2}{200} + \frac{(60 - 14)^2}{14} + \frac{(30 - 36)^2}{36} + \frac{(10 - 50)^2}{50}$$

$\chi^2 = 230.17$
$df = (r - 1)(c - 1)$
$df = (2 - 1)(3 - 1)$
$df = 2$

Table 11-5. Expected frequencies calculated for Table 11-4

	Confluent	Abundant	Sparse	Total
Vaccinated within 10 yr of attack	$\dfrac{(400 \times 70)}{500} = 56$	$\dfrac{(400 \times 180)}{500} = 144$	$\dfrac{(400 \times 250)}{500} = 200$	400
Never vaccinated	$\dfrac{(100 \times 70)}{70} = 14$	$\dfrac{(100 \times 180)}{180} = 36$	$\dfrac{(100 \times 250)}{250} = 50$	100
TOTAL	70	180	250 =	500

vaccination in this example had a significant effect.

With chi-square, we deal with one variable but test its occurrence in a number of different situations. This comparison of categorical type information is the type of problem for which χ^2 is best suited. In a sense, therefore, we are really dealing with two variables, although values for the second variable need not be related to the other in any recognizable pattern.

Correlation

Correlation analysis allows us to deal with another type of problem, quite commonly found, in which there are two variables, each measuring some different characteristic. Each unit in the data we are testing consists of a pair of measurements and our objective is to determine the strength of the relationship. One measurement in the unit is for the first variable and one is for the second variable. Correlation is best applied when the number of pairs is very large, since the larger the number, the more reliable the results. The relationship between pairs is easiest to grasp using what is called a scatter diagram (Figs. 11-4 and 11-5).

In Fig. 11-4 there appears to be no relationship between the two variables and no way to predict the value of Y from a value of X. In Fig. 11-5, however, a relation becomes apparent, not perfect, but recognizable: as one variable changes the second variable changes in the same direction.

The measure of the direction and strength of the relationship between two variables is summarized by the *correlation coefficient*. Fig. 11-4 has a correlation coefficient of 0; Fig. 11-5 has a correlation coefficient of +0.87. A correlation of +1 would mean that all the points in Fig. 11-5 were located exactly on the ascending diagonal line. Values for X would thus increase as values for Y increased (though the ratio need not be

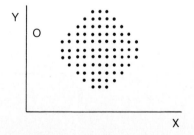

Fig. 11-4. Hypothetical scatter diagram showing correlation coefficients of 0.0.

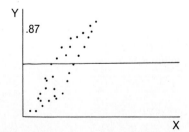

Fig. 11-5. Hypothetical scatter diagram showing correlation coefficients of +0.87.

one to one), and for every possible value of X it would be possible to predict exactly the corresponding value for Y. Inverse or negative correlation would imply a descending line, with values for X decreasing as values for Y increased. If the correlation coefficient were -1, then all points would be located exactly on this descending straight line. The plus or minus sign indicates the direction of the relationship, same or inverse respectively, while the absolute value indicates the strength of the relationship. The closer the coefficient is to 1, the stronger the relationship. Confidence can seldom be given to a correlation coefficient built on less than a dozen pairs of observations unless the correlation is almost perfect, that is, where r approximates either $+1$ or -1. Often 30 cases is used as the recognized minimum number of pairs and most researchers believe that using 100 pairs produces stability and confidence in the correlation coefficient.

Student's t-test

The t statistic is used to compare two means to determine the probability that the difference between means is greater than that expected by chance. Note that if more than two means are to be compared, then another statistical procedure such as analysis of variance (ANOVA) is indicated and not the t-test. Before proceeding, the student is cautioned against performing analyses or accepting results that have more than two means and proceed to calculate a large series of t-tests using different combinations of means, two at a time. This is blatantly incorrect statistical application, although it may be found in many published articles.

The theoretical distribution for testing statistical significance is Student's t distribution. The t distribution varies. Graphs for t distributions with different degrees of freedom are pictured in Fig. 11-6 in three examples. As the degrees of freedom approach 30, the curve begins to closely approximate the normal curve.

A calculated t value can be positive or negative. The following example will help clarify the use of the t-test.

	Group X	Group Y
No. of individuals	10	10
$\overline{X}$	14.8	8.8
Variance	22.84	25.96
Standard deviation	4.78	5.09

Based on the information presented in the

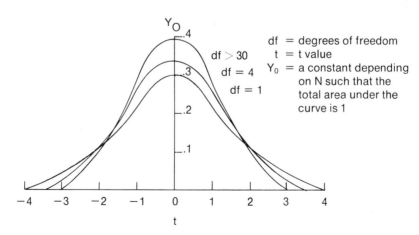

Fig. 11-6. Distribution of t for several different degrees of freedom.

example, the t-test is the statistic of choice. Assume the level of significance is 0.05, since no level is specified and after calculation, a $t = 2.101$ is produced. One more step remains before the determination can be made as to the degree of difference between means: calculation of the degrees of freedom. The number of degrees of freedom is equal to the number of independent scores that are used to estimate a parameter. For the t-test, the parameter estimated is the standard error. For each sample a standard error is estimated. Thus, for most examples with 2 samples, $df = n_1 + n_2 - 2 = 18$.

The previous discussion has dealt primarily (with the exception of the chi-square) with statistical tests called parametric tests. The user of these tests must accept the following two assumptions:

1. Normal distribution. Scores are equally distributed (systematically) around the mean. There are an equal number of low and high scores and most scores are found within three standard deviations of the group mean.

2. Continuous equal interval measures. A score must be a whole number or a fractional part, that is, 1, 2, 3, 6.9, or 7.1. This is not a situation where the only possible scores are whole numbers.

One final type of statistical test is nonparametric. This test is used in situations where the data clearly do not fit the two assumptions just indicated. These tests have minimal assumptions specific to each test, but generally these assumptions are less rigorous than those for parametric tests. Again, the student is directed to standard statistical tests for an expanded discussion of these and other statistical topics.

BIBLIOGRAPHY

Boyer, E.M.: Basic statistical concepts and techniques applied in dental health, Des Moines, 1975, University of Iowa.

Darby, M.L., and Bowen, D.M.: Research methods for oral health professionals—an introduction, St. Louis, 1980, The C.V. Mosby Co.

Dunning, J.M.: Principles of dental public health, ed. 2, Cambridge, MA, 1975, Harvard University Press.

Emory, C.W.: Business research methods, ed. 3, Homewood, IL, 1985, Richard D. Irwin, Inc.

Hill, A.B.: Principles of medical statistics, ed. 7, New York, 1961, Oxford University Press.

Richards, L.E., and LaCava, J.L.J.: Business statistics: why and when, New York, 1983, McGraw-Hill, Inc.

Snedecor, G.W, and Cochran, W.G.: Statistical methods, ed. 6, Ames, IA, 1971, Iowa State University Press.

CHAPTER 12

Program Evaluation in Health Care

PURPOSE OF PROGRAM EVALUATION

Program evaluation is concerned with finding out how well programs work, using social science research techniques to assess information of importance to program practice and public policy. The fundamental purpose of program evaluation is to provide information for decision making. At its basic level, evaluation is a judgment of merit or worth about a particular person, place, or thing. Such judgments may be abstract and general, as is often the case in basic research, or they may be highly concrete and specific as in demonstration or applied research.

EVALUATION VS. RESEARCH

Terms such as *grading, measurement,* and *assessment* are often used interchangeably to describe activities mistaken for evaluation. However, the term most often mistakenly used to describe evaluation is *research.* Since research and evaluation are so frequently confused, the similarities and differences between the activities of researchers and program evaluators will be discussed briefly.

Researchers and program evaluators possess many similarities. They both engage in scientific inquiry. They both use tests, questionnaires, and other measurement devices. They both collect and analyze data systematically using common statistical procedures. And finally, they both can be found describing their outcomes in formal reports.[6] At first glance, even the expert could not differentiate the activities of the evaluator from that of the researcher. Yet, upon further examination, one will notice several differences among the activities of the two individuals. When gathering information, researchers and evaluators differ in the use they wish to make of materials. Researchers want to draw conclusions. Evaluators want to make decisions. Understanding phenomena is often the sole purpose of researchers, while evaluators want to understand phenomena so that they may better influence someone's actions regarding those phenomena.

Another important difference between research and evaluation stems from whether or not results can be generalized. Researchers study the relationships among activities so that, ideally, findings can be generalized to a wide variety of similar situations. The more able they are to generalize results, the more successful researchers feel. Evaluators, on the other hand, focus on a particular program. Most program evaluators have no intention of generalizing results to other situations.

To elaborate for a moment on this distinction between researcher and evaluator, consider the role each individual might have played in the testing of fluoride rinse. In examining the value of fluoride rinse, the basic science researcher was probably concerned with the effects of fluoride on teeth, the strength of the solution necessary to produce a reduction in caries, and whether his/her conclusions could be generalized across the population. The evaluator was interested in determining whether the program, initiated to test the researcher's conclusion, was run correctly and followed the objectives it stated. The evaluator's concern for the fluoride rinse was only superficial. Once the evaluator judged whether the program was an accurate test of the fluoride rinse, his/her secondary results probably related to the positive or negative effects of fluoride rinse. In other words, that particular program's operation was of prime importance to the evaluator and the effect of fluoride was only important in terms of its results as applied to a realistic, monitored program.

Determining the value of things is another difference between evaluation and research. Evaluation eventually comes down to making a decision about what should be done or which course of action is best. Researchers only strive to obtain accurate, truthful information. There is no requirement to attach assesments of merit to the discovered relationship.[6] Basically, the researcher's job is not dependent on a value decision whereas the evaluator's job is.

FOCUS OF EVALUATIONS

To evaluate the effectiveness of health programs, it is necessary to develop a systematic approach that examines a program's objectives, materials, and finances. Whenever evaluation is undertaken to serve as a basis for future decisions, questions arise: Whose decisions will determine the ultimate fate of a program? At what level should the evaluation be directed? What kinds of decisions will be made? Individuals interested in the results of evaluation may include program developers, direct program staff, program directors, policy makers (state or federal bureaucrats), program directors in other similar agencies, or epidemiologists.[10] Each group seeks different information about the same program. Program developers seek all kinds of information about ways to improve specific parts of the program that affect them directly. The director of the program is usually interested in knowing the overall effectiveness of the basic program, although he/she is generally more concerned with finding out what specific modifi-

cations will be needed to improve the organization and operation of the program. Financial issues are usually of concern to policy makers, who question whether a program should be continued as is, given more resources, or cancelled. Staff from other programs are interested in whether the program can be generalized for possible adaptation. Epidemiologists may seek to compare the effect of different program principles and generalize about the factors responsible for success. Out of these competing interests, which questions should an evaluation try to answer? To answer questions relative to the evaluation of health programs, it is best to first distinguish between different types of evaluation. Scriven used the terms *formative* and *summative* to describe two types of evaluation.[8]

Formative evaluation

Formative evaluation refers to the internal evaluation of a program. It is an examination of the processes or activities of a program as they are taking place. It is usually carried out to aid in the development of a program in its early phases.

The following situation is one in which formative evaluation may be conducted. A fluoride rinse program is initiated at a neighborhood health center in which paraprofessionals are trained to administer three types of fluoride rinses under a strict sequence of procedures. After 3 days of operation, the work of the paraprofessionals is observed to determine the extent to which the strict sequence of procedures is being adhered to. The observation and determination of correct or incorrect procedure sequence provide an example of examining the activities of a program as they are occurring— formative evaluation. If the sequence is incorrect, formative evaluation allows the program to make remedial changes at that point, without waiting until the end of the program. Formation evaluation is used primarily by program developers and possibly program staff concerned with whether various components of a program are workable or whether changes should be made to improve program activities.

Summative evaluation

Summative evaluation, on the other hand, judges the merit or worth of a program after it has been in operation. It is an attempt to determine whether a fully operational program is meeting the goals for which it was developed. Summative evaluation is aimed at program decision makers, who will decide as to a program's continuation or termination, and also at decision makers from other programs who might be considering adoption of the program.

Different evaluation designs are needed to carry out the two evaluation purposes, as well as different types of measures and time schedules. Since most programs are ongoing and change simply as a result of trial and error, they may never finish but will continue to grow and develop while in operation. In such cases, the dichotomy between formative and summative evaluation may not be as precise as described previously, and formative evaluation may continue to be important as the program develops and matures.

Most health programs can be divided into four phases of implementation, which should occur in sequence: (1) the pilot phase, whose development proceeds on a trial and error basis, (2) the controlled phase, where a model of a particular program strategy is run under regulated conditions to judge its effectiveness, (3) the actualization phase, where a model of the program strategy is subjected to realistic operating conditions, and (4) the operational phase, where the program is an ongoing part of the structure. Often this ideal progression from phase 1 to phase 4 does not occur, and a program becomes lodged at one state of development. Each phase has different objectives to be met and thus different evaluation designs by which to best assess achievement of program objectives. Formative evaluation plays an important part in both the pilot and controlled phases of program implementation. Summative and formative evaluations are used during the actualization phase, while the final operational phase is evaluated using a summative evaluation design.[9]

SPECIFYING HEALTH PROGRAM OUTCOMES AND INPUTS

One generalization that can be made of health program evaluation is that it is primarily concerned with how well a program is meeting its goals, either at some formative stage (so that the information can be fed back into the program) or at the end. The first step in evaluation, then, is to discover what the program goals are and to then restate them as clear, specific objectives written in measurable terms.

The first step is often a formidable task. Many program directors and staffs have very general goals expressed as vague abstractions. They find it difficult to translate them into concrete specifications of the changes in behavior, attitude, or knowledge that they hope to effect. Programs often have multiple goals. Some are more important than others, some are closer in time, some are easier to study, and some may be incompatible with others. Yet each program director and staff member must establish a sense of goal priorities in order to be able to study significant program issues. Program directors and staff may find it useful to work actively with consultants, if available, to sort out program priorities.

The frequency of ambiguous and unclear goal statements has led some observers to speculate about the underlying reasons for this state of affairs. One speculation is that it usually requires support from diverse groups and individuals to get a program accepted. Program goals have to be formulated in ways that satisfy the diversity of interest represented. Another speculation is that program planners lack experience with expressing their thoughts in measurable terms and concentrate mainly on the specifics of program operation. In one sense, ambiguous goal statements serve a useful function: they hide differences among diverse groups by allowing for a variety of interpretations. However, such differences between groups and staff or within the staff could be disruptive if the program is implemented. Once a program has been initiated, if there is lack of true consensus as to what the program is specifically attempting to achieve, progress is difficult. Each staff member may be pulling in a different direction trying to implement his/her interpretation of the goal. The area of clear goal formulation is one component of program development where evaluation can make a substantial initial contribution.

Evaluation attempts to measure program outcome. If a program's goals cannot be operationalized (stated in a precise, measurable manner), it becomes nearly impossible to determine whether or not the desired outcomes of a program have been achieved. In other words, without clearly stated goals and objectives, evaluation becomes an imprecise tool and is of questionable usefulness. Evaluation also plays a significant role in setting priorities among goals and in the reconciliation of divergent viewpoints.

One common difficulty in specifying desired objectives is that objectives usually lie far in the future. Often it would take decades to find out whether certain goals were in fact achieved. In the interim, evaluation is conducted by relying on surrogate measures of attitudes, knowledge, skills, or behaviors that presumably are related to the ultimate objectives.

This is a problem that is not unique to evaluation but is basic to program design as well. A program may be designed to produce certain intermediate changes on the assumption that they are necessary for the attainment of ultimate goals. In such cases, probably the best that evaluation can do, at least under the usual time constraints, is to discover whether intermediate goals are being met. It is up to other more intensified research efforts to investigate the relation between these goals and desired final outcomes.

Measuring outcomes

To evaluate the effectiveness of health programs, specific measurement instruments must be set up to systematically collect data on the attainment of each program objective and program goal. These procedures follow accepted principles of biostatistical and research design, which are discussed in Chapters 11 and 13.

The establishment of an effective health program evaluation requires specific description and measurement of each objective of a program. Usually, multiple instruments are required. If a program has several objectives, the use of a simple summary instrument is likely to be superficial and misleading. If measurement instruments that are relevant to program intents are available, they should be used, thus moving the evaluation process several steps ahead. Time is saved, and the program and evaluation benefit from tested and validated instruments. Use of the same measurement instruments makes it easier to compare the relative effectiveness of one program across many programs and adds significantly to the overall body of research knowledge. However, if existing instruments are not relevant to the program objectives, new measures that are constructed for the specific needs of the program must be developed.

Instrument reliability and validity

Measurement instruments used to assess program objectives and materials must be valid and reliable. Briefly, a valid measurement instrument is one that provides a score that accurately describes the characteristics it is intended to measure. A reliable instrument consistently or repeatedly produces the same score. Validity and reliability are important because no test or other measurement instrument is perfect. Each time a test is administered, a range of scores will result. Each score will be mostly accurate but also will contain a small amount of error because of testing procedures. If the procedure is repeated 10 times for 10 separate components of a health program, one can see how the amount of error can build, thus reducing the ability of the evaluation to accurately assess program effectiveness. The greater the reliability and validity, the more accurate will be the information collected during the evaluation process.

A simple example of a test that might be reliable but not valid would be the dental hygiene board examination administered to first-year dental students. Results of that test might prove to be highly reliable, consistent, yet not valid. One might guess that if first-year dental students took the dental hygiene board examination a number of times, their individual scores would not fluctuate much higher or lower from the scores they received at the first administration. Thus, the test would be considered highly reliable. It repeatedly produced the same or nearly the same score. This test would not be considered valid because it measured material totally foreign to the first-year dental student. The test is designed to measure skills of graduate dental hygienists, not first-year dental students. Thus the test is reliable but not valid.

As a second example, let us assume a course is offered in which four tests are administered during the course of the semester. No one test was found to be perfectly reliable, thus error as a result of testing would result with each administration. Assume student A received the scores indicated:

	Score	Reliability	Testing error	Range
Test 1	80	0.80	5	75 to 85
Test 2	70	0.63	8	62 to 78
Test 3	80	0.55	12	68 to 92
Test 4	90	0.92	2	88 to 92
AVERAGE	80			73 to 87

In this example student A obtained an average

of 80 and probably would receive a course grade of B− or B. Yet, because of normal error associated with the unreliability of the four tests, that student's true performance may be between 73 and 87. These scores indicate that student A's course grade could actually be between C− and B+, a substantial difference for most students. The more reliable the test, the smaller the error. Compare the reliability scores with the test error. The test with high reliability (0.92) has the smallest error (2), while the test with low reliability (0.55) has the greatest amount of error.

Difficulties in obtaining necessary information

After considering what measurement instruments to use and when to measure outcomes, a final concern must be how to measure. In this area two problems are particularly important: bias and sampling. The possibility of bias is great if one evaluates his/her own work. Bias may be avoided by using objective measures rather than subjective measures and also by using several people to measure outcomes rather than a single person. Sampling is used in evaluating a health program when it is not possible or practical to obtain information from every person involved in an activity or when it is not possible to assess every activity that a program initiates.

Sample size depends on the activity to be studied. The student is advised to consult a standard research design text for a more formal discussion of bias and sampling problems related to evaluation and research.

Constant intrusions into the program in order to collect data can be a source of friction with program staff. The evaluation is a service to the program, not vice versa; therefore, evaluation activities should be limited to only those found essential to furthering program effectiveness. One thoughtfully constructed test or questionnaire is often better than three imperfectly conceived ones. When the evaluation is clear about what is needed and why, measures can be constructed and data collected with a minimum of disruption.

Programs may intend to bring about changes not only in people but in agencies, larger social systems, or the public at large. Measures have to be relevant to such changes. Cost-benefit analysis is another measurement technique. Cost-benefit analysis is not a suitable substitute for usual methods of evaluation but a logical extension of it. Evaluation defines the program's benefits; cost-benefit analysis adds consideration of the value of the benefits. Costs of the program are compared with benefits as a way of judging whether the program is a worthwhile investment.

How does one decide which program activities to measure? Difficulties arise when theory and knowledge are inadequate to define the factors that affect success. In most program areas, the general rule of thumb is that each stated objective of the program should be measured. A clearly stated objective will indicate what achievement is sought, and thus such an objective will aid in the identification of what procedures to use for measuring program outcomes.

Table 12-1 indicates six general factors where evaluation of health programs may begin. Below each general factor are listed specific areas in which various program members would find evaluation information of interest. This list is not intended to be all inclusive, but it should provide a few ideas to an individual who is not sure where to begin.

To conclude this section on measurement instruments, a summary outline to aid in the selection of instruments is presented below. The outline identifies three factors to consider in instrument selection: importance, statistical adequacy, and feasibility.[7]

1. Importance

   Is the information that is gained by administering the instrument the measure that is needed to assess health status or health program effectiveness?

   Does the program require this information to perform its function?

2. Statistical adequacy

   a. Validity: Does the instrument accurately assess what you are trying to measure?

   b. Reliability: Will repeated application of the computational method for the measure yield similar results? How reliable are the data used to calculate the results?

   c. Sensitivity: Can the instrument adequately distinguish among levels of performance?

3. Feasibility

   a. Clarity of measure: How precise is the measure? Is the wording understandable? Are its limitations explained?

   b. Data availability and cost: Does the program have the information needed to assess the objective? Are the instruments appropriate for their specific use within the program?

   c. Compatibility: Can data collected for this program be compared with similar data on a statewide or national basis? Can they be compared with similar data from different types of programs?

   d. Ease of use and interpretation: Can collection and interpretation of data for implementation of the measure be done without specialized or statistical knowledge?

STUDY DESIGNS APPROPRIATE FOR SPECIFIC PROGRAMS

In the broadest sense, evaluation research designs are divided into two groups: experimental and nonexperimental. Experimental design has long been considered the ideal for evaluation. The design requires that people, objects, and so on be randomly assigned either to the program or to a control group. A control group is a group of individuals in an experiment whose selection and experiences are identical in every way possible to the program participants except that they are not part of the program. The control group may receive a pseudoprogram (the social science equivalent of the laboratory placebo), the standard program (the traditional rather than the innovative program), or no program at

Table 12-1. Component factors of health system characteristics

Availability	Accessibility	Cost	Quality	Continuity	Acceptability
Supply of services: Existing service capacity Utilized capacity Supply of resources: Personnel Equipment Facilities Financial resources	Ability to obtain services in terms of the following factors: Economic Out of pocket cost Health insurance coverage and benefits Opportunity cost to patient/client, family and others Temporal Travel time Waiting time Locational Architectural Cultural Organizational Informational Utilization of services by specified population sub-groups	Service cost: Costs incurred by providers Costs incurred by financing mechanisms Sources of payment for services	Structure Competence and qualifications of resources Existence and extent of review and assurance mechanisms Minimal volume of specialized services Process: Accuracy of services Appropriateness of services Documentation of treatment Outcome: Health status Behavior Environment	Coordination of within settings among health system components and to/from other nonhealth systems: Regular source of care Degree of interruptions or delays in service plan given a logical sequence of services Patient transfer Medical and health information transfer Follow-up	Consumer satisfaction with: Availability Accessibility Cost Continuity Courtesy and consideration Provider satisfaction

Modified from Hadley, S.A., and Gillespie, J.F., Jr.: Operational measures: indicators of health system performance, Am. J. Health Plan. 3(1):44, 1978.

all. Relevant measurements are taken before and after the program. If the program recipients show greater positive change than the controls, the outcome can clearly be attributed to the program. Experimental design is the study design all researchers will choose if given a choice.[2]

Toothbrushing studies are a perfect example of the true experimental design model. For illustration purposes, the study shown in Table 12-2 is designed to demonstrate the effectiveness of a fluoride toothpaste for the reduction of new carious lesions. The study is of 3-year duration and of longitudinal design. Both experimental and control groups brush daily under supervision. The study is double blind; all experimental materials are color coded and look and taste are identical. All participants use the same brand and model of brush, with the type of paste (that is, fluoride paste and nonfluoride paste) being the one variable examined in the study. Results of the study show a significant reduction in the numbers of new lesions, thus allowing the researcher to assume the reduction was a result of the one differing variable (that is, fluoride vs. nonfluoride).

One major problem arises when one tries to implement experimental procedures in health programs. It is nearly impossible to implement the design in the busy day-to-day activities of the program. One must question how random services can be tested on people who come to drop-in, multiservice, or neighborhood health centers. In addition, there is resistance from the program staff, and difficulty resulting from the very nature of the recipient groups, and to outside events that "contaminate" the controls placed on the study. These contaminations reduce the validity of the evaluation.

There are two types of validity that affect the ability to implement evaluation research designs according to strict experimental requirements: *internal validity* and *external validity*. These kinds of validity are different from the

term used earlier relating to measurement instruments. A program has internal validity if its outcomes are a result of the approach or techniques being tested rather than a result of other causes that have nothing to do with the program being implemented. Internal validity determines whether or not the results can be accepted based on the evaluation design of the program.[2]

A program has external validity if the results obtained would be generalizable everywhere to similar programs or approaches. External validity affects one's ability to credit the evaluation results with generality based on the procedures used.[2]

The process of conducting an experimental evaluation design by its nature exercises some degree of control over the program, thus contributing to internal validity while producing some limitations in external validity. A Catch-22 situation is produced. As the circumstances of a program are controlled, the chances increase that what happens in the program will be exactly what the evaluator hopes to find (internal validity). However, the more conditions are controlled, the less chance there is that the pro-

Table 12-2. Longitudinal results of 3-year fluoride toothpaste study

	Randomly assigned groups	
	Experimental (fluoride paste)	Control (nonfluoride paste)
Baseline examination (DMFS) (prior to beginning testing of paste)	97.4	97.5
After 1 year	91.5	95.0
After 2 years	86.3	93.4
After 3 years	80.0	90.3
Difference	17.4	7.2

gram will continue to work when the controls are removed (external validity).

The constant struggle between external and internal validity is an important one; external validity is of little value without some reasonable degree of internal validity to provide confidence in the conclusions. There is no advantage in being able to generalize results that are based on invalid or inconsistent program activities. The two sets of validity demands must strike a balance. There should be enough internal validity so that an experiment can be conclusive and yet sufficiently realistic to be generalized. In program evaluation, internal validity becomes the major concern since most programs attempt only superficially to generalize results beyond their program.

Perhaps "the source" in the area of research design is Donald T. Campbell. Campbell suggests that experimental design is possible in most health programs with careful planning and administrative backing, and control groups can be used in somewhat turbulent programs.[1]

In reality it is often impossible to fully apply rules relating to internal validity. To evaluate programs in such situations, the evaluator must choose some approach other than experimental. If circumstances eliminate experimental design situations, Campbell and Stanley[2] have developed quasiexperimental designs that are often suitable. Campbell offers three types useful in evaluation: interrupted time series, control series, and regression discontinuity designs.[1] While the results do not provide the certainty and the potential for generalization of experimental designs, they guard against most of the important threats to valid interpretation. Again, for the interested student, a standard research methods text is suggested for more comprehensive discussion of research design. It should also be noted that evaluation is concerned with making decisions about specific programs. Therefore, internal validity is often more important than external validity to the evaluator.

CONSTRAINTS ON USING THE RESULTS OF EVALUATION

Once the evaluation is completed, the logical expectation is that the results will be used to make rational decisions about future programming. All too often, however, the results are ignored. With all the money, time, effort, skills, and irritation that went into the acquisition of information, why does it generally have so little impact? One reason may be that evaluation results do not match the informational needs of decision makers.

Individuals responsible for conducting evaluations should have a better understanding of decision processes and of informational requirements relevant to decision making. An allied issue is that of timing. Evaluation results should be ready in time to be considered, not after the decisions on future programming have been reached. Moreover, the evaluation results may not be relevant to the level of the decision maker who receives them. For example, overall assessments of program merit may be most useful to directors in other agencies who want to know whether or not a new program strategy works, and under what conditions. Such people may never receive the report or may receive it in a nearly unreadable form.

Another constraint on the use of results may be a lack of clear direction for future programming. Results may be ambiguous, implications unclear. They have to be translated into terms that make sense for pending decisions and that delineate alternatives that are indicated. There seems to be a large void between the findings of program evaluation and the planning of future programs. Someone is needed to translate the evaluation results into explicit recommendations for future programs.

In practice, evalaution is sometimes undertaken for dubious reasons. Evaluation may be used by program decision makers to delay a decision, to justify a decision already made, to pass the responsibility of future decisions to others, to vindicate a program in the eyes of its observers, or to satisfy funding conditions of government or foundation agencies.[9] These noninformational reasons for evaluation are not rare, and individuals conducting evaluation should be forewarned if they learn that one of these is the underlying purpose of evaluation. It is as important to spend enough time investigating who wants to know what, and why, as it is to carry out the evaluation activities. Evaluations for political ends or where there is no commitment to using the data for decision making might well be eliminated rather than waste the talents of the individuals involved.[4]

External evaluators (persons called in who are not part of the program) are often reluctant to draw conclusions from their data. However, judgments and recommendations for action have to be made somewhere. Unless the evaluator plays a leading role in the process, it may not get done.

A further constraint on utilization of results is that organizations are comfortable with the status quo. When presented with negative results, their prestige, ideology, and even resources are threatened. They frequently react by rejecting the results.

Campbell suggests that one way out of this dilemma is for reformers to change their stance. Instead of committing themselves to new programs as though they were proven solutions, they would do better to commit themselves to seeking solutions to the problem. Then they could run a series of experimental programs until genuine solutions were found.[1]

The prevalence of negative findings in a wide range of program fields is not something to bemoan or cover up, even when it provokes political controversy or organizational resistance. Rather, the evidence that so many programs are having little constructive effect represents a fundamental critique of current approaches to social programming. This is a matter to which society will, in time, have to respond.

SUMMARY

Evaluation is not only a look at a program after it is in operation; evaluation also is placing value on something done every day of the week on specific objective evidence available. It includes at least four steps: formulating objectives, specifying criteria used in measuring success, determination and explanation of the degree of success, and recommendations for future program activity.[5]

Evaluations are not undertaken simply to reveal success or failure. If that were the case, most evaluations of programs would reveal lack of total success in attaining goals and objectives. Evaluation does more, however, than demonstrate degree of attainment. It also identifies where problems exist, and, ideally, identifies options to correct programs and improve program efficiency. The evaluation of programs assumes that (1) programs have been planned to expend funds to enable materials to be developed and activities to be performed and that (2) the activities are intended to cause the achievement of program goals.

A program may not achieve its goals for several reasons[3]:

1. Resources were not used as planned
2. The assumptions linking resources to activities were invalid
3. Activities were not performed as planned
4. The assumptions linking activities to objectives were invalid
5. The assumptions linking objectives to the program goals were invalid

Locating program difficulties requires measuring each of three program variables: objectives, materials, and finances. If evaluation can identify the problems, subsequent program planning should proceed more effectively than it could in the absence of evaluation. Thus, a successful evaluation in the hands of a thoughtful administrator can improve planning of programs and thereby increase program effectiveness.

REFERENCES

1. Campbell, D.T.: Reform as experiments in evaluating action programs, Boston, 1972, Allyn & Bacon, Inc.
2. Campbell, D.T., and Stanley, J.C.: Experimental and quasi-experimental design for research, Chicago, 1966, Rand McNally & Co.
3. Deniston, O.L., Rosenstock, I.M., and Getting, V.A.: Evaluation of program effectiveness, Public Health Rep. 83(4):323, 1968.
4. Elinson, J.: Effectiveness of social action programs in health and welfare, assessing the effectiveness of child health services, Report of the Fifty-sixth Ross Conference on Pediatric Research, Columbus, OH, 1967, Ross Laboratories, p. 77.
5. Glossary of administrative terms in public health, Am. J. Public Health 50:225, 1960.
6. Popham, J.W.: Educational evaluation, Englewood Cliffs, NJ, 1975, Prentice-Hall, Inc., p. 1.
7. Schulberg, H.C., Sheldon, A., and Baker, F.: Program evaluation in the health fields, New York, 1969, Behavioral Publications, Inc.
8. Scriven, M.: The methodology of evaluation. In Tyler, R.N., Gagne, R.M., and Scriven, M., editors: Perspectives of curriculum evaluation, AERA Monograph Series on Curriculum Evaluation, No. 1. Chicago, 1967, Rand McNally & Co., p. 39.
9. Suchman, E.A.: Action for what? A critique of evaluation research. In O'Toole, R., editor: The organization, management, and tactics of social research, Cambridge, MA, 1970, Schenkman Publishing Co.
10. Weiss, C.H.: Evaluating action programs: readings in social action and education, Boston, 1972, Allyn & Bacon, Inc.

BIBLIOGRAPHY

Baker, E.L.: Formative evaluation. In Popham, J.W.: Evaluation in education: current applications, Berkeley, CA, 1974, McCutchan Publishing Corp.

Bloom, B.S., Hastings, S.T., and Madaus, G.F.: Handbook on formative and summative evaluation of student learning, New York, 1971, McGraw-Hill Book Co.

FitzGibbon, C.T., and Morris, L.L.: How to design a program evaluation, Beverly Hills, CA, 1978, Sage Publications, Inc.

FitzGibbon, C.T., and Morris, L.L.: How to present an evaluation report, Beverly Hills, CA, 1978, Sage Publications, Inc.

Goodman, H.: Evaluation activities of curriculum projects: a starting point, AERA monograph series on curriculum evaluation, no. 2, Chicago, 1968, Rand McNally & Co.

Guba, E.G.: Development, diffusion and evaluation. In Eidell, T.E., and Kitchell, J.M., editors: Knowledge production and utilization in educational administration, Eugene, OR, 1968, Center for the Advanced Study of Educational Administration, University of Oregon, p. 37.

Guba, E.G.: Failure of educational evaluation, Educ. Tech. 9(5):29, 1969.

Polit, D.F., and Hungler, B.P.: Nursing research: principles and methods, ed. 2, Philadelphia, 1983, J.B. Lippincott Co.

Rosenstock, I.M.: Evaluating health programs, Public Health Rep. 85(9):835, 1970.

Rosenstock, I.M., Welch, W., and Getting, V.A.: Evaluation of program efficiency, Public Health Rep. 83(7):603, 1968.

Stufflebeam, D.L., and others: Educational evaluation and decision making, Itasca, IL, 1971, F.E. Peacock Publishers, Inc.

Suchman, E.A.: Evaluation research: principles and practice in public service and action programs, New York, 1967, Russell Sage Foundation.

Tuchman, B.W.: Conducting educational research, ed. 2, New York, 1978, Harcourt Brace Jovanovich, Inc.

Wholey, J.S., and others: Federal evaluation policy, Washington, DC, 1970, The Urban Institute.

Worthen, B.R.: Toward a taxonomy of evaluation designs, Educ. Tech. 8(15):3, 1968.

CHAPTER 13

Research in Community Dental Health

If it can be said that biomedical research falls into one of two categories—basic (laboratory) research or applied (clinical) research—there is no doubt that research in community dentistry is predominantly applied research. The research invariably involves people, who are not only the experimental subjects but often the immediate as well as the long-range beneficiaries. Not until a new material or technique has been tested on a human population is a researcher able to say with some degree of certainty, "This method really works," or "This method clearly does not work." It is unfortunate that a procedure or a material sometimes slips into the standard armamentarium of the clinician or educator without having been tested adequately in controlled research. A case in point is the assumption that a rubber cup prophylaxis *must* precede the application of topical fluoride. The clinician has always believed that this is indeed the case, but it is so? Clinical research is only beginning to apply rigid criteria to research regarding this and other firmly held, and often arbitrary, assumptions.

This chapter will deal with several aspects of research in community dentistry:

1. Various types of research commonly carried out in this field
2. Role of the federal government in supporting such research
3. Ethical issues related to research involving human subjects
4. Techniques for designing research studies and writing protocols (for example, a typical clinical trial and a questionnaire survey)

5. Methods for reading and critically evaluating the published dental research literature

In a detailed discussion of research methodology one cannot avoid the troublesome subjects of epidemiology and biostatistics; these disciplines are basic tools of the clinical investigator. However, there is serious danger of an introductory discussion of research becoming submerged in epidemiological and statistical jargon. In the interest of making this chapter readable to the widest possible audience, we will not deal explicitly with these topics, and jargon will be kept to a minimum. For detailed discussions of biostatistics and epidemiology, the student is referred to Chapters 11 and 7, respectively.

TYPES OF RESEARCH IN COMMUNITY DENTISTRY

Community dentistry research falls into three different areas: (1) clinical trials and tests of techniques and of therapeutic agents, (2) research in educational techniques and the behavioral sciences, and (3) research related to the administration and evaluation of community dental programs.

An increasing awareness of the importance of cost in relationship to effectiveness has recently developed. This awareness has permeated all aspects of community dental care research and has become, to a great extent, the yardstick by which research outcome is measured. No longer is it sufficient to say that a therapeutic agent works: that it prevents some proportion of dental disease. The critical question becomes, "How much does it cost to prevent this dental disease, and are there other techniques that can accomplish as much at a lower cost?"

Table 13-1 shows several different methods for preventing dental caries, all of which are well proven in the research literature. However, from the point of view of community dentistry, one must ask the question, "What are the relative costs of these methods?" Although the *clinical* effectiveness of the various techniques is somewhat comparable, the *cost* effectiveness (cost of preventing one carious tooth surface) covers a wide range, from the very high cost-effectiveness of community fluoridation, to the very low cost-effectiveness of the individual daily topical fluoride application. Although the more costly techniques may be acceptable in a private office where the patient is paying the bill, they may not be acceptable in a community situation where society is paying the cost.

Clinical trials of techniques and therapeutic agents

Clinical trials of techniques and therapeutic agents usually follow as the practical applications of laboratory (in vitro and animal) research, epidemiological observation, or both. A case in point is the clinical use of fluorides for the prevention of dental caries. Although the student is referred to other sources for a definitive history of fluorides,[11] the subject will be summarized briefly here.

In the early 1900s, the observation was made that populations in certain parts of the United States, for example, eastern Colorado, displayed teeth with severe staining and mottling. Concurrently, it was observed that this disfigurement invariably was accompanied by relatively low dental caries prevalence. It was not until the 1930s that the observational techniques of epidemiology and the analytical techniques of chemistry were able to establish the connection between mottling of the teeth and fluoride content in the drinking water. The inferential step from the mottling-fluoride observation and the mottling–low caries observation is obvious. In the late 1930s and early 1940s clinical researchers began asking two questions: (1) If the presence of fluoride in drinking water reduces dental caries and causes mottling of the teeth, might there be some optimum concentra-

Table 13-1. Efficiency and practicality of fluoride procedures in nonfluoridated community

Agent	Procedure	Caries reduction (surfaces/year)	Cost of saving (each surface)
0.5% APF gel	Supervised daily, self-applied	1.6	$21.30
8% SnF	Annual, professionally applied	0.7	$ 6.00
0.6% APF solution	Five times/year supervised brushing	0.4	$ 5.60
2% NaF solution	Knutson multiple application	0.7	$ 2.95
0.2% NaF	Weekly rinse	0.5	$ 1.00
Various fluoride compounds	Community water fluoridation	1.2	$ 0.17

Modified from Burt, B., editor: The relative efficiency of the methods of caries prevention in dental public health, Proceedings of a workshop at the University of Michigan, June 5-8, Ann Arbor, 1978.

tion of fluoride in the drinking water that would minimize mottling while maximizing the anti-caries effect?[8,10] (2) If fluoride in drinking water inhibits dental caries, might not a prepared fluoride solution applied topically to the teeth have a similar effect?[4,6,16]

The first question was answered by careful evaluation of the amount of mottling and the level of dental caries in communities having varying concentrations of fluoride in the drinking water.[9] The optimum amount was found to be approximately 1 part per million of fluoride ion. In the mid-1940s this epidemiological conclusion led directly to the controlled addition of fluoride compounds to the drinking water in several communities in the United States and Canada.[1] These clinical "community dentistry" research projects have demonstrated conclusively over the past four decades that drinking water fluoridated at the proper concentration can prevent approximately 65% of dental caries in a population.

The second question led directly to laboratory research measuring the effect of topical fluoride applications on incidence of dental caries in laboratory animals.[3] Those studies were quite successful, and application of topical fluorides to the teeth of human subjects was first attempted in the early 1940s.[4,6,16] Ultimately the technique gained wide acceptance within the profession and today is used almost universally in private dental offices and in community, programs, not only professionally applied but self-applied as well.[17]

Before beginning a clinical trial of some therapeutic agent (for example, a toothpaste with a new form of fluoride or a mouthrinse containing a chemical that could inhibit plaque formation—in short, any drug that has not previously been used in that manner in human populations), the investigator may need to consider certain federal regulations. For instance, a license to use the new drug in a human population may frequently be required from the federal Food and Drug Administration. Further information regarding this license, called an IND (Investigative Exemption for a New Drug), can be secured from the Food and Drug Administration, 5600 Fishers Lane, Rockville, Maryland 20852. Also the research study probably needs to be approved by the Institutional Review Board for Studies Involving Human Subjects (IRB) of the institution where the investigator is employed or is a student. These issues will be discussed in more detail later in this chapter (see Ethics of Dental Research p. 236). Finally, the drug or chemical compound may be protected by a patent as, for instance, are some of the formulations incorporated in therapeutic toothpastes.

Having conceived a worthwhile clinical study based on favorable research in laboratory studies or on well-established epidemiological observations, and having dealt with the federal and institutional guidelines previously described, the investigator is ready to design and implement his/her research study. The design of a clinical trial will be dealt with in more detail later (see Research Design p. 240).

Educational and behavioral research

Educational and behavioral research are frequently carried out by undergraduate dental students and dental hygiene students. Both types of research have the advantage of not usually requiring large numbers of study subjects, and often the study can be carried out in a relatively short period of time. Typically the study deals with applying some behavioral or educational technique to the oral hygiene practices of an individual or a group.

Experimental subjects can be approached on several different levels involving changes in knowledge, attitudes, or behavior. Much traditional dental health education and accompanying research has been based on changing the level of knowledge regarding dental health and disease in a population. Recent evidence firmly establishes that, although increases in levels of knowledge may be easy to accomplish, this approach is probably of little value in terms of improving dental health.[13] Most persons, when asked what they *should* do in order to maintain good dental health, verbally respond with the correct answers, although intraoral evidence may show that this knowledge is not being put into practice. If persons are not able to link their knowledge of dental health to their own personal dental health needs, their behavior will not change.[13] Ultimately permanent changes in behavior are essential for improving dental health. These issues and their resolution are discussed in more detail in Chapter 7.

Administrative and evaluative research

Administrative and evaluative research typically deal with the way in which a program (for example, a school-based clinical dental program) operates and how it can be improved, or with how some innovation (for instance, use of pit and fissure sealants) has been accepted in the professional community. Administrative and evaluative research involvement in evaluation of programs is discussed in detail in Chapter 12.

The questionnaire survey. An important tool of administrative and evaluative research is the questionnaire survey. Carefully designed questionnaires can be extremely effective for securing information from a population under study. The questionnaire itself, referred to as the survey instrument, requires a great deal of thought and careful planning. Not only is the content itself important, but equally significant are the structure and appearance of the questionnaire. A method for designing and carrying out a questionnaire survey will be discussed in detail later (see Research Design p. 240).

Government role in community dentistry research

For the past few years the federal government has played an increasingly important role in dental research. A great deal of this research falls within the scope of community dentistry. With an operating budget in excess of $117 million (1987), the National Institute of Dental Research is able to exert an enormous amount of influence on the dental research community. Although many individual researchers may object to this influence, there is no doubt that the effect over the past few years has been largely positive. This influence has been of three types: (1) defining research priorities, (2) conducting intramural research, and (3) funding extramural research.

Defining research priorities. Areas of potentially fruitful research are identified and published primarily through the mechanism of sponsoring conferences of recognized experts in some particular field. These research areas subsequently tend to become areas for which funding is available.

Intramural research. Some agencies (particularly the National Institute of Dental Research, located in Bethesda, Maryland) carry out a great deal of intramural research with staffs of highly competent researchers.

Extramural research. The bulk of dental research is conducted by means of extramural funding mechanisms. A contractual arrangement is made between the federal agency and some institution competent to carry out the research in question. Funding of extramural research is of two basic types: grants and contracts.

A *grant* is awarded either to an institution or to an individual for the purpose of attaining some research goal that has been defined by the individual or the institution. Although the general area of research may previously have been suggested by the federal agency, the research design is developed by the grantee. On the other hand, so-called *contract* research evolves from a research protocol that has been designed and stipulated in detail by the federal agency.

Most government research in dentistry is

sponsored by the Department of Health and Human Services through the National Institute of Dental Research of the National Institutes of Health. The approval and funding processes, regardless of the agency involved, are generally the same. Initially the agency issues an announcement to appropriate institutions. These announcements are of two types: requests for proposal and requests for applications.

The *Request for Proposal* (RFP) is a device used when contract research is anticipated. The RFP is a detailed definition of the goals and parameters of the research project. Institutions that are interested and feel competent to carry out the research are invited to submit detailed proposals in which they describe exactly how they would meet the terms of the proposal (the Scope of Work). Responses to RFPs must meet all the conditions of the RFP, and any deviation from the defined protocol must be submitted as an alternative proposal.

The *Request for Applications* (RFA), on the other hand, suggests a general area where the federal government places a high research priority. Applicants are invited to submit grant applications (as opposed to contract proposals) that are addressed to this general area or priority. In the resulting grant application the researcher defines his/her own research goals and develops his/her own protocol.

In either case, whether for a grant or a contract, the proposal is submitted to review by a group of experts who are peers of the principal investigator of the proposal. For proposals that meet the standards of excellence defined by the peer group, there is a final negotiation process and ultimate funding of the project, assuming funds are available.

ETHICS OF DENTAL RESEARCH

To the extent that proposed research involves human subjects, an elaborate system of safeguards has evolved out of concern for the welfare of human beings and the protection of the rights of persons who could be victims of inappropriate or poorly conceived research.

The Nuremberg Code of Ethics for Medical Research grew out of the deliberations of the Nuremberg War Crimes Tribunal and the revelations regarding biomedical research that was carried out by the Nazis during World War II. The principles established were reinforced by the Declaration of Helsinki, which was adopted by the World Medical Association in 1966.[14]

In the early 1950s the Department of Health, Education and Welfare (now called the Department of Health and Human Services) became involved in establishing guidelines for the design and conduct of research involving human subjects at the federal level. For any institution using Department of Health, Education and Welfare funds, these guidelines became mandatory in 1974.[14]

The formal mechanism for monitoring research that uses humans as experimental subjects is the Institutional Review Board for Studies Involving Human Subjects, established according to federal regulations at all institutions conducting research paid for by federal funds.

Minimally the institution must have a committee consisting of five members including both males and females. It should represent a variety of professions, include at least one nonscientist, and include at least one person who is not associated with the institution.[10] The IRB must review all research involving humans, whether or not it is to be supported with federal funds. No project involving humans is to be approved unless evidence is presented that the rights of the human subjects have been protected adequately. In the case of federally funded projects the institution must submit a form that indicates that the appropriate review has been carried out.

Concept of informed consent

In order for a person to be involved legitimately as an experimental subject in a research project, he/she must have given free and informed consent to the researcher. Although this discussion is directed to informed consent in relation to research studies, the same principles prevail in regard to consent for receiving clinical treatment.[2,18]

Informed consent (over and above that informed consent required for regular clinical care) is required whenever a person will receive some treatment or be involved in some technique of physical or psychological manipulation that is regarded as experimental in nature. Informed consent may not be required if the individual is not directly involved in the research, for instance, if patient records, radiographs, or previously extracted teeth are used in a situation where the patient is not directly identified. However, if the records or radiographs were collected for the purposes of the research informed consent would be required. Assume, for instance, a patient is scheduled for extractions for orthodontic reasons. If prior to the extractions some experimental treatment is to be carried out, even if it will be absolutely harmless, consent is required for the procedure. In general, if a patient or experimental subject is manipulated in any way for experimental purposes, even though the manipulation be minimal and the risk or inconvenience be inconsequential, consent is still required.

The following case studies illustrate what may often be the thin line between requiring and not requiring informed consent for participation in experimental research. The issue of informed consent prior to routine treatment or therapy is not considered here.

Case study 1. A clinician wishes to determine which of two commonly used methods for educating patients in plaque control, A or B, is more effective. In order to help answer this question, clinical records of 100 patients previously exposed to each of the two methods were examined. Routinely, a plaque measure has been recorded on a patient's chart prior to exposure to the educational program and then at regular intervals after this exposure. These data were collected for each of the

patients in the two groups, as well as other data such as age, sex, educational level, and socioeconomic background. All of these data become a part of the patient's regular record. The data are tabulated according to the identified variables, and the clinician determines that method A produces better results than method B.

Informed consent is not required for this study for the following reasons:

1. Only existing patient records were used.
2. The patients, within the context of the research, became experimental subjects but were not manipulated in any way beyond the normal treatment procedure.
3. The patients' confidentiality (their right to privacy) was not invaded by the research since no data were used that could serve to identify them.

Case study 2. A research protocol is conceived precisely the same as that described in Case Study 1, except that it is conceived before the fact of the regular care and the research subjects are placed randomly in two groups, one group to receive program A and the other to receive program B. In all other respects the project is exactly the same.

Informed consent is required for this project for the following reasons:

1. It is decided a priori that the patients would be part of a research project.
2. The patients are manipulated to the extent that they are each placed arbitrarily and randomly in one of the two experimental groups.
3. Even though the outcome is the same, and even though there is no invasion of the patients' privacy, the prior intention of the activity is to collect research data and the patients are being manipulated to that extent.

Several elements are necessary in a properly designed informed consent document.[7]

1. A fair explanation of the procedures to be followed and their purposes, including identification of any procedures that are experimental

EFFECT OF PRENATAL FLUORIDE SUPPLEMENTS IN PREVENTING DENTAL CARIES

Consent form

Dear _____ :

The Center for Community Dental Health at the Maine Medical Center, the Eastman Dental Center in Rochester, New York, and the National Institute of Dental Research (National Institutes of Health) are cooperating in conducting a study to determine the value of using fluorides during pregnancy in preventing tooth decay in the baby teeth of offspring. As an expectant mother, you are being asked to consider participating in this study.

If you participate you will be asked to consume a daily tablet, beginning during the fourth month of your pregnancy and continuing until the birth of your baby. In order for the study to yield valid data, one-half of the women will consume a tablet containing one milligram of fluoride and the other half will consume a tablet which will look and taste the same, but will not contain fluoride. This is called a "blind" study and it is the only way that we can measure a difference in effect between consuming, and *not* consuming, fluoride during pregnancy. Assignment to group will be random, so you will have a 50/50 chance of being in the fluoride group. At the completion of the study, five years from now, all subjects will be told which group they were in.

After your child is born, you will be given (free of charge) fluoride for him/her to take until the age of five. The fluorides will be in the form of drops during the first two years and chewable tablets after that. If your child is receiving a vitamin supplement from his/her physician/pediatrician, it should not contain fluoride since this prescribed dosage is adequate. All children will receive fluoride, regardless of which group the mother was in.

At the age of three your child will receive a dental examination (without x-rays) and at the age of five he/she will receive another dental examination, including a single x-ray on each side of the mouth. If any dental problems are found you will be notified immediately. In any case, your family dentists will be given the exam results, if he/she so requests. There is no charge for the dental examinations. You, as the parent, would be responsible for seeking any dental care that might be necessary.

Risks

There are no known risks involved in this study. The amount of fluoride you consume during pregnancy will be approximately the same amount you would consume if you lived in a community with fluoridated water. If you should move to a fluoridated community while either you or your child is taking daily fluoride supplements you should discontinue the supplements, as the drinking water will contain the amount of fluoride needed for prevention of tooth decay.

Regarding the dietary fluoride supplement for your child, this procedure is used routinely and probably would have been recommended by your pediatrician when your baby was born.

Consent form—cont'd

The dental examinations are routine and as recommended by most dentists, although you should take your child to your family dentist for regular checkups, in addition to participation to this study.

Benefits

Your child will derive the benefit of daily fluoride supplements (at no cost to you) and two dental examinations. Additionally, if you are in the fluoride group, there is a possibility of even greater prevention of tooth decay. If this study should show a benefit from prenatal fluorides, children everywhere will have the opportunity to have fewer cavities.

If you have any question regarding this study you may call Ms. Vaughan at (207) 874-1025 or Dr. Leverett at (716) 275-5007 (call collect, if long distance). Also, you are encouraged to discuss the study with your family dentist, obstetrician or pediatrician.

Of course, this study is entirely voluntary, and if you elect not to participate, or withdraw before completion of the study you will not jeopardize the status of your child or of you as patients in any of the participating institutions.

Whenever possible, the father of the child should be aware of the nature of this project and give his consent to your participation. If this is not possible, please so indicate on the line marked "Father's Signature."

☐ I *DO* consent to participate in the prenatal fluoride study. Also, I have discussed the study with my obstetrician and he has no objection to my participation.

Signature	Date
Print name	Your birthdate
Street	Expected date of birth of child
City/town	
Phone number	
Father's signature	Name of obstetrician or prenatal clinic

☐ I *DO NOT* consent to participate in the prenatal fluoride study.

Signature	Date
Print name	

2. A description of any attendant discomforts and risks reasonably to be expected
3. A description of any benefits reasonably to be expected
4. A disclosure of any appropriate alternative procedures that might be advantageous for the subject
5. A statement describing the confidentiality of records
6. For research involving more than minimal risk, an explanation as to whether compensation and medical treatment are available if physical injury occurs and, if so, what they consist of and where further information may be obtained
7. An explanation of whom to contact for answers to pertinent questions about the research and research subjects' rights and whom to contact in the event of a research-related injury to the subject
8. A statement that the person is free to withdraw his/her consent and to discontinue participation in the project or activity at any time without prejudice to the subject

The box on p. 238 is an example of a consent form used in a research project. The necessary elements described previously are clearly evident.

The use of placebos

A placebo is an agent that is known to have no physiological effect on the patient and can have an extremely beneficial effect with a patient whose problem is basically psychological rather than organic. One of the important elements of research design is to compare an experimental drug or technique to some other drug or technique, the efficacy of which is known with a great degree of accuracy. It is quite understandable, therefore, that the most common comparison in biomedical research has been to the placebo, the physiological efficacy of which is known to be zero. Typically a study population would be divided in half, with one group taking

the experimental drug and the other group taking a placebo that looks, smells, and tastes like the experimental drug. The degree to which the experimental-drug group is different from the placebo-drug group in its outcome is a measure of the efficacy of the experimental drug.

With the growing armamentarium of effective drugs, for example, fluorides for the prevention of dental caries, it is considered unethical to design a study in which one half of the study population is denied a preventive treatment of known efficacy.[5] However, in a situation where a drug or technique of known efficacy is available (this is commonly the case) the dilemma is dealt with easily by the use of an *active* control, rather than a *placebo* control. Practically speaking, this presents no problem because the clinical value of the experimental drug or technique ultimately must be measured against previously accepted alternatives.

RESEARCH DESIGN

This section will consider the design of two types of research common in community dentistry: the clinical trial and the questionnaire survey. Typical examples of these genres will be presented, together with accompanying discussions.

The clinical trial

Probably the most frequently conducted form of research in community dentistry is the clinical trial. Reasons for carrying out clinical trials and the essential antecedents to such research have been discussed earlier in this chapter. The clinical trial can be quite elaborate, involving several thousand research subjects and extending over a period of 2 or 3 years or more. The major clinical trial used to test the Salk polio vaccine, for instance, involved over 400,000 children.[12] A typical clinical trial intended to test the efficacy of some caries-preventive agent, for example, a fluoride mouthrinse, would begin with several hundred children in the caries-prone age range of 11 to 13 years and continue for 2 to 3 years. This population size and time frame are made necessary by the fact that differences in dental caries increment manifest themselves slowly and in relatively small numbers. However, a clinical trial that is intended to measure what is anticipated to be a large difference occurring in a short time could require much smaller numbers and a considerably shorter period of time.

The box on pp. 242 and 243 exemplifies the large-scale clinical trial. A typical brief protocol for a study that was presented for approval to the Institutional Review Board of the Eastman Dental Center is shown. This protocol, which should be considered as a summary protocol, is brief and concise, although it contains all of the elements of good study design and protocol writing. A typical grant application or contract proposal submitted to a federal agency for funding would be considerably more detailed. The consent form attached to this protocol has been described and evaluated earlier.

The questionnaire survey

Typically, the notion to conduct a questionnaire survey begins with the identification of a population containing individuals who possess what the researcher thinks may be useful information. The problem, of course, is to facilitate the willingness of the individuals to share this information in a useful and measurable manner. This section will describe a technique for developing and carrying out a questionnaire survey.

Let us suppose, for the sake of illustration, that we are concerned with the relative efficacy of undergraduate dental curricula in private and state-supported schools and we decide that one method for beginning to address this issue is to conduct a questionnaire survey.

Selection of study population. For a study of this type we would select equal numbers of dentists who have graduated from the two types of

dental schools. The number of subjects selected would depend on the number and complexity of questions asked in the survey and on the proportion that we expect to respond. The decision regarding sample size can best be handled by a statistician and will not be dealt with in this discussion. However, let us say that we decide to select as the study population 200 to 300 subjects from each of the two types of dental schools. Further, we should select subjects who are as much alike as possible, except for the variable under study (source of funding for school). Other differences, which are called confounding or intervening variables, could be minimized by selecting subjects from among graduates of American dental schools during a given 1-year or a 2-year period—say 1982 and 1983. By contacting appropriate dental schools we could secure lists of names and addresses of graduates during those 2 years. If this procedure results in more subjects than are required for the study, some technique for randomly selecting from among the potential population would be instituted in order to end up with the desired population of 400 to 600 graduates.

Defining the goal of the study. The goal of the study would be to determine whether there are any measurable differences between the two study groups.

Hypotheses. The null hypotheses for this study would be that, when looking at dental graduates from the two types of schools, there are no differences in terms of (1) the structure and outcome of dental practice, (2) the performance of these persons as students in dental school, (3) involvement in professional activities outside the dental office, and (4) other similar measures that we may care to identify. At this point, we will focus on hypothesis 1, using it as an example of a way in which the questionnaire can be developed.

Core area objectives. In dealing with one of the hypotheses, we should make a statement, from which measurable questionnaire items can

EFFECT OF PRENATAL FLUORIDE SUPPLEMENTS IN PREVENTING DENTAL CARIES

Background

There has been interest for many years in the use of dietary fluoride supplements prenatally. Since calcification of primary teeth begins in utero, it has been suggested that the ingestion of fluoride supplements by women during pregnancy could result in increased protection for these teeth in the offspring, enhancing the benefit derived from the use of supplements postnatally, as commonly prescribed. Although there is a reasonable amount of clinical evidence to support this practice, virtually all of the published studies of prenatal fluoride supplementation have major shortcomings in design or execution that compromise their value.

The insufficiency of clinical evidence was noted by the U.S. Food and Drug Administration in 1966. As a result, the FDA banned the marketing by manufacturers of fluoride products that made claims of caries prevention in the offspring of women who used the supplements during pregnancy. While questioning the efficacy of prenatal fluoride supplements, the FDA did not challenge the safety of the procedure, since the amount of fluoride prescribed was approximately equivalent to the quantity consumed daily by persons residing in areas with optimally fluoridated drinking water.

Although the FDA action is still in effect, additional studies have been conducted since 1966, which have demonstrated the placental transfer of fluorides in humans, and clinical studies have also offered further support for the efficacy of prenatal fluoride supplementation in preventing dental caries. However, prenatal studies are still few compared with those that form the basis of the more well-established caries-preventive procedures, such as water fluoridation or postnatal fluoride supplements, and most of the prenatal studies that exist are deficient in some important respects.

Thus, it cannot be concuded from currently available data that prenatal fluoride supplementation should be recommended for the prevention of dental caries. Acceptance and promotion of any preventive procedure should be based upon scientifically sound and conclusive clinical data, and the available data are neither. However, the positive trend in the data clearly offers suggestive evidence that the procedure might benefit primary teeth. Hence, further research to determine efficacy is indicated.

Objective

The objective of this study is to determine whether children whose mothers regularly ingested fluoride supplements during pregnancy have a lower incidence of dental decay than children whose mothers did not ingest fluoride supplements during pregnancy.

Population

The population of this study will be women who are in the first three months of pregnancy and who reside in a community with a low level of fluoride in the drinking water (0.3 ppm or less) within York and Cumberland Counties, Maine.

EFFECT OF PRENATAL FLUORIDE SUPPLEMENTS IN PREVENTING DENTAL CARIES—cont'd

Method

After having the study explained to them, women who are interested will be asked to sign a consent form (see sample attached)* and will be assigned randomly to one of two study groups. Subjects in Group I will consume one tablet containing 1 milligram of fluoride as sodium flouride each day during their pregnancies, beginning during the fourth month. Subjects in Group II will consume a tablet identical in appearance and flavor but containing no fluoride, beginning during the fourth month and continuing the remainder of their pregnancies.

Assignment to the two groups will be entirely random and "blind" (neither the study personnel nor the study subjects will know which group is which).

Upon completion of the term of pregnancy all offspring, regardless of group assignment of their mothers, will receive daily fluoride supplements. Initially, the supplements will be in the form of drops and will be replaced by chewable tablets at approximately two years of age. These supplements will continue until each of the children reaches five years of age.

At three years of age each child will receive a thorough dental examination, without x-rays. At five years of age, each child will receive a second dental examination including a single x-ray on each side of the mouth. The results of all dental examinations will be made available to family dentists, upon request.

Risks

There is no known risk to the procedures described. The amount of fluoride consumed by the mothers-to-be is approximately the same amount that would be consumed by a person residing in a community with a fluoridated public water supply. The use of dietary fluoride supplements of this type is widespread. For example, in southern Maine the Center for Community Dental Health, the Portland Health Department and the State Office of Dental Health have been instrumental in establishing several community programs for using dietary fluoride supplements which have been in operation for up to seven years.

Benefits

A certain benefit of this program is that all children participating will have provided to them dietary fluoride supplements for the first five years of their lives, which should result in less decay than in children not using fluoride supplements. Additionally, all children will receive two thorough dental examinations during that time. There also is a possibility that the children whose mothers consumed fluoride supplements during their pregnancies will have even less dental decay.

Obviously, there is also a substantial potential benefit to society-at-large, should the procedure prove to be efficacious.

*See Consent form on p. 238.

be developed. For instance, "Graduates of private and publicly-funded schools who enter private practice will not differ with regard to the ultimate structure and outcome of their dental practices."

Subgoals. The example of a core area objective refers to both structure and outcome of dental practice; therefore a more specific subgoal is required. Obviously, a rather specific statement is ultimately required and, if the core area objective is sufficiently specific, the statement of the subgoal may not be necessary. In terms of the example, the subgoal might be "Graduates of private and publicly-funded schools who enter private practice will not differ with regard to the form of their dental practices."

At this point we have a statement that is sufficiently specific and that represents a small enough chunk of our study goal that we can begin to make a quantifiable statement which, when converted to actual questionnaire items, will solicit the information we seek.

Subgoal statement. Graduates of private and publicly-funded schools who enter private practice will not differ with regard to the form of dental practice. Specifically, they will:

1. Have the same proportion of general practitioners.
2. Have the same distribution of specialty practices.
3. Be as likely to enter solo or group practice.
4. Have similar patterns of utilization of auxiliaries.
5. Delegate clinical responsibilities to auxiliaries in the same manner.
6. Have the same patterns of referral for specialty care.
7. Have the same number of operatories.
8. Have similar configurations of dental equipment.

You may wish to add other statements of the same type.

Items. The student will notice that by a very careful process of refining we have reached the point where we have defined quite specifically the quantifiable information that we wish to secure. Our next task is to write the actual questions, or *items*, that the respondent will be asked to answer. However, before taking this step, it would be worthwhile to explore the various formats used for questions.

The *dichotomous-response* type question is characterized by the "yes/no," "true/false," and "present/absent" type of response. For example:

Do you have a recall system?	Yes/No
Are you in general practice?	Yes/No

This type of question is desirable in a questionnaire, since it is very easy to answer accurately and the response is easy to analyze.

A *multiple choice* question is necessary in a situation where there is a list of possible responses:

Do you have any of the following equipment in your office?

Panoramic x-ray	Copying machine
Ultrasonic cleaner	Computer

When *quantifiable items* are involved, questions may lend themselves to a specific number as a response:

With how many other dentists do you practice? ____

How many operatories do you have? _____

How many continuing education courses did you take

   during the last year? _____

Occasionally, it may be necessary to ask a question that requires a *written response:*

   List all dental organizations of which you are an active member.

However, this type of question is best avoided, since it is very difficult to tabulate the completed data. You should, in a case such as this, provide a list, albeit a long one, of potential options and thereby convert the question to a multiple-choice type of question.

Sometimes, particularly in situations where one is attempting to elicit feelings rather than facts, a question that resembles a multiple choice question may be asked:

How successful have you been in maintaining low turnover of office personnel?
Very successful
Moderately successful
Neither successful nor unsuccessful
Moderately unsuccessful
Very unsuccessful

Arranged in the above format we are specifically soliciting one of five responses. However, the same responses can be arranged horizontally as follows:

/	/	/	/	/
Very success- ful	Moder- ately success- ful	Neither success- ful nor unsuc- cessful	Moder- ately unsuc- cessful	Very unsuc- cessful

In this case, a respondent can make a mark anywhere along the scale, either at one of the five points or somewhere between. This type of scale is somewhat more difficult to score and should be avoided in most cases.

Occasionally, a combination of a dichotomous response and some other form may be indicated. For example:

15. Do you have a recall system?   Yes/No
    If No, please skip to question 16.
    If Yes, when is the appointment scheduled?
    ☐ At the time of the visit
    ☐ By mail, near time of recall
    ☐ By phone, near time of recall
    ☐ Patient reminded to call for appointment
    With your recall system, what percent of patients respond affirmatively? _____

Some questions fall conveniently into a *matrix format:*

16. Which of the following clinical responsibilities do you delegate and to which auxiliaries?

	Hygienist	**Assistant**
1. Prophylaxis		
2. Fluoride treatments		
3. Taking radiographs		
4. Impressions for study models		

Now, returning to the example, here are some questionnaire items that are intended to derive specific quantifiable information suggested by the subgoal statements.

1. Are you a general practitioner?   Yes ☐   No ☐
   If no, which specialty do you practice?
   ☐ Orthodontics
   ☐ Periodontics
   ☐ Pediatric dentistry
   ☐ Other (specify) _____
2. With how many other dentists do you practice?
3. How many operatories do you have in your office:

	Fully equipped including x-ray	**Partially equipped (list equipment)**
For dentist(s)		
For dental hygienist (2)		
Other (specify)		

Demographic and baseline data. Assuming that the questionnaire responses are anonymous (and this is absolutely imperative for maintaining a high response rate), we will want to include questions that establish certain characteristics about the respondent: (1) year of birth, (2) year of graduation from dental school, (3) name of dental school, and (4) other useful data.

Data collection and evaluation. This topic is extremely important to the successful conduct of a questionnaire survey, but it is beyond the scope of this discussion. Since the method of collecting, tabulating, and analyzing data is dependent on the type of computer facilities available, the advice of persons at a local computer facility should be sought prior to establishing the final design of the survey instrument.

Pretesting. After the final design of the survey has been established, it should be tested on a small number of persons who are not in the selected study population but who have similar backgrounds. A final item on the pretest survey should solicit comments and criticisms (relating to the questionnaire itself) from the respondent. In this way errors and ambiguities can be corrected and the length of the questionnaire altered if it is too time-consuming.

Maximizing response to the questionnaire. No questionnaire survey can be successful if a significant proportion of the population does not respond. Here are a few suggestions for improving the rate of response:

1. Use a cover letter that is signed or cosigned by a person who represents authority and prestige to the study population, for example, a dean of a dental school, a president of a dental society, or a noted authority in the area under investigation. This letter should be brief but should emphasize the importance of the study and describe direct and indirect benefits to the respondent.
2. Have an esthetically pleasing questionnaire.
3. Provide a self-addressed, stamped envelope.
4. Provide some sort of follow-up reminder for nonrespondents.

If the questionnaire is truly anonymous, follow-up is not possible. However, there are ways to short-circuit the anonymity in this type of questionnaire. One method, not to be recommended, is to code the return envelope in order to identify the respondent. In this case the cover letter would contain a promise not to link the envelope with the questionnaire. A better method is to include a self-addressed postcard on which the respondent's name is printed. He is instructed to return the postcard several days after returning the questionnaire. In that way he

can be identified as a respondent, although still maintaining the anonymity of his response. When the flow of responses has diminished to an average of about 1% per day (usually after approximately 2 weeks) a postcard reminder can be sent to nonrespondents. This usually will generate an increase in the rate of response and when the flow again returns to about 1%, a mailing identical to the first mailing should be sent to each nonrespondent, with the word *reminder* written at the top of the cover letter. Further follow-up will probably be unproductive, and the investigator should be satisfied with a response rate in excess of 60%. Certain demographic characteristics of nonrespondents, for example, year of birth, dental school, year of graduation, and specialty practice, can be secured from the latest edition of the American Dental Association Directory, and this information can be useful in determining to what extent the respondents differ from nonrespondents.

READING THE RESEARCH LITERATURE

In 1985 over 17,000 articles were published in the dental periodical literature.[15] A substantial proportion of these articles report original dental research. A list of some of the more important journals publishing original research in community dentistry may be found at the end of this chapter.

One would be foolish to believe that all journals maintain the same standards of quality or that all published dental research is of equal value and quality. Following are a few general guidelines that the student can use to identify the better and more reliable published dental research.

Date of publication. Of course there are a few "classic" articles in the literature, articles that probably will always represent preeminent contributions to the body of knowledge. The general rule, however, is that research tends to become dated and a contribution that was valid and useful a few years ago may be obsolete or even misleading when interpreted within the context of the current "state of the art." One should give greater credence to more recently published research.

Reputation of the journal. The more respected, or so-called refereed, journals accept articles for publication only after they have been reviewed and critiqued by eminent researchers in the field. This *peer review* process tends to reject inadequate research and provide useful criticism of basically sound research.

Reputation of the author(s). Evaluation on this point may be beyond most casual readers who are not familiar with the important people in the field. However, a review of the "Author Section" of the *Index to Dental Literature* can give some idea of the publishing frequency of the authors and the subject areas in which they publish most often. The sequence of authors' names can be important. When a well-known researcher's name is not first in authorship, it may mean that he/she did not contribute substantially to the research.

Source of financial support. Usually the source of financial support, whether a government or commercial grant, will be acknowledged with the published research. One should accept cautiously favorable findings reported in research sponsored by a commercial source having a vested interest in the results.

Corroborations from other sources. Although the findings of a single study on a particular subject, even though quite dramatic, need to be accepted with caution, repeated corroboration from other sources substantially increases the reliability of the original report.

Quality of literature review. A careful researcher will be thoroughly familiar with other research done in the area under investigation, and this will be reflected in the quality and completeness (not to be confused with the quantity) of his/her literature review. This is, of course, another area in which the less-informed reader will have difficulty making a sound judgment.

However, one could seek the advice of a colleague or teacher. As a general rule-of-thumb, government-supported research published in refereed journals will have a high-quality literature review as part of the introduction.

Characteristics of study design. Characterizing the difference between good research and bad research in just a few words is impossible. However, there are a few characteristics of the protocol that should be noted.

1. Is the study design adequately described? Although it need not be long, the description should be complete enough that another investigator could replicate the study.
2. Is the sample size adequate? Samples may be both too small or too large. If a sample is too small, modest differences between groups may not reach the level of statistical significance and thus important findings may be overlooked. If sample size is too large, very small differences may reach levels of statistical significance. In the latter situation, it is not unusual for investigators to report that a difference was "statistically significant," while ignoring the fact that the difference was so small that it was not "clinically significant."
3. Was the data analysis adequate? Were appropriate statistical tests used? Were *any* statistical tests used?
4. Are the conclusions based solidly on the data? Does the author avoid generalizing beyond the limitations of the study?

Style of writing. This criterion is probably (and unfortunately) the least reliable of those listed. It is painfully true that some of our finest researchers are terrible writers, and the converse is probably also true—that some of our worst researchers are good writers. Nonetheless, good research that is well written should be considered better than excellent research that is poorly written because it is communicated better to the rest of the scientific world.

JOURNALS PUBLISHING ORIGINAL RESEARCH IN COMMUNITY DENTISTRY

Journal of Public Health Dentistry
Journal of the American Dental Association
American Journal of Public Health
Journal of Dental Research
Public Health Reports
Journal of Dental Education
Community Dental Health
Community Dentistry and Oral Epidemiology
Clinical Preventive Dentistry
Caries Research

REFERENCES

1. Ast, D.B., and Fitzgerald, B.: Effectiveness of water fluoridation, J. Am. Dent. Assoc. **65**:581, 1962.
2. Barber, B.: The ethics of experimentation with human subjects, Sci. Am. **234**(2):25, 1976.
3. Bibby, B.G.: Use of fluorine in the prevention of dental caries. I. Rationale and approach, J. Am. Dent. Assoc. **31**:228, 1944.
4. Bibby, B.G.: The use of fluorine in the prevention of dental caries. II. Effect of sodium fluoride application, J. Am. Dent. Assoc. **31**:317, 1944.
5. Bok, S.: The ethics of giving placebos, Sci. Am. **231**(5):17, 1974.
6. Cheyne, V.D.: Human dental caries and topically applied fluorine: a preliminary report, J. Am. Dent. Assoc. **29**:804, 1942.
7. Code of Federal Regulations 45 CFR 46, revised as of March 8, 1983, U.S. Government Printing Office, Washington, D.C.
8. Dean, H.T.: Endemic fluorosis and its relation to dental caries, Public Health Rep. **53**:1443, 1938.
9. Dean, H.T., Arnold F.A., Jr., and Elvove, E.: Domestic water and dental caries. V. Additional studies of the relation of fluoride domestic waters to dental caries experience in 4,425 white children, aged 12 to 14 years, of 13 cities in 4 states, Public Health Rep. **57**:1155, 1942.
10. Dean H.T., and Elvove, E.: Studies on the minimal threshold of the dental sign of chronic endemic fluorosis (mottled enamel), Public Health Rep. **50**:1719, 1935.
11. Dunning, J.M.: Principles of dental public health, ed. 4, Cambridge, MA, 1986, Harvard University Press.
12. Francis, T., and others: An evaluation of the 1954 poliomyelitis vaccine trials, Am. J. Public Health **45**(5, part 2): XIV-63, 1955.
13. Frazier, P.J.: A new look at dental health education in community programs, Dent. Hyg. **52**(4):176, 1978.
14. Horowitz, H.S.: Ethical considerations of study participants in dental caries clinical trials, Community Dent. Oral. Epidemiol. **4**:43, 1976.
15. Index to dental literature, 1985, Chicago, 1986, American Dental Association.
16. Knutson, J.W., and Armstrong, W.D.: Effect of topically applied sodium fluoride on dental caries experience, Public Health Rep. **58**:1701, 1943.
17. Miller, A.J., and Brunelle, J.A.: A summary of the NIDR community caries prevention demonstration program, J. Am. Dent. Assoc. **107**(2):265, 1983.
18. Morganstein, W.M.: Informed consent—the doctrine evolves, J. Am. Dent. Assoc. **93**:637, 1976.

SECTION SIX

MANAGEMENT AND ETHICS
IN DENTAL CARE

The dental student or dental auxiliary student has ahead of him/her 40 or 45 years of dental practice. For some, it will be a "private practice," for others, a career in education, public health, group practice, or community health. Yet all practitioners of dentistry are faced with certain inevitable challenges—how to lead a happy, successful life—being one of tantamount importance.

As dental practice changes, as evidenced in Chapter 2 of this book, the skills of the practitioner must also change. Gone are the days of the solo practitioner working alone in the little office over the corner drugstore; here today is the team practice. Management of personnel may be the key to a successful practice, whether it be in a dental office providing care or in a health department administering government programs. As Dr. Moosbruker states in Chapter 14, "Effective management of job functions, communications, decision-making, problem-solving, finances, and interpersonal relations improves productivity and saves money."

Dental professionals are faced with ethical decisions throughout their practicing lives. Issues such as breach of confidentiality, iatrogenic disease, paternalistic behavior toward patients as well as paternalistic public health laws are common. Chapter 15 discusses ethical principles in health care and the responsibility professionals have toward society. Several ethical dilemmas and a decision-making model are presented.

CHAPTER 14

Team Management in Dental Practice

The practice of dentistry has changed dramatically during the past decade. The field of community dental health is now concerned with the efficient delivery of dental care as well as the traditional concerns for preventive dentistry and dental health education. This chapter deals with the team approach to dental care and the skills and philosophy necessary to manage a modern dental practice. As the number of people who must interact on a regular basis increases, the need for management increases. Households require management, one's social life requires management; indeed any situation where a number of people are involved in complex processes requires management.

Although the dentist has traditionally been the team leader, it is likely that as dentistry moves into the 1990s other dental health professionals will also emerge as team leaders. The independently practicing dental hygienist, for instance, must acquire the skills of management if he/she is to be an efficient practitioner. Whether one is the manager or the managed, the fundamental principles enumerated in this chapter will be of importance. Effective management of job functions, communications, decision-making, problem-solving, finances, and interpersonal relations improves productivity and saves money.

The most useful way of thinking of a group of people whose activities must be managed is as a team. This chapter focuses on the various processes that a successful team leader must be able to manage and some of the methods through which he/she can accomplish the task.

It begins with a brief working definition of a team. A discussion of two alternate theories of management follows, together with the principles derived from these theories. Next, the major interpersonal and group processes that the team leader must be able to manage are described: communication, problem-solving, and decision-making. Since an understanding of the dynamics of functioning groups is also extremely helpful in managing a team, there is a discussion of what to observe in an ongoing group process. Additional team management issues that are discussed include team roles and role negotiations, the supervisory function, conflict management, and team building.

WHAT IS A TEAM?

The definition of a team that is used here is "a group of interdependent individuals, usually with different roles and functions, whose combined efforts toward a mutually shared goal are required for the successful completion of a task."

A number of problems commonly occur when team functioning is attempted. Some of the reasons for the problems include:

1. Absence of clear and shared goals
2. Lack of a specified decision-making mechanism
3. Use of a decision-making mechanism that attributes more to educational background and professional status than to having the most relevant information
4. Lack of clarity over responsibilities of each team member

5. Closed or only partially open communication channels
6. Absence of a time and method for problem identification, analysis, and solution
7. Insufficient planning time or an inadequate planning process
8. Lack of a mechanism for resolving team conflicts
9. Inadequate selection procedures for team members

Unresolved team problems can be extremely costly. Friction between team members can be felt by patients and can result in inadequate care of patients, loss of patients, and high personnel turnover. Team rapport is needed to keep the dentist in touch with patients. In a busy practice, auxiliaries serve as a communication bridge. Continuity of care may depend on their relationship with the patient and their ability to bring the dentist into the relationship to share the ongoing conversation and learn the patient's concerns.

A question for any dental team's consideration is the extent to which the patient is regarded as a member of the team for discussion of and decisions about his/her own treatment. What is meant here is more than a brief description of the situation by the doctor and a rapid and uninformed decision by the patient. Ideally at least one meeting would take place between dentist, auxiliaries, patient, and hygienist, if appropriate, concerning the specific problems of the patient with the patient *not* sitting in the dental chair.

Including the patient in the team to this extent will probably result in better rapport, more cooperation with the treatment plan, and perhaps even an earlier payment of bills. However, taking the additional time for the team to talk with the patient may also result in decreased earnings or in higher fees to compensate.

THEORIES OF MANAGEMENT

Underlying assumptions, values, and beliefs are guiding factors in our behavior but are often not identified as such. The manner in which someone goes about managing or participating on a team is also determined in large measure by his/her underlying beliefs about people: what motivates them, what they need, how they function. McGregor described two very different theories of management, outlining the underlying assumptions about people on which they are based and the principles of organization that logically follow.[4] The theories are designated simply "X" and "Y." Theory X's assumptions about average people are the following:

1. They are lazy, preferring to work as little as possible.
2. They dislike responsibility or are incapable of handling it.
3. They prefer to be dependent on others, to be led.
4. They are incapable of self-control and therefore must be controlled by others.
5. They cannot find satisfaction of important needs in work and must, therefore, seek basic satisfaction outside the work setting.

These assumptions lead to an organizational structure that has a very clear chain of command, where the top of the hierarchy both directs and controls the bottom. For example, each level directs the actions of the level below it by making assignments, coordinating activities, and perhaps explaining procedures. The top controls the bottom through allocation and distribution of resources including money, time, and materials, and through specifying behaviors. There is usually little communication up the line, with the result that the person directing does not know the effects of his/her directives. For example, beginning the day at 8:15 AM rather than 8:30 AM may mean an auxiliary has to catch an hourly bus that arrives at 7:30 AM rather than at 8:30 AM. The dentist may then wonder why he/she is so tired at 4:30 PM but never ask about it.

A second outcome of accepting Theory X's assumptions about people is that one builds an organization with narrow task specialization.

The assignments are made so that each individual has a small and narrowly defined task that he/she will do well. Further, each person has responsibility for a relatively small segment of the organization's work. The result is that they cannot substitute for each other, even though tasks are within the scope of their competence. More important, they often do not understand each other's jobs, so that needless conflicts can arise because of lack of knowledge and awareness. The best example of task specialization is the assembly line, but it has parallels in the dental office. For example, one auxiliary always sterilizes the instruments or takes the x-rays, and no one else but the dentist knows how to operate the equipment. If the knowledgeable individual is sick or very busy, a slowdown occurs.

The assumptions that Theory Y makes about people are quite different. They include the following:

1. They prefer to be active rather than passive.
2. They are capable of assuming responsibility and find satisfaction in doing so.
3. They prefer being independent, finding greater satisfaction in not having to look to others for direction.
4. They are capable of finding basic satisfaction and self-fulfillment in their work.
5. They are capable of self-control, not needing control from outside.

Acceptance of these assumptions about people leads to the formation of an organization with minimum hierarchy. If people find greater satisfaction in assuming responsibility and in being independent and are capable of self-control, then greater productivity and satisfaction will result from fewer people being in superior-subordinate relationships with one another. The integrative force in the organization is mutual confidence rather than authority. There is shared responsibility in a Theory Y organization through wide participation in decisions rather than centralized decision-making. The basic unit of organization is the small group rather than the individual. People plan task performance and assign jobs according to qualifications and interest. The role of the supervisor is as an agent for maintaining intra- and intergroup communication rather than as an agent of higher authority.

The basic philosophy of management in Theory Y and Theory X organizations may be summarized as follows:

Theory X. Since the average person is lazy, dislikes or is incapable of assuming responsibility, is dependent, prefers to be led, is incapable of self-control, and cannot find basic satisfaction in his/her work, it is important that management create a system in which higher supervisory levels:

1. Direct the efforts of their subordinates
2. Provide the motivation for their subordinates (rewards and punishments)
3. Control the action of their subordinates

Theory Y. Since the average person prefers to be active, is capable of and wants to assume responsibility, prefers to be independent, is capable of self-control, and is capable of finding satisfaction and self-fulfillment in his/her work, then it is important that management provide a climate in which:

1. Self-direction and self-control are encouraged through minimizing superior-subordinate relationships
2. People are encouraged to use and develop more and more of their abilities

It is also true, however, that the theories in operation are probably never absolute; nor would they be completely effective if they were. The individual worker and supervisor lend their own personalities to the functioning of any organization. It is possible for an employee, for example, to be so conditioned to Theory X principles that he/she believes its assumptions about himself/herself and acts accordingly, thus undermining Theory Y organization. Other employees may believe Theory Y assumptions about themselves, demanding more and more freedom, yet perform in a manner that causes management to treat them on the basis of Theory X principles.

McGregor's organizational theory[3] parallels the development of psychological theories of human motivation. Freud's "drive reduction" theory dominated the literature for years. People were thought to be motivated solely to decrease their drives for food, drink, and sex. Given satisfaction of these basic needs and the absence of pain, no one would do much of anything, similar to Theory X's assumptions. The 1950s saw the emergence of new theories about intrinsic motivation, competence motivation,[8] and research to support them. It appeared that even chimpanzees "preferred" a little stimulation and would solve puzzles for the "reward," not of food, but of looking into a busy laboratory at people working.[1] Here we have the basis for Theory Y.

There do seem to be different types of people, however, some fitting one theory and some the other. Maslow explained this in a developmental framework, suggesting that different people operate on the basis of different needs but are capable of being motivated by higher order needs as the more basic ones are satisfied.[3] Thus one part of motivating people involves helping them to satisfy lower order needs such as physical needs (providing a job with a living wage in a safe environment), security needs (insurance, pension, and sick leave plans), and social needs (a supportive working group). Of course, work is not the only part of people's lives. Outside difficulties such as illness or family problems may be working against an individual's progress.

The most motivated employees from an employer's viewpoint are probably those operating at the level of ego needs. They are willing to be different from the group, to take risks in order to achieve, and are responsive to praise and criticism. Some management practices that facilitate an employee's reaching this level and

working effectively in it are joint goal setting for future performance and frequent feedback on performance. Involvement in group decision-making and attention to the individual's career development ensure continued high performance. Motivational issues will be discussed again under Leadership and Decision-Making and The Supervisory Function.

COMMUNICATION

Communications are necessary for any team's functioning; therefore ways or processes through which they are achieved will have a large impact on efficiency, energy expended, quality of care provided, and satisfaction level of the team. Time is a major requirement for effective communication processes. That is, the team members need a set period of time, preferably daily, during which they can all share information, identify problems and issues, and give and receive feedback on their interactions. This can occur in the form of a *debriefing session* at the end of the day or at a specified time each day. The issues identified and worked through in this daily session can range from the discovery of a series of patients returning with sensitivities, to the auxiliaries' feelings that they are being ordered around and not appreciated by the team leader. Fifteen minutes set aside at the end of the day for debriefing could improve the effectiveness of most dental teams.

The manner in which a team discussion is led can determine the amount of information that is actually shared. For example, compare, "I did not see anything worth discussing occur today, did you?" with, "What did you observe about the way I handled Jimmy's fears this morning?" If you are the team leader there are several rules of thumb for getting group members to participate in a discussion:

1. Do not state your opinion first.
2. Ask an open-ended question that requires some thought, not one that can be answered by a "yes" or "no."

3. Wait for a response, even if it seems like an interminably long time.
4. Do not do a lot of the talking yourself; make your point once and then stop to give the others a chance.

Team members can be most facilitative of each other's growth and development on the job if they ask for and give each other feedback on their daily functions. The question, "What did you observe about the way I handled Jimmy's fears?" is a direct request for feedback. The kind of feedback designated here has two components: an objective observation of behavior and a subjective reaction to the observations. An auxiliary might respond that he/she had seen the dentist try to convince Jimmy to "take it like a man" and not be a "crybaby." Then the auxiliary would describe his/her feeling reaction. It might be something like, "I felt very close to you because that is just the way my father used to talk to my little brother;" or he/she might say, "I felt very sorry for Jimmy and wanted to tell him I understood his being frightened, that everybody was afraid sometimes." These are both specific feeling reactions to the dentist's behavior and avoid the global noninformative value judgment of "I thought it was good (or bad)." After either of the first two reactions, the dentist might ask, "Can any of you think of another way to deal with Jimmy?" The pros and cons of the alternatives can then be discussed along with supporting data. For example, one of the auxiliaries may have seen Jimmy interact with his father or mother and could report the technique he or she uses and the results; or the auxiliary may have tried something that was successful.

The discussion thus far may suggest that only children have significant enough problems during dental care procedures to warrant a team discussion. Such is clearly not the case. Fear of going to the dentist is widespread. It is the subject of many jokes and stories and the bane of most dental professional's existences in that it is the major cause of the reactions they receive on announcing "I work in a dental office." It is possible that careful discussions of patient management, with team members giving feedback to each other on their styles and skill development, could eventually change the image of dentistry.

A major issue in the communication between any two people or groups of people is the degree of openness that is considered acceptable. A particularly appropriate example for a dental office is telling someone that his/her breath smells. Generally people do not trust each other's intentions sufficiently. If I think you are telling me my breath smells because you have my best interests at heart and do not want me to offend patients, I will accept the feedback. If, on the other hand, I think that you wish me ill, do not like me, or talk about me behind my back, then I will be offended by your feedback. Trust is an element that must be carefully fostered and protected in any group. Its development requires the freedom to check out one's perceptions, to ask questions about motivation, and to share feelings, which are all part of being open. The conditions of trust and openness are interactive: trust is built through openness, and openness develops in a trusting environment. The team's task, then, is to constantly strive for more trust and openness, pushing the boundaries as far as they will go at any moment by being willing to take a risk.

Effective feedback tends to increase the trust level in the group. Feedback is more likely to be heard by and be useful to the person receiving it if it is:

1. Descriptive: tells what you saw and heard
2. Specific: not global, but concrete and detailed
3. Objective: nonjudgmental; not "good" or "bad" or "right" or "wrong"
4. Well-timed: close to the event, unless time is needed for calming down
5. Contracted for: the person says he/she

wants to hear the feedback

6. Owned: "This is my feedback and nobody else's; I cannot speak for anybody else"

7. Involves a personal risk: the giver puts himself/herself on the line by sharing his/her personal reactions and feelings; judgmental feedback puts the receiver on the line

8. Checked out: the giver makes sure the receiver understands what the giver means to say

Communication is difficult. There are more misunderstood or half-understood messages than there are complete understandings. The difficulty occurs because people assume that they have understood and that communication is easy. If you doubt this point, try checking out all of the communications you receive in a day. Not only are you likely to discover that your first perception of the message was at least partially inaccurate, either because you missed part or read in too much, but you will probably also be regarded as dimwitted for even suggesting that simple communications could go awry. The difficult can be described in terms of a filter system, such that each of us screens in and out those messages to which we are especially attuned. The content heard and understood vs. that screened out is determined by our own life experiences, knowledge, attitudes, values, and psychological makeup. For example, if I am a very religious person and you are sending messages about your negative attitudes toward religion, I may not hear those messages, especially if I like you and if it is also important to me to have my friends believe the way I do. "Hearing" in this sense could mean either not picking up the sound waves, not processing them mentally, or adding extenuating factors to the processing. The filters, then, are our perceptual system, which includes more than just sensory receptors. It includes mental processing of the information received.

PROBLEM-SOLVING

If it is true that a good communication process requires an amount of time to be set aside for that purpose alone, then it is doubly true of problem-solving. Many individuals have at least a moderate degree of difficulty in admitting that they even have a problem, particularly one that cannot be blamed on nature or other circumstances beyond their control, for example an interpersonal problem. It is easier to ignore or avoid problem areas than to confront them openly. There seems to be an underlying belief that to have problems is weak or wrong. It would benefit us greatly if we could change that belief to one that held the failure to acknowledge problems to be wrong, but the process of working to solve problems to be strong and right. The time most individuals are willing to work at solving a problem is when it has been festering for so long that the pain is very severe and potential solutions are blocked by layers of hurt feelings and resentments. Accepting that any group of people working together will have problems is the basic ingredient of an effective problem-solving process. Once that is achieved, there are many ways of finding solutions.

A second difficulty that groups often face in problem-solving is approaching solutions before the problem has been clearly defined. It is important to begin with a statement of the problem with which everyone can agree, in order to ensure that the whole team is really working on the same problem. Often the problem is stated as a solution, for example, "to synchronize our timing." It is not clear from this statement what is the real problem, and further analysis is prevented by a premature goal statement. The problem might be, "Each member of the team has a lot of lag time." Such a statement allows for an analysis of the problem to ascertain who has lag time, for instance, when, how do they feel about it, is money being lost because of it, and what procedures could be changed with what cost. The analysis phase in problem-solving includes data collection about the problem and determination of the ways in which it is a psychological (feelings and needs), sociological (attitudes and norms), economic (dollars and cents), and/or political (power and influence) problem. For example, the questions might be asked, "What negative feelings result from whom from this situation?" "Whose feelings are operating to keep this problem in place and what, specifically, are those feelings?" For the economic analysis, "What does it cost (us, society, the organization) in dollars and cents to have this problem?" Costs of a solution cannot be determined until a solution approach is clearly defined.

In one particular situation, a problem arose in the university dental clinic because intake procedures for all patients were standardized, and initial diagnosis was performed by persons other than those carrying out the treatment procedures. This turned out to be primarily a psychological problem, in that the long waiting time between diagnosis and treatment and the multiple contacts interfered with the patient's need to feel cared for and frequent desire for immediate treatment. It thwarted the dental student's need to determine the treatment plan that he/she had to carry out. Occasionally, it became an economic problem, in that when the student decided or discovered that the plan was wrong, time and money were lost through an incorrect beginning. Had the team decided to try to change the clinic admission procedures, political factors would have to have been considered. As it was, they decided to allow an extra fifteen minutes preplanning time for each new patient, to check the diagnosis against the patient's actual needs.

A thorough analysis of the problem facilitates solution finding. As added preparation for the hard work of deciding on a solution agreeable to all, a brainstorming session can be used. The process is one wherein each person says what outcome situation he/she would like to see "in the best of all possible worlds." No contradictions, objections, or presentations of barriers are allowed. The group just brainstorms their fantasies of an ideal solution. It is a helpful process because it builds solidarity within the group and promotes a creative solution. People are generally in more agreement about what they would like to see happen than about how to get there or what is possible.

The next step in problem-solving is the difficult one of suggesting alternative solutions. Each proposal must be fully explored before a final decision is made. The suggestions are tested for desirability of the outcome, likelihood of the outcome, and feasibility in terms of the motivation and capability of those involved. Known and potential barriers must be analyzed along with known and potential assets. When the solution approach is decided on, there remains the task of planning the steps of its implementation. A clear assignment of tasks, time frames, and check points for evaluation needs to be built in. The major work is done, but the goal can be lost through inadequate planning and follow-through. The following model summarizes the steps that are likely to be necessary for an adequate problem-solving process (see the box on p. 258).

The model, or part of it, is appropriate for any situation arising in a dental practice that requires more than mere fact-finding or improved communication between the people involved. For example, in a three-dentist group practice with a hygienist and several auxiliaries, patients have been raising objections to the practice of charging fees on the basis of time per visit, claiming that the dentists differ in their degree of speed and thoroughness. In a one dentist, one hygienist, one assistant, and one receptionist/bookkeeper practice, a certain group of patients is always breaking appointments. Either

---

PROBLEM-SOLVING MODEL

Step 1. Define the problem.
Step 2. Collect data about the problem (all known information, plus a list of information that must be obtained).
Step 3. Problem analysis: In what sense is this a(n)
    a. Psychological problem?
    b. Sociological problem?
    c. Economical problem?
    d. Political problem?
Step 4. Redefine the problem, if necessary.
Step 5. Brainstorm fantasy solutions, "in the best of all possible worlds."
Step 6. Suggest and test alternate solutions.
Step 7. Decide on a solution approach.
Step 8. Plan implementation of the solution.
Step 9. Plan to evaluate the solution.

---

of these situations lends itself to utilization of the problem-solving process by the whole team.

LEADERSHIP AND DECISION-MAKING

The decision-making mechanism adopted by team members is integrally related to the theory of management under which they are operating and to the leadership style of the team leader. At the far end of the Theory Y continuum, every member of the team would participate in every decision. The leader's style would be represented by the right-hand side of the diagram in Fig. 14-1. At the extreme Theory X end of the continuum, the leader would make all the decisions by himself/herself, the style represented by the left-hand side of the diagram.[5] There are numerous positions along the continuum, both with respect to the leader's style as indicated in the diagram and also with respect to the type of decision being made. Some decisions are more appropriately made by the team leader, either with or without first collecting data from the other team members, and other decisions are more appropriately made by the entire group.

Problems are most likely to occur when the team is not consciously aware of its decision-making process, operating instead in some haphazard fashion largely dependent on the mood of the leader. In that situation, people do not know how they can have influence, and unless the team is in perfect agreement or most members are extremely apathetic, dissatisfaction builds. A conscious awareness of how decisions are made opens the mechanism to review and possible change. The first decision a team must

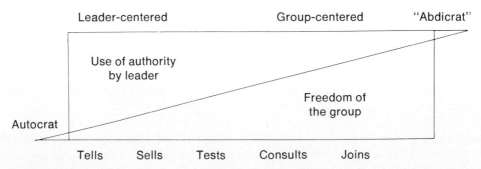

Fig. 14-1. Leadership continuum. (Developed by Tannenbaum, R.T., and Schmidt, W.H.: How to choose a leadership pattern, Harvard Business Rev., March/April 1958, p. 95.)

face in order to operate logically is, "How are we going to make decisions?"

Some criteria for determining how the decision should be made have been suggested by Vroom.[6]

1. The importance of the quality of the decision, for example, to what extent is there a "right" and "wrong" decision?
2. The extent to which the leader possesses sufficient information/expertise to make a high quality decision himself/herself.
3. The extent to which the problem is structured, for example, is it known what information is needed and where it is located?
4. The extent to which acceptance or commitment on the part of subordinates is critical to effective implementation of the decision.
5. The prior probability that the leader's autocratic decision will receive acceptance by subordinates.
6. The extent to which subordinates are motivated to attain the group or team goals explicitly involved in the particular problem, for example, quality patient care when working overtime is involved.
7. The extent to which subordinates are likely to be in conflict over preferred solutions.

The decision-making processes available include autocratic—decision-making by the leader; consultative—decision-making by the leader after sharing the problem and getting input from subordinates; and consensus—the group makes the decision.

In general, the decision is made in the manner that takes the least amount of time, providing certain rules are not violated. Some examples follow:

1. If a quality decision is required (one solution is more "right" than another) and either the leader does not possess enough information himself/herself or the problem is unstructured, then the leader cannot make the decision by himself/herself. In the dental office, the decision might be whether the amount of discomfort caused a patient by placement of a rubber dam is worth the advantage of a dry field. The dentist cannot make this decision alone because he/she does not know how much discomfort the patient experiences. In this case, he/she needs to consult both the patient and the auxiliary for the most complete information.

2. If the acceptance of the decision by subordinates is critical to effective implementation, and if it is not certain that an autocratic decision by the leader would receive acceptance, then he/she cannot make the decision alone. An example here would be whether sick days are actually time an employee can take off or for emergency use only. If employees do not agree to the latter interpretation, they can continue to use their sick days as vacation time without the team leader's knowing.

3. If the employees do not share the team goals involved in the decision, then the group cannot make the decision by itself or with the leader merely acting as a member. For example, auxiliaries who do not share in the gross profits of the office ought not to be allowed to decide the number of hours they will work.

4. If subordinates are likely to be in conflict over the appropriate decision, and if commitment is crucial for implementation, then group discussion is needed. For example, if the bookkeeper/receptionist and the dental assistant are both trained dental auxiliaries who were both hired for that role, and both strongly prefer assisting to bookkeeping, then the whole team needs to discuss and decide who will play what role when. An arbitrary decision by the dentist without hearing the feelings of those involved and having them hear each other's feeling would be likely to be rejected with the result of poor desk work and continuing conflict.

PROCESS OBSERVATION

Managing the group processes of communication, problem-solving, and decision-making is greatly facilitated by an understanding of group dynamics. Observing an ongoing group (for example, a dental team's planning or debriefing session) is a good way to build that understanding. Some of the dimensions to be observed include:

Participation: Did everyone participate? Did some participate more than others? Did certain individuals only participate on certain issues? Was an effort made to draw people out? Did a few people dominate? Did some people appear to be excluded from the discussion?

Leadership: Was there a designated leader, or did one emerge? Was leadership shared? What leadership functions were exhibited, for example, initiating ideas, polling the group, summarizing?

Roles: Who proposed tasks, goals, or action? Who gave information? Who expressed feelings? Who clarified issues or interpreted ideas? Who attempted to reconcile disagreements? Who facilitated the participation of others? Who blocked the group's movement for personal or unstated reasons? Who distracted the group from its task?

Communication: Did people appear to feel free to talk? Did they listen to others? Was there any interrupting or cutting people off? Did people take responsibility for their own statements by saying "I" and "me," rather than "they" or "one"?

Decision making: Were a lot of ideas suggested or only one? Was there thorough discussion before a decision was made? Was everyone's opinion considered in making the decision? Who influenced the decision? How?

Nonverbal: Who was looked at when speaking? Who was not? At whom did the speakers look? What postures were observable? What gestures? What facial expressions? What was the seating arrangement in the room? Did people move around at certain points in the discussion?

Climate: What was the group temperature: cool and distant, warm and friendly, or hot and heavy? What was the tempo: lively, slow? What was the emotional tone: supportive, hostile, depressed, anxious, resentful?

It is more difficult to observe an ongoing group process when one is involved in the content of the discussion. Providing an opportunity to observe without being involved greatly facilitates learning. The next skill level is to be able to participate in the discussion while still being aware of the process or dynamics of the group. The final skill is successful intervention into the process. "Successful" here means helping the group accomplish its task to the greater satisfaction of its members. The same general rules for giving feedback to individuals apply, particularly the one about being nonjudgmental. The group's "process" is not a concrete fact; that is, there is no objective truth about what was really going on. The dynamics of the group are understood, or the group is "processed" by having each individual present express his/her opinion about what was happening and share his/her feeling-level reactions. Examples of the latter are "I was bored," "I was angry at Dr. Williams for interrupting me twice," or, "I was depressed about our inability to stay on topic."

These same observation skills can be applied to the flow of the technical operation of the team and to interaction with the patient. An opportunity to observe another team's functioning may prove valuable. A word of caution, though—learning through observation requires a lot of concentration. The role itself can be somewhat trying, for example, standing quietly in a corner while others are active. There is a temptation to start a conversation with a fellow observer or to join the action in some way to avoid the tension of the observer role. What is needed is careful attention to overall flow and the details of what is occurring and an active attempt to form hypotheses, collect data to test them, and make connections to other experiences and knowledge bases.

ROLES AND ROLE NEGOTIATIONS

Team planning is particularly necessary in determining who is to do what. For example, what specific role functions are going to be performed by which member of the team? Since each individual needs to be aware, not only of his/her own functions, but of the functions of each other member of the team, one-to-one planning will not contribute to as much team efficiency as a team discussion of each other's roles.

The way in which people carry out their particular duties and functions is also an important aspect of their roles. For example, instruments can be put in a sterilizer quietly or noisily, gently or roughly, accompanied by singing or cursing. It is perfectly reasonable to have a personal reaction to the way others play out their roles. Sometimes there are even disagreements about the definition of a role. In these cases the process of role negotiation may be very appropriate.[2] Role negotiation consists of working out agreements among the members of the team regarding what activities each individual is to perform, such as what decisions they can make, what information they need to transmit to whom and how often, who can legitimately tell them what to do and under what circumstances. The process has four steps.

The first step of a role negotiation process consists of each member of the team writing down for every other member a list of those things they would like to see the other person: (1) do more or do better, (2) do less or stop doing, and (3) keep on doing the same way. These should be things that would enable the sender to do his/her job more effectively; for example, giving feedback on speed and quality of operations, sharing important information about the patient, explaining procedures to the patient, or on the other hand, disappearing for 5- to 10-minutes without notice.

In step two of the process each person makes a master list containing all the messages he/she received in each of the three categories. The

lists are printed large enough to be posted and seen by the other team members.

In the third stage members ask each other questions for clarification or additional information about the messages they have received. Defenses, rebuttals, and negotiations for changes are not allowed at this time. Nothing else is attempted until everyone fully understands all of his/her messages. The reasons for controlling the process at this point are to avoid misunderstandings and to avoid escalations of potential conflicts. Free expression of feelings at this point might lead to hostility, which would be hard to undo later.

Step four begins with persons marking on their own chart those behaviors that they are willing to, and feel they can, change. Each person marks on the charts of others those behaviors that he/she most desires to have changed. Thus the most negotiable issues become clear. The rule of thumb for step four is that a quid pro quo provides the motivation for lasting change. That is, changes in behavior are negotiated: "I will make the coffee if you will stop complaining whenever I take a coffee break," or, "I will stop yelling at you if you will keep the appointment book neater."

Whenever an agreement is reached between two or more persons, it is written down in order to give it the status of a formal contract. Participants to the agreement also discuss what incentives or sanctions they are willing to bring to bear on the agreement. The negotiating process continues until all agreements that participants are willing and able to make have been reached. Pressure is not exerted to go beyond what they think is possible. It is most helpful to have a behavioral science consultant available to guide the group through this process of role negotiation. He/she could be useful in orienting the group toward constructive processes, adding the importance of an outside-the-group presence to the agreements, and reorienting potentially harmful conflicts.

THE SUPERVISORY FUNCTION

There are usually two goals of supervision: monitoring of performance and staff development. Achieving a balance between the two often presents difficulties. It is easy to fall into a pattern of only helping or only policing. The substantive issues in supervision can be described as quantitative and qualitative. For purposes of this discussion, quantitative relates to *how often* and *when* the supevisor checks; qualitative refers to the quality of the intervention or supervision, not quality standards for the operations themselves. If the team has afforded itself a time for communicating about problems and issues, supervision becomes much easier. The time can be used to discuss what checkpoints are most appropriate. Most people have a fairly good idea of their strengths and weaknesses and, when consulted, will probably have an opinion about what aspects of their work they would appreciate having checked. With this kind of an agreement, the whole process of supervision becomes a pleasant one.

The supervisors can now feel free to observe, but what happens when he/she thinks the quality of work is not sufficient? The answer depends on whether or not the supervisee agrees with the supervisor. If the supervisee thinks the work is not up to par, then the process is one of helping him/her to do it more effectively in the future. If he/she feels it is adequate or better, then a process of confrontation must occur before any help can be negotiated. Both are complicated interpersonal processes. The remainder of this section will focus first on confrontation and then on help.

Confrontation is a type of communication in which differences are acknowledged and dealt with. What is confronted is the fact that there is a disagreement or a difference of opinion. It is also possible that one of the parties has been unaware of the difference in perspective. Confrontations need not be full of anger and resentment. They can, instead, be motivated by caring for the other person and for the relationship. Angry feelings tend to build when confrontations are avoided beyond people's tolerance for frustration. The first couple of times someone slams a door, for example, it is easy enough to say, "You know it really jars me when you slam the door. I jump every time. Could you please close it more quietly?" When the frustration engendered by the slamming has built up for weeks or months, it is more likely that if you say anything, you will scream rather than speak calmly, substituting anger for reasonableness.

The confronting of differences of opinion and perspective in order to resolve them or keep an open discussion going helps to maintain a good relationship. The energy required to start the discussion is an investment in the other person. It is unfortunate that the word confrontation has negative connotations because a confrontation can truly be an act of love and caring. Our cultural biases may tell us that differences imply inequality or other negatives, but different does not have to mean that one is better than the other or even that one is right and the other is wrong. Differences openly confronted can provide energy and stimulation.

The helping part of supervision also requires a certain amount of skill. The tendency in offering help is to give advice or to take over the situation before fully understanding what the problem is and why the person needs help. In order to help a person in such a way that he/she can do a better job in the future, it is necessary to understand his/her peception of the situation. One of the most useful things a helper can do is to ask open-ended questions.

For example a dentist supervising a hygienist may notice some calculus remaining in a patient's mouth. It is possible that the hygienist is aware of what he/she has missed but decided that with this particular patient and at this time it was better to avoid trauma and pain. The hygienist may be planning to have the patient come in for another appointment when he/

she can be more thorough. The dentist, in this situation, will not facilitate the hygienist's development without asking questions before evaluating. Appropriate questions might help the hygienist to evaluate whether he/she did, in fact, make the right decision.

The helping situation requires mutual trust, a recognition that helper and helpee are engaged in a joint exploration, and good listening on both sides, but particularly on the part of the helper. Disparaging or making light of the problem by the helper may cause the helpee to feel inferior or to lose trust. Defensiveness on the part of the helpee requires patience from the helper, not added pressure.

The helpee has a part in the process too, such as giving the helper feedback on what is helpful, not trying to take the focus away from him/herself, not just looking for sympathy, not responding in terms of "yes, but," but being ready to accept help and change behavior when it is appropriate and necessary.

Confrontation and helping are two components whenever there is a need felt on someone's part (supervisor, employee, patient) for an employee to do something differently.

CONFLICT UTILIZATION

"Conflict management" was a potential heading for this section. "Utilization" was chosen because it highlights the positive effects of openly discussing different viewpoints. For example, open articulation of opinion forces one to think, thereby increasing understanding of one's own position. Further, a diversity of viewpoints leads to increased innovativeness and an increase in motivation and energy in the group or organization.

Walton's model for third party intervention in a two party conflict situation includes many helpful ideas and will be the basis of much of what follows.[7] The discussion of a conflict is called a confrontation. The purposes of a confrontation can vary; the purpose might be to diagnose the conflict, to attempt to de-escalate the conflict, to increase the authenticity in the relationship, or to increase commitment to improve the relationship. The phasing of the discussion moves from substantive issues to emotional issues and back, depending on the level of emotion and the degree to which substantive issues can be worked. The pair might begin by talking about policies and practices, resources, role conceptions, or role relationships. The process for these substantive issues is one of problem-solving. When blocks become apparent (when, for example there is no further progress being made), the third party suggests that the principals discuss their feelings toward each other. Underlying feelings may include any number of emotions, such as, anger, fear, scorn, resentment, distrust, rejection. Misperceptions about feelings often exist and are seldom discussed. A restructuring of perceptions and working through of feelings is likely to liberate energy for further work on substantive issues.

The model for confrontations suggests that a number of factors be in balance between the two parties, such as position or status in the organization, articulateness, ability to express feelings, and having allies or supporters in the group or organization. Total situational power can be in balance, even if a "boss" and subordinates are confronting each other. For example, the subordinate may have a higher degree of verbal ability, or the meeting may take place in his/her territory (office), or he/she may be paired with an ally during the meeting.

Motivation to work out the issues must be nearly equal between the two parties as well as their distance from and trust in the consultant. In other words, the third party must either be a neutral but respected figure to both or be a close friend of both parties. A consultant who is close to one person and does not know the other may create an imbalance. Minimum requirements for the consultant's role are that both parties agree to the person's playing that role and feel they can trust him/her.

The actual functioning of the third party is similar to that of an orchestra conductor but is more subtle. Ideally, he/she functions as an unobtrusive facilitator making suggestions to each of the principals but always encouraging them to talk directly to each other and not to the consultant. Interventions are concerned with getting the information out about the substantive matters, keeping both parties talking about the issues, or balancing the amount of talking being done so that each has equal time. The consultant may intervene to present his/her diagnosis of the conflict, to repeat what has been said as a way of clarifying the messages, or to give feedback to the principals. The consultant might also ask for feedback, particularly as to whether the clients are finding him/her helpful. Ending the meeting at an appropriate and agreed-on point is part of the third party's responsibility. It is almost always necessary to plan another meeting. Even if it appears that all of these issues have been resolved, knowing that there is some checkpoint in the future will strengthen the new agreements. The discussion often will be a first step and is best understood that way; utilizing conflict is an ongoing process.

A confrontation meeting might be used in a situation where two of the dentists in a group practice have some ongoing disagreements about use of office space, hours of covering the practice for each other, and fee schedules. In addition, there are some underlying feelings of distrust and resentment of unclear origin. Both dentists like, trust, and talk to the hygienist about their mutual difficulties. They feel that he/she understands their positions but is impartial. At some point, several hours of either the working day or after-hours time could be scheduled for the purpose of airing all the differences of opinion between the two with the help of the hygienist. He/she might watch, for example, to see that each has an equal amount of talking time, that one does not overpower the other, that they do not pile on issue after issue without attempting to problem-solve any one of them, and that they do not engage in unsupported assertions or labeling of each other.

The example of the hygienist as consultant is used here purposefully because the third party should not be an authority figure but merely a facilitator. If the dentist plays this role between two employees, there is a danger that they will look to him/her for a solution, and the dentist will have to make it clear that he/she is there to help them work out their own problems, not to tell them what to do.

The confrontation meeting is appropriate whenever there is an ongoing conflict between two persons who are willing to talk about it and whenever a third neutral person is available to help them.

TEAM MEMBERSHIP GUIDELINES

The team leader cannot be held solely responsible for the team's success or failure since this responsibility is, by definition, shared. There are several requirements necessary to be an effective group member. Most important is a willingness to participate, to open up and share what is on your mind. Team members must also listen to each other, not just in a pro forma way, but actively for understanding. These first two guidelines have even more impact when there are disagreements among team members. The most effective way to deal with differences in perceptions, values, and opinions is to talk them through.

A spirit of cooperation is also very helpful. There is such a thing as "healthy competition," for example, trying to do something better than someone else in the interest of better overall team performance. But when the attempt is to look good or make the other person look bad, it can become destructive competitiveness.

Another guideline is to attempt to solve problems rather than to establish blame. Helping each other and providing support toward doing a better job are effective team behaviors. Giving and being willing to accept feedback is an important component of that process. Finally, inclusion of all team members is necessary for good team performance. Exclusiveness or scapegoating one or more members can decrease overall productivity.

TEAM BUILDING

All of the processes described in this chapter are potential "team builders." That is, joint decision-making, problem-solving, and working through conflicts are likely to strengthen mutual commitment as well as individual skills. What is meant by team building, then, is both the development of the individual team members and the improvement of their interdependent functioning.

When a new member joins a team, it might be appropriate to add some specific team-building exercises or processes to the usual team meeting. These might include each member sharing background information about himself/herself, sharing favorite activities, places to go on vacation, or sharing values like "the person I most admire" or "what I want most out of life." Values discussed might also be work-related, such as "the most important thing to me about dentistry is. . . , or, "the reason I chose dentistry as a field is. . . ." Exploring these questions in a group can often build or add to career commitment. If doubts about the choice are shared, that too builds support and understanding among team members and could suggest areas where people may need help in the future.

SUMMARY

This chapter has focused on the individual as a member of a team. Theories of management derived from social science literature formed the foundation for many of the guidelines presented. Whether we are talking about a private dental office, a community health center, or a major corporation, people function in similar ways. Successful team management requires the effective utilization of a number of ongoing interpersonal and group processes, such as communication, problem-solving, decision-making, role negotiation, supervision, and conflict resolution.

Whether one is the manager or the managed, it is important to practice personal skills of observation of interpersonal and group interaction, giving personal feedback, confrontation, and helping. A dental office is a small organization, yet few dentists or dental hygienists have had formal education in management. This chapter has provided a few helpful suggestions on how to manage and participate in an organization. The preceding team membership guidelines should be particularly useful for members of the dental team. It is hoped that this overview proves helpful for dentists, dental hygienists, and educators in furthering their understanding of the human aspects of team management.

REFERENCES

1. Harlow, H.F.: Mice, monkeys, men and motives, Psychol. Rev. **60**:23, 1953.
2. Harrison, R.: Role negotiation: a tough minded approach to team development. In Burke, W., and Hornstein, H.A., editors: The social technology of organization development, Fairfax, VA, 1972, NTL Learning Resources Corporation, Inc.
3. Maslow, A.H.: Motivation and personality, New York, 1954, Harper & Row, Publishers, Inc.
4. McGregor, D.: The human side of enterprise, New York, 1960, McGraw-Hill Book Co.
5. Tannenbaum, R.T., and Schmidt, W.H.: How to choose a leadership pattern, Harvard Business Rev., March/April 1958, p. 95.
6. Vroom, V.H.: A new look at managerial decision making, Organizational Dynamics, Spring 1973, p. 66.
7. Walton, R.E.: Interpersonal peacemaking: confrontation and third party consultation, Reading, MA, 1969, Addison-Wesley Publishing Co., Inc.
8. White, R.W.: Motivation reconsidered: the concept of competence, Psychol. Rev. **66**:297, 1959.

CHAPTER 15

Ethical Issues in Dental Care

The practice of dentistry is governed by rules of conduct that are stated in law. In the United States these laws are generally assembled in the dental practice acts of each state. These acts specifically define the practice of dentistry and describe the duties that may be performed by dental auxiliaries. Federal laws may also apply to dentistry, such as in the regulation of controlled substances or of advertising.

A more subtle regulation of conduct, however, lies in the ethics of a profession. Whereas laws are written and generally clearly defined, ethical rules of conduct are not always so clear. Laws are enforced by an arm of government, but ethical rules are generally only weakly enforced by professional societies such as the American Dental Association and the American Dental Hygienists' Association.

This chapter will discuss some of the concepts of bioethics that form the foundation for the healing professions. Several case studies will be presented and a framework for ethical decision making will be developed.

PROFESSIONAL RESPONSIBILITY

Dentistry is treated by society as a learned profession, and as such, dental professionals have a responsibility to society. Contemporary professions arose during the Middle Ages and are represented by fields such as medicine, law, and the ministry. All professionals have four common requirements: (1) a distinct body of knowledge generally requiring education beyond the usual level, (2) a component of service to society, (3) the right and responsibility to be self-governing, and (4) a code of ethics.

The special status that society confers upon professionals requires professionals to behave in an ethical manner. The professions such as dentistry determine their own standards for licensure: they control the numbers of entering professionals, the length and conditions of education, the distribution of services, and to a great extent the cost of services. It is society's belief that professionals place the welfare of the patient above their own welfare, which supports the independence of the professions in a regulated society. It is this covenant with society that requires professionals to practice in an ethical manner if society is to continue to accord these special privileges. Although the public-at-large is not aware of the details of the professional code of ethics of the American Dental Association or the American Dental Hygienists' Association, it does expect that the professionals will behave in an ethical manner. In a 1981 Gallup Poll the public ranked the dental profession third among all professions in respect to ethical behavior.

Each of us establishes our own set of ethical standards. These standards may be higher or lower than those set by our respective professional groups. These standards are determined by our value and belief systems and are rarely at a conscious level. When we are confronted by an ethical question or dilemma, we may draw upon our belief system to find an answer. This chapter is designed to help dental professionals with those difficult questions.

ETHICAL PRINCIPLES

Ethics is the part of philosophy that deals with moral conduct and judgment. In order to provide a common basis for ethical reasoning, certain principles and terms will be discussed in this chapter. There are several principles that health care professionals must be aware of in the practice of their profession. Knowing the names of these principles will not make us more ethical, but understanding the basis for certain behaviors may help us make more carefully reasoned decisions when confronted with ethical dilemmas. Although many ethical principles can be traced to early Greek physicians and philosophers, they appear in many early Eastern philosophies too. The major principles that will be discussed in this chapter are: to do no harm (nonmaleficence), to do good (beneficence), autonomy, justice, veracity or truthfulness, and confidentiality.

To do no harm or nonmaleficence is generally attributed to Hippocrates and is considered to be the foundation of social morality.[5] It is clear that although dental care professionals support this principle in theory they are at times guilty of transgressions. *Iatrogenic disease* is the name we give to doctor-induced illness, and all of us in the dental field have seen overhanging restorations cause periodontal disease or failure to sterilize instruments cause an infection. One example of a typical dilemma is whether a dental hygienist should use instruments that have not been adequately sterilized if the dentist employer tells the hygienist that it is not necessary to sterilize. Since the dentist is ultimately responsible, is it the hygienist's concern? Each of us is responsible for our own actions. If we knowingly do harm to our patients, excusing our acts because *someone else* is legally responsible, we have still behaved in an unethical manner. The decision is not an easy one, since refusing to use the instruments might cost the hygienist his/her job, but clearly there is a "right" answer

in this case if we follow the ethical principle of *do no harm.*

To do good or beneficence, a concept also traced to Hippocrates, is required of all health care providers.[6] It should be the role of dentists and dental hygienists to benefit patients, as well as not to inflict harm. The expectation of the patient is that the care provider will initiate action that will benefit him/her and that there is an agreement between the doctor and the patient that some good will occur. It is not enough to say "Well, it won't hurt the patient if I do this procedure." What is important is: Will it help the patient? A dentist who feels pressured to produce more work in order to meet expenses might be tempted to recommend replacing a basically sound restoration in a patient who needs no work, using the argument that "it won't hurt the patient to have the filling replaced, and it would probably have to be done some time in the future anyway." The question is whether it will do the patient any good, and certainly when examined closely there would be a number of "harms" to the patient—unnecessary anesthesia, potential loss of some sound tooth structure, extra time in the chair, and of course paying for something that is unnecessary.

Autonomy is a principle that dictates that health care professionals respect the patients' right to make decisions concerning their own treatment.[5] Informed consent is an essential component of a patient's right to autonomy. This consent requires that the following four elements be present:

1. Disclosure of appropriate information including risks and benefits involved in treatment, consequences of nontreatment, alternative treatments when applicable
2. Comprehension of the information by the patient
3. Voluntary consent
4. Competence to consent[5]

Dentists sometimes attempt to direct a patient toward a particular mode of treatment by stressing certain advantages and not mentioning disadvantages. The dentists may believe that it is in the "best interest" of the patient to have the treatment, but it is a breach of ethics to mislead or misinform patients. In addition, it may well become a legal issue. Dentists are often trained in a paternalistic setting, and therefore they practice in a paternalistic way after graduation from dental school. Paternalism is defined by the Oxford English Dictionary as the principle of government as by a father, that is, a dictatorial "father knows best" attitude. Paternalism in health care can take the form of withholding information, restricting choices, or making the choices for the patient. Paternalism may also be expressed in laws that protect people from themselves rather than protect people from other people, as in most laws. An example might be a law requiring motorcyclists to wear crash helmets. This public health law is designed to protect those cyclists who might choose to ride without helmets. Another example is the law mandating fluoridation of community water supplies. This law protects those people who might not avail themselves of self-administered fluoride drops or tablets. We may be able to justify paternalistic laws as being in the public 's interest, but we should recognize that these laws limit the rights of a segment of the public because we judge that it is in their "best interest."

Justice is often described as fairness or equal treatment, giving to each his right or due. An oath often attributed to the Jewish physician Maimonides states: "Preserve the strength of my body and of my soul that they ever be ready to cheerfully help and support rich and poor, good and bad, enemy as well as friend. In the sufferer let me see only the human being."[6] In providing dental care it is difficult to distribute services to all who are needy, but it should be the concern of health care professionals to see to it that as even a distribution as possible occurs.

Dentists often complain that they cannot treat Medicaid patients because the fees are too low or that the patients break too many appointments or they cannot treat the mentally retarded because it takes too long. The question still must be answered, Who will treat the poor and needy since only dental professionals can provide dental care?

Truthfulness or *veracity* is an ethical principle that one would expect to go unquestioned, yet many health care professionals practice in a less than truthful way.[5] Lying fails to show respect for persons and their autonomy, violates explicit agreements, and threatens relationships based on trust. As discussed above, the dentist may feel that it would be better if the patient took a certain course of action and therefore manipulates the information that is given to the patient. Whatever the reason, the relationship will ultimately suffer and the dentist will be guilty of transgressing on a major ethical principle.

Another example of the failure to be truthful relates to the use of placebos. The following case study suggests a possible scenario.

Case study. A middle-aged patient who has been treated at Dr. Jones' office for a number of years complains of a pain in her upper molar area. When Dr. Jones reviews the patient record, he notices that Mrs. Carter has complained of pain numerous times over the past several years. In most cases the record indicates that nothing substantive was found. After a detailed clinical examination and radiographs, Dr. Jones can find nothing wrong. He tells Mrs. Carter that it may be a sinus problem but if the pain persists she should return next week. Mrs. Carter returns still complaining of the pain. She is a very noisy person and irritates most of the office staff. Since Dr. Jones can find nothing wrong, he decides to provide a "nontreatment" or placebo. He writes her a prescription for a sugar pill, tells her that it will reduce the pain, and that he will adjust her bite because this is probably the problem. He pretends to grind her teeth, but merely runs the high-speed drill without touching her teeth. Mrs. Carter leaves "feeling better" and calls the next day to say that the pain has gone away. Dr. Jones tells his staff that she is just a faker and his nontreatment clearly shows she had no real problem.

The use of placebos can be argued against both scientifically and morally. Studies indicate that 30% to 40% of persons with pain of organic origin may show an analgesic response to a placebo. There is little evidence to suggest that pain relieved by a placebo is not real.[10] From an ethical point of view, the use of placebos transgresses the principle of veracity.

Confidentiality is the last ethical principle that we will discuss in this chapter. It is a principle that can be traced to the Hippocratic oath[4] and that exists today in the International Code of Medical Ethics, the Principles of Ethics of the American Dental Association, the American Dental Hygienists' Association, and the American Dental Assistants' Association. The patient has the right to expect that all communications and records pertaining to his/her care will be treated as confidential. It is very natural to want to gossip about a patient, particularly if it is someone famous or possibly a neighbor, but to do so would break a bond of trust between the dental professional and the patient. Another case where confidentiality might be broken is when a dental hygienist uses another patient as an example, such as "Look, Connie, you really should do a better job with your flossing. My last patient has a terrible case of gingivitis, lots of bleeding, bad breath, and she may lose some of her teeth." At this point your patient might wonder, "Will she use me as an example with her next patient? I don't want everyone to know I have gingivitis." With the exception of required reportable diseases and extreme cases where "disclosure is necessary to avert danger to others," confidentiality must be maintained.[4]

ETHICAL REASONING IN DECISION-MAKING

The principles outlined above can be used as tools to solve our ethical dilemmas. Ethicists cannot give us answers, only insight into different ways of looking at issues or words of caution about potential moral traps. Decision-making on ethical issues is similar to any decision-mak-

ing,[7] and the model provided by Harron and others[9] may be useful.

1. *Analyzing:* dividing a problem into its leading alternatives
2. *Weighing:* assessing the strengths and weaknesses of alternatives by balancing one against the other
3. *Justifying:* providing a compelling and sufficient moral reason that appeals to an established moral principle, such as to tell the truth
4. *Choosing:* selecting one or more of the alternatives for which some justification can be made
5. *Evaluating:* reexamining the choices and their justifications based on one's exposure to other similar moral cases

In the following case studies let us consider whether this model can assist in reaching the best decisions.

Case study. Ms. Johnson, a dental hygienist, has been working in a large group practice for 2 weeks and has been very happy in the new job. Her present patient, Susan Carter, is a 16-year-old with no history of caries. Ms. Johnson has just completed a prophylaxis and had bitewing radiographs made. Dr. Smith enters the operatory, completes the clinical examination, and finds no caries or gingival problems. As he leaves the operatory he asks Ms. Johnson if she has done a topical fluoride treatment. Ms. Johnson responds that since the patient has never had any caries, is presently caries free, and lives in a fluoridated community, she felt that a fluoride treatment was unnecessary. Dr. Smith states that it is office policy that all patients under age 21 routinely receive topical fluoride treatments. Ms. Johnson says that she knows the policy and that she had just applied fluoride to the patient's two younger siblings, also caries free, but that the patient's mother had told her that they were having some difficult financial problems and could she please see to it that only necessary work was done. Mrs. Carter's bill already totals $205 for the examinations, prophylaxes, and bitewing radiographs for the three children and the fluoride treatments for Susan's two siblings. The fluoride treatment for Susan would add $20 more to the bill. Dr. Smith states that he is the dentist and he knows best. He further states that if Ms. Johnson wants to keep her job she had better take a more positive attitude toward office policy.

Ms. Johnson has a dilemma—should she "follow orders" and do the topical fluoride treatment that she believes is unnecessary, or should she follow her own conscience and not do the treatment?

Looking at the model for decision-making, we should begin by *analyzing*. What are the alternatives? 1. Do the fluoride treatment. 2. Refuse to do the treatment. 3. Tell Mrs. Carter that the treatment is probably not necessary for Susan but that it is office policy and it would be easier on her (Ms. Johnson) if Mrs. Carter would just tell the receptionist that she had to leave right away because she was already late and that she would make another appointment later for the fluoride. There are probably other alternatives. Try to think of a few.

Weighing is the next step. What are the strengths and weaknesses of each alternative? Doing the treatment could be considered "doing harm" because if it lacks any benefit or has very little benefit to Susan, the $20 it costs Mrs. Carter is a form of harm. In this case Mrs. Carter has specifically asked that only important work be done, and Ms. Johnson would be breaking faith if she did the treatment when she believed it would not be beneficial. However, doing the treatment would put her in the good graces of Dr. Smith, and Ms. Johnson likes her job. Alternative 2, refusing to do the treatment, could get her fired or at least cause problems with Dr. Smith. She might not get much support from others in the practice because this is not an absolutely clear professional decision, and there are probably some members of the profession who would support doing a topical fluoride treatment. Alternative 3 would seem to be the easiest because it would save Mrs. Carter the $20 without Mrs. Johnson having to directly confront Dr. Smith. It might, however, cause Mrs. Carter to lose faith in the practice and possibly make her question the necessity of the fluoride treatments for her other two children and past fluoride treatments. It would also place Mrs. Carter in the position of having to tell a lie.

Justifying requires that we find a compelling moral reason for each decision. Although there may be some reasons for "following office policy," (for example, it is generally helpful to have office policies so that patients are treated uniformly and employees will know what to do in most situations), there appears, in this case, to be no strong moral reason for alternative 1—doing the treatment. Alternative 2 could be justified on the basis of "doing no harm." Alternative 3 could also be justified on the basis of "doing no harm" and possibly "doing good" because Mrs. Carter would have some new information to aid her in making future decisions about topical fluoride treatments. The negative side of the alternative is that it encourages Mrs. Carter to lie in order to help Ms. Johnson and causes Mrs. Carter to distrust Dr. Smith.

Choosing means selecting one of the alternatives and giving your justification *or* finding another alternative that you can justify.

Evaluating becomes easier as you face more and more ethical dilemmas because you will improve your decision-making powers and will have more experience to draw from. It is important to discuss your dilemmas with others and draw upon their experiences. You will find that you are not alone in these dilemmas and that many of your colleagues will have faced similar dilemmas in their professional lives. Making a decision is often difficult, but indecision itself is a decision and just "going along" with something may not lead to the outcome you really want. You must make the best decision that you can at the time.

Case study. A young man comes to the office of a dentist and asks to have a tooth "pulled" because of a toothache. After taking a radiograph and conducting a clinical examination, the dentist determines that there is a small carious lesion in the lower first molar. A careful history of the type and intensity of the pain clearly supports the diagnosis of an early carious lesion on the occlusal surface penetrating the enamel but with only minimum penetration into the dentin. The dentist explains to the patient that the tooth can easily be restored with a silver filling. The patient, however, wants the tooth extracted because he "had a tooth filled once and the drilling drove him crazy with pain." He insists that the dentist pull the tooth.

The dentist explains that the tooth is a very important one because it performs 60% of the chewing on that side of the mouth. If it is lost, the other teeth around it will shift and cause other problems. A bridge or partial denture might be needed, and this will be costly and require several visits. The filling will take about a half an hour, and after the injection of a local anesthetic there should be no pain. The cost of the filling will be $40.00, the same price as an extraction. The patient is restless throughout the talk and persists in his desire for an extraction.

What should the dentist do? Does patient autonomy override the dentist's feelings about "good dentistry"? Can a patient dictate treatment or should the professional make the decision?[3]

Use the decision-making process to reach a decision. In this case try to develop as many alternatives as possible—whether to extract the tooth or not. For instance, the dentist might convince the patient to have a temporary filling placed in order to sedate the tooth and allow the patient to make the decision when he is not in pain. There are often more alternatives than immediately come to mind.

CODES OF ETHICS

As stated previously, a fundamental requirement for the status of profession is a formal code of ethics. All professional organizations have a published code to which members of the profession are expected to adhere. These codes have been developed over long periods of time and reflect the customs and beliefs of current members of the profession and provide a historical link with the past. Some modern codes can trace their origins to statements made by Hippocrates or Hammurabi long before the birth of Christ. Professional codes often state basic moral or ethical principles such as *not doing harm* or *injustice*, but in essence these codes provide a pattern of behavior for how professionals should

behave toward other professionals—a code of etiquette. In dentistry the code is the American Dental Association's Principles of Ethics and Code of Professional Conduct.[1] This code contains five major sections:

1. Service to the public and quality of care
2. Education
3. Government of a profession
4. Research and development
5. Professional announcement

Sections 2, 3, and 4 each consist of one paragraph defining the principle, for example, "Section 3, Government of a Profession—Every profession owes society the responsibility to regulate itself. Such regulation is achieved largely through the influence of professional societies. All dentists, therefore, have the dual obligation of making themselves a part of a professional society and of observing its rules of ethics." In addition, section 4 has two brief paragraphs on inventions, patients, and copyrights. Sections 1 and 5 are much longer and consist of detailed codes of conduct related to each principle, such as statements on patient selection, patient records, community service, emergency service, consultation and referral, use of auxiliary personnel, and justifiable criticism. Some of these items of conduct relate to specific moral principles, such as the statement "While dentists, in serving the public, may exercise reasonable discretion in selecting patients for their practices, dentists shall not refuse to accept patients into their practice or deny dental service to patients because of the patient's race, creed, color, sex, or national origin," which can be attributed to the principle of *justice*. Some statements relate laws to cultural norms of the profession, such as "Use of Auxiliaries". Dentists shall be obliged to protect the health of their patients by only assigning to qualified auxiliaries those duties that can be legally delegated. Dentists shall be further obliged to prescribe and supervise the work of all auxiliary personnel working under their direction and control. Other statements, however, are more closely related to cultural norms of the profession, which tend to restrict competition, such as "Dentists who choose to announce specialization should use 'specialist in' or 'practice limited to' and shall limit their practice exclusively to the announced special area(s) of dental practice, provided at the time of announcement such dentists have met in each approved specialty for which they announce the existing educational requirements and standards set forth by the American Dental Association."[1]

The statements that clearly relate to universal moral or ethical principles are likely to remain in the code over time, whereas the more limited cultural norms are likely to change as society changes. A case in point relates to the statement restricting advertising that appeared in the code until 1979.

Case study. *Ethics vs. Professional Cultural Norms.* The following case illustrates that professional codes of ethics do not necessarily espouse true ethical principles. Prior to 1977, professionals such as lawyers, physicians, dentists, and pharmacists were constrained from advertising by the code of ethics of their professional societies. The then-current 1962 American Dental Association's Principles of Ethics and Code of Professional Conduct specifically stated: "The dentist has the obligation of advancing a reputation for fidelity, judgment, and skill solely through professional services to patients and to society. The use of advertising in any form to solicit patients is inconsistent with this obligation." State dental society bylaws very clearly spelled out the size and types of signs dentists could have outside their offices and the type of professional announcements dentists could send.

In the mid-1970s, as the consumer movement gathered strength, court cases encouraging competition appeared. In the 1975 *Goldfarb vs. Virginia State Bar* case, the court ruled that "learned" professions, including dentistry, were subject to the federal antitrust laws. Subsequently a 1976 ruling, *Virginia State Board of Pharmacy vs. Virginia Citizens Consumer Council*, permitted pharmacists to advertise prescription drug prices. Finally, in 1977, in the case of *Bates and O'Steen vs. State Bar of Arizona*, the U.S. Supreme Court ruled that the legal profession's restriction on advertising by its members was in restraint of trade. In January 1977

the Federal Trade Commission (FTC), a regulatory arm of the federal government, issued a complaint against the American Dental Association and several of its constituent societies alleging violation of antitrust laws and section 5 of the FTC Act, which prohibits "unfair methods of competition in commerce and unfair or deceptive acts or practices in commerce." Some specific allegations were that restrictions on advertising resulted in:

1. Prices of dental services being stabilized or fixed
2. Competition among dentists in the provision of services being hindered, restrained, and frustrated
3. Consumers of dental services being deprived of information pertinent to the selection of a dentist and of the benefits of competition
4. Dentists being restrained in their ability to compete and make dental services readily and fully available to consumers
5. Development of innovative systems for the delivery of dental services being hindered and restrained[11]

In 1979 the ADA entered into a consent decree with the FTC to allow dentists to advertise. The ADA revised its Principles of Ethics and Code of Professional Conduct to read: "Although any dentist may advertise, no dentist shall advertise or solicit patients in any way that would be false or misleading in any material respect." Thus in 1979 the century-old restriction on advertising by professionals was ended. The courts did hold that professional associations could regulate advertising under their codes of ethics if they had a *reasonable* basis to believe that the advertising was false or misleading in a material respect.[2]

In the wake of the Supreme Court ruling and the FTC complaint, state dental practice acts were changed and restrictions on advertising were removed. An example is the 1981 amended Massachusetts Dental Practice Act, which states: "Unfair, misleading, deceptive and fraudulent advertising is prohibited. A dentist may advertise truthful and accurate information pertaining to dental services."[8]

Professional Codes of Ethics serve a useful purpose in that they assemble in a single document many of the cultural norms of a profession as well as promote some of the universally held principles of biomedical ethics. The professions must be careful, however, that they continue to remember that a professional is one who places the interests of the patient above his/her own.

Professions exist only at the pleasure of society; if professions fail to promote the good of society, they will cease to exist since society can regulate and thus limit the autonomy of professions at will.

IN CONCLUSION

Dental care professionals have an obligation to practice in an ethical manner. Based on our individual backgrounds we have internalized values and standards by which we behave. Although this chapter has not tried to teach you to be ethical, it has attempted to present some ethical principles that health care practitioners over the past centuries have held to be important and to provide you with a method for finding answers to ethical dilemmas. When we are faced with an ethical dilemma, a debate goes on in our heads. The more puzzling the question, the longer the debate. It is important that this debate occur. For example, a patient needs a three-unit bridge to replace a missing upper first molar tooth. The patient has dental insurance that will pay 50% of the cost of the bridge, but the insurance runs out next week when the patient loses his job. The patient asks you to file for the bridge as if it were completed this week and then do the work, thus saving the patient $750.00. The patient states that he cannot afford to pay the entire fee and therefore could not have the work done unless the insurance payed half.

At first you are tempted to say yes. An inner debate begins: "It would mean a $1500 case and I can certainly use the money." A second voice says, "It's unethical. It would mean lying on the insurance form." The first voice says, "The patient needs the bridge, so I would be doing a good service." You think again, "Am I going to turn into the kind of dentist I'm always complaining about, the kind I'd like to see thrown out of the profession?" A resounding "NO" ends the debate. You tell the patient that you cannot do what he asks, but you would be happy to do the bridge and could help him work out a plan to budget the costs over time. You also mention that, although the bridge should be done soon, a short delay until he gets dental coverage again would probably not be too harmful. You feel good about the decision and realize that the temptations are always there, but each time it seems to get a little easier to resist.

REFERENCES

1. American Dental Association Principles of Ethics and Code of Professional Conduct, J. Am. Dent. Assoc., 109:81, July 1984.
2. AMA v. FTC, 636 F. 2nd 443 (2nd Cir. 1980).
3. Aronoff, G.M.: Evaluation and treatment of chronic pain, Urban & Schwarzenberg, Inc., Baltimore/Munich, 1985.
4. Beauchamp, T.L., and Walters, L.: Contemporary issues in bioethics, Belmont, CA, 1978, Wadsworth Publishing Co.
5. Beauchamp, T.L., and Childress, J.F.: Principles of biomedical ethics, New York, 1983, Oxford University Press, Inc.
6. Bok, Sissela: The tools of bioethics. In Reiser, S.J., Dyck, A.J., and Curran, W.J., editors: Ethics in medicine, Cambridge, MA, 1977, The MIT Press.
7. Brody, H.: Ethical decisions in medicine, Boston, 1981, Little, Brown & Co., Inc.
8. Commonwealth of Massachusetts, Revision of 234 CMR 200, Vol. 10, p. 312, May 29, 1981.
9. Harron, F., Burnside, J., and Beauchamp, T.L.: Health and human values, New Haven, CT 1983, Yale University Press.
10. Stimmel, B.: Pain, analgesia, and addiction: the pharmalogical treatment of pain, New York, NY, 1983, Raven Press.
11. Stock, F.: Professional advertising, Am. J. Public Health 68:1207, 1978.

Index

A

AADS; *see* American Association of Dental Schools

Accreditation, Southern Association of Schools', 173-174

Acid etching technique of pit and fissure sealants, 130-132

Acidulated phosphate fluoride (APF), 134-135, 233

Action for Children's Television, 173

Actualization phase of implementation of health programs, 223

Actuarial analytical tools for insurance, 97

Acyclovir, 35

ADA; *see* American Dental Association

ADAA; *see* American Dental Assistants' Association

ADAMHA; *see* Alcohol, Drug Abuse and Mental Health Administration

ADHA; *see* American Dental Hygienists' Association

Administrative research, 235

Administrator and geriatric dental program, 82-83

Adrenergic inhibitors, 28

Advertising, profession of dentistry and, 36, 63, 91, 92, 272

Advisory dentist in nursing facilities, 81

AFDC; *see* Aid to Families with Dependent Children

Agent factors, epidemiology of dental disease and, 115

Aging
  changes in, elderly and, 73-74
  of U.S. population, 70-71
  utilization of health services and, 60

Aid to Families with Dependent Children (AFDC), 7, 88

AIDS-related complex (ARC), 34

Alabama Dental Association, 174

Alabama Nutrition Council, 174

Alcohol, Drug Abuse and Mental Health Administration (ADAMHA), 6

Allowances, maximum, in insurance, 19

Alzheimer's disease, 73, 77, 79-80

American Academy of Pediatrics, fluoride supplementation recommendations of, 127-128

American Association
  of Dental Examiners, 46, 47
  of Dental Schools (AADS), 46, 47
  of Public Health Dentists, Research Committee of, 172
  of Retired Persons, 17

American Board of Dental Public Health, 3

American Cancer Society, 159

American Dental Assistants' Association (ADAA), 40, 47, 48, 269
  Certification Board of, 40, 41
  Education Committee of, 40
  National Curriculum Committee of, 40

American Dental Association (ADA), 4, 12, 16, 37, 40, 45, 47, 67, 129, 132, 159, 266, 272
  Annual Report on Dental Auxiliary Education, 42
  Bureau of Health Education and Audio Visual Service, 174
  Code of Professional Conduct, 271, 272
  Commission on Dental Accreditation, 40, 41, 42, 52
  Council on Dental Care Programs, 174
  Council on Dental Education, 40, 42, 45, 46
  Council on Dental Health and Health Planning, 6, 174
  Council on Dental Therapeutics, 128
  fluoride supplementation recommendations of, 127-128
  Health Foundation Research Institute, 174
  House of Delegates of, 40, 45
  Meritorious Award in Community Preventive Dentistry, 163
  Principles of Ethics of, 269, 271, 272
  Special Committee on the Future of Dentistry, 4